FIERCE
CHEMISTRY

FIERCE
CHEMISTRY

A HISTORY OF UK DRUG WARS

HARRY SHAPIRO

AMBERLEY

For Kay, my bedrock.

First published 2021

Amberley Publishing
The Hill, Stroud
Gloucestershire, GL5 4EP

www.amberley-books.com

Copyright © Harry Shapiro, 2021

The right of Harry Shapiro to be identified as the Author of this work
has been asserted in accordance with the Copyright, Designs and
Patents Act 1988.

British Library Cataloguing in Publication Data.
A catalogue record for this book is available from the British Library.

ISBN 978 1 4456 6544 3 (hardback)
ISBN 978 1 4456 6545 0 (ebook)

1 2 3 4 5 6 7 8 9 10

Typesetting by Aura Technology and Software Services, India.
Printed in Malta.

Contents

Glossary

ACMD	Advisory Council on the Misuse of Drugs
ACPO	Association of Chief Police Officers
ASBO	Anti-Social Behaviour Order
BFC	Board of Film Censors
BZP	benzylpiperazine
CARAT	Counselling, Assessment, Referral, Advice and Throughcare
CDCU	Central Drugs Coordinating Unit
CDRPs	Crime and Disorder Reduction Partnerships
CIDA	Concerted Inter-Agency Drug Action Group
CND	Campaign for Nuclear Disarmament (see below)
CND	Commission on Narcotic Drugs (a United Nations agency)
CSJ	Centre for Social Justice
CSR	Comprehensive Spending Review
DAT/s	Drug Action Team/s
DDA	Dangerous Drugs Act
DEA	the United States' Drug Enforcement Administration
DfEE	Department of Education and Employment
DH	Department of Health
DIP	Drug Interventions Programme
DORA	Defence of the Realm Act 1914
DTTOs	Drug Treatment and Testing Orders
FOI	Freedom of Information
HASC	Home Affairs Select Committee
LGDF	Local Government Drug Forum
INCB	International Narcotics Control Board (a United Nations agency)
ISDD	Institute for the Study of Drug Dependence

MDMA	3,4-methylenedioxymethamphetamine
NA	Narcotics Anonymous
NPS	novel psychoactive substances
NTA	National Treatment Agency
NTORS	National Treatment Outcomes Research Study
OST	opioid substitute therapy
PSA	Psychoactive Substances Act
SCODA	Standing Conference on Drug Abuse
SCRAs	synthetic cannabinoid receptor agonists
SKF	Smith, Kline & French (manufacturers of Benzedrine)
Spads	Special Advisors
SSOT	Society for the Suppression of the Opium Trade
TDT	Tackling Drugs Together
UKADCU	UK Anti-Drugs Coordinating Unit
UNODC	United Nations Office on Drugs and Crime

Preface

I joined the Institute for the Study of Drug Dependence (ISDD) as an information officer back in 1979, so you could say that this book has been 40 years in the making. I have often been asked how I got into the field in the first place. Having trained as a librarian, I was working in the information service of an international firm of architects and engineers. At the same time, I was embarking on my first book, a biography of Graham Bond, a legendary musician on the British blues scene. Graham had a serious heroin habit about which I knew nothing, so I started reading around that subject. Meanwhile life was getting rather dull cataloguing building trade literature on cladding and aluminium doors until I saw an advert for the job at ISDD in *The Guardian*. Armed with my newly minted wealth of drug knowledge I applied and was appointed, apparently over seventy other applicants.

ISDD began life in 1968 during the first wave of public and political concerns about drugs in the UK with heroin, amphetamine, LSD and cannabis use all on the rise. Frank Logan, a former Home Office and UN Narcotics Division official who had just retired from the Royal Institute for International Affairs, was searching in vain for sound, objective information about drugs for an article he planned to write. He decided to set up an institution to solve the problem. On 1 April 1968, ISDD opened for business from the attic of the Royal Society of Medicine premises near Oxford Circus with a library you could fit into a cupboard. ISDD moved around various parts of London with the library growing all the time to become one of the largest of its kind in Europe and probably second only to the library of the US National Institute on Drug Abuse. In 2000, DrugScope was formed from the merger of ISDD with another charity, the Standing Conference on Drug Abuse (SCODA), an umbrella body supporting voluntary sector drug services. DrugScope finally closed its doors in 2015.

For all of its history spanning nearly half a century, both ISDD and DrugScope stuck to the principles that the organisations would only provide information (whether through the library, publications or our internationally respected policy unit) that was current, non-judgemental and, well before it became common currency, evidence-based. This example will suffice: I recall one day in the ISDD library when seated at one end of the table was the Legalise Cannabis Campaign and, at the other, officers from the Metropolitan

Police Drug Squad. Neither were aware of the others and they were treated the same in providing them with the information they needed.

And here I am still doing it, remaining true to that objective, running a small online information service called DrugWise in partnership with my former ISDD/DrugScope colleague Jackie Buckle. Why? The fame? The money? A superficial answer would be that it is an endlessly fascinating subject; the scene, the politics, the people are all in a constant state of flux and in drug terms, you never know what is coming around the corner. Going a bit deeper, I have always been attracted to the outsiders in society, the people who really don't want to play by the rules. Make no mistake, in this world, there are plenty of outsiders, and I don't just mean people who use or deal drugs. I have known police officers, academics, civil servants, drug treatment CEOs and their teams, doctors and nurses and many other professionals who were more than happy to be 'flexible' in their interpretation of rules, regulations, procedures and whatever the current political and policy zeitgeist on drugs happened to be.

I think it is in my DNA to want to challenge myth, stereotypes, ignorance and prejudice and what are euphemistically called these days 'alternative facts', 'post-truths', 'fake news' and all the other nonsense we used to call lies and propaganda. No doubt few groups in society have suffered more in this respect than people who use drugs. So, once I started writing about the subject, I hoped to do my bit in support of a particular group of marginalised and stigmatised people who are the victims of injustice of one sort or another and among whom I have found some of the most thoughtful and intelligent individuals it has been my pleasure to know.

Although the phrase 'war on drugs' is commonplace, it is both nonsensical and sinister while at the same time has its uses. Throughout our history, anything we don't understand or want to relate to more closely, we tend to humanise – everything from ancient civilisations translating natural disasters into angry gods who need to be appeased, to the mundane naming of our pets Reg, Fergus or Tess. We even try it on inanimate objects; remember the famous scene in *Fawlty Towers* when Basil attacks his broken-down car with a branch having 'warned you time and time again'. But of course, you cannot wage war against a pile of powder or plant material. Talking about a war against drugs is a political smokescreen hiding the real war against everybody from seriously dangerous international traffickers to farmers struggling to make a living and young people landed with a criminal record for simple possession. Moreover, under that disingenuous mantra of 'unintended consequences', there are the absolutely intended consequences: extrajudicial murder in Thailand and the Philippines; the incarceration of thousands of young black Americans for non-violent drug offences; compulsory drug treatment in some Far East Asian countries involving chaining people to radiators; and the denial of life-saving harm reduction interventions in Russia. These are just by way of example. What lies beneath is a global horror story of crimes against humanity.

I was once in a 'civil society' meeting in Vienna – the quote marks are deliberately ironic. Drug user activists were calling for harm reduction to be included as a phrase in United Nations drug control documents on the grounds of human rights and civil liberties. American groups (of the Parents Against Everything persuasion), being coached in the room by a US State Department official, were genuinely mystified at the idea that drug users had any human rights. The top line argument was that they were lawbreakers, but then so are corporate banking fraudsters who can wreck the lives of millions yet few would deny them their basic human rights. The subtext of their outrage was – how can somebody who is a drug user and therefore subhuman have human rights?

That said, the subject of this book is the UK and there are far worse places in the world to be a drug user, but a few that are arguably better if your drug of choice is cannabis. In another sense, however, the phrase 'drug wars' might be more applicable to the UK than many other countries because we are not just talking about cops and robbers, enforcement versus traffickers. The approach to drug treatment which has been left largely in the hands of those delivering the services (as opposed to being primarily driven by political diktat) has also left the door open for battles royal to be fought between users and doctors over drug prescribing, the medical establishment versus those doctors whose prescribing was considered unethical, those in support of interventions to reduce harm versus those who believe abstinence is the only option. More broadly and in keeping with other countries, law reformers battle prohibitionists, politicians argue over strategies, ministers fight to preserve fiefdoms and perhaps underlying the whole scramble for the moral high ground is the idea that the drug war is a proxy war, a fight against some of society's deepest fears.

Could the term 'drug war' have any utility? From the above, it should be clear where my general sympathies lie. Even so, I have always believed that in this subject, clouded and refracted with so much smoke and so many mirrors, there has to be a place for the 'demilitarised zone', that area which allows for evidence to be evaluated and dispassionately presented and where stories can be told with some level of balance and objectivity. I am reminded of a remark I heard by the British journalist and writer Robert Peston that balance does not mean giving equal weight to opposing views, but grounding conclusions on the evidence.

So, I have been accused of sitting on the fence by those who come from the perhaps enviable position of cast-iron certainty. Actually, I quite like the view from up here.

What about the book then? I have tried to shine a light into most areas of this perennially complex and controversial aspect of British culture. Because I have broadened the concept of 'drug war', I have shied away from too much detail about enforcement activity and the careers of the big names in British drug smuggling history as these stories have been amply covered in other accounts and are listed in the bibliography. Instead, I have focused more on the political aspects of enforcement.

There have been many fine detailed histories of periods or aspects of the UK drug scene from excellent writers such as Virginia Berridge, Terry Parssinen, James Mills, Marek Kohn, Geoffrey Pearson, Susanne MacGregor, Gerry Stimson, Alex Mold and Bing Spear. But this is a first attempt to chronicle the whole period from the first laws against recreational drug use in 1916 to the Psychoactive Substances Act of 2016 and beyond, a narrative of drug law from nothing banned to everything banned.

My knowledge and opinions have been shaped and informed by the work of the authors mentioned above, most of whom I am glad to say I have got to know personally over the years, along with Don Aitken, Mike Ashton, Julian Cohen, Griffith Edwards, Mark Gilman, Anthony Henman, Lorraine Hewitt, Richard Ives, Roger Lewis, Michael Linnell, Tim Malyon, John Marsden, Lyn Matthews, Ethan Nadelmann, Maia Szalavitz, David Turner, Ian Wardle, Adam Winstock, Jasper Woodcock and Rowdy Yates.

Specific to this book, I would like to thank: John Ashton, Philip Bean, David Blunkett, Alex Boyt, Gill Bradbury, Terry Byrne, Bob Campbell, John Corkery, Julian Critchley, Annette Dale-Perera, Nicholas Dorn, Steve Easton, Jim Fitzpatrick, Chris Ford, Norman Fowler, Nick Goldstein, Chris Green, Lee Harris, Paul Hayes, Roger Howard, Keith Humphreys, Jules Hunt, Ken Hyder, Les King, Peter McDermott, Sara McGrail, Susanne MacGregor, David MacIntosh, David Marjot, John Marks, Sara Mars, Peter Martin, Alan Matthews, Tim Millar, Martin Mitcheson, Geoff Monaghan, Denis Moran, Tim Morrison, Simon Morton, Joy Mott, Dennis Muirhead, Russell Newcombe, Brian Paddick, Richard Phillips, John Ramsey, Rick Rutkowski, Ruth Runciman, Sue Smith, John Strang, Ken Stringer, Gary Sutton, Mike Trace, Alan Travis, Ric Treble and Tony White.

Nods and winks too, to former government civil servants who provided candid insights but who wished to remain anonymous. Thanks also to my agent Peter Buckman at Ampsersand, the good folk at Amberley Publishing and Tom Burgess.

However, despite all the enormous influences over 40 years that have been brought to bear on this book and the specific assistance given in the writing – it goes without saying but I'm going to say it anyway – I am totally responsible for all that follows, although I'll probably find somebody to blame if pushed.

But no list of thanks will ever be complete without heaps of gratitude to my partner Kay Waddilove, my rock and my compass over all the years, who keeps me pointing in the right direction and grounded in the realities of life even as I fend off the fan who beats a path to my door.

Introduction

We have a very narrow view of what constitutes a 'drug'. When a friend asked about the next book I was writing, she immediately understood what I meant by the UK drug scene – that seedy, criminal and violent world of illegal drugs. Then I said that although the story of illegal drug use in the UK was indeed the focus of the book, I wanted to set this in a wider context at the beginning of the narrative. She had no problem with opium, knowing as she did that the drug was widely and legally available as a medicine in past centuries. Nor did she have a problem (unlike the drinks industry) tagging alcohol with the label 'drug'. However, she genuinely looked askance when I added tobacco to the list (she is a heavy smoker) and even more quizzically at the mention of tea, coffee and sugar. Expanding the list still further includes other psychoactive drugs: opioid painkillers, tranquillisers, sleeping pills and antidepressants swallowed in the UK every day in their millions. Yet most patients would be horrified if you called them drug users or, worse still, addicts.

Even so, by any scientific definition, they are all drugs which impact on the central nervous system – albeit with effects ranging from the subtle to the dramatic. In other words, any substance you ingest for the purpose of changing the way you feel is a drug for whatever reason you are taking it – as a medicine, to celebrate, escape, relax, work, study, enhance performance, to delve into your psyche or commune with your gods. They are all of a piece.

The need to alter our mood and perceptions is so universal across all time periods, in all geographical areas and throughout myriad cultures and religions, that it seems hardwired into our DNA. Thomas Hobbes' belief that human life is 'nasty, brutish and short' sums up why we try to take the edge off. So enthusiastic are we to trace this lineage that some have let their imaginations run away with them. The writer Terence McKenna in his book *Food of the Gods* posited the idea that humans learnt to speak through experiencing the mind-expanding properties of magic mushrooms, taking us from grunting in a variety of pitches to 'I say, Godfrey, look, a sabre-toothed tiger!' The red-and-white spotted fly agaric psychedelic mushroom is supposed to explain why Santa Claus is kitted out in red and white as he flies across the sky and why Viking Berserkers went into battle stoned out of their helmets. In truth, you don't need to go to the edges of possibility to realise just how much human time, money and effort goes into satisfying this hunger to alter our state of consciousness, to change the way we feel and look at the world.

As the addiction psychiatrist Professor Griffith Edwards often observed, if you took a bird's-eye view of the planet you would spot thousands of acres devoted to the different crops used in the production of alcohol, tea and coffee plantations and sugar beet and cane fields. You would see vineyards in Europe and right across the southern hemisphere; huge tobacco plantations in China, Brazil, India, the USA and Indonesia; South American coca bushes; poppy fields across the Middle East and Asia; and cannabis just about anywhere. You would see how mood-altering plants exist in the most extreme and contrasting environments from peyote cactus in the desert to hallucinogenic vines in the steaming jungle of the Amazon.

Fly over our urban landscapes and beneath you would see factories producing vast amounts of synthetic mind-altering drugs, tranquillisers, antidepressants, sleeping pills and painkillers, and the chemicals used to produce all the synthetic recreational drugs such as amphetamine, LSD, ecstasy and ketamine. Moving away from large-scale industrial sites you could see the widespread domestic growing of cannabis, kitchen-sink drug production and indications of underground drug laboratories.

Beyond basic cultivation, there is all the infrastructure that brings the products to market. Taking alcohol as an example, there are companies manufacturing alcohol, managing processes such as brewing, distillation, and bottling. There are companies supplying products and services such as farm machinery, distillation equipment and freight services. Distribution and wholesaler intermediaries connect producers and vendors, typically storing and transporting the product. Then there are the sellers, both on licence (where drinks are bought and consumed on the premises such as pubs, clubs and restaurants) and off licence (where the drinks are bought in stores and supermarkets for consumption elsewhere). Finally, alcohol companies employ agencies for marketing, consultancy and lobbying. Now multiply that whole infrastructure across all the other globally available legal drugs. The world of organised international drug trafficking also needs all the subsidiary business activities and infrastructure that bring drugs from field or laboratory to the street.

The total global value of all those psychoactive drugs is calculated at nearly $1.4 trillion. Only oil generates more revenue – the top ten oil companies earn around double at $2.8 trillion. By contrast, the global arms trade is valued at around $100bn. Next to oil, incidentally, coffee is the most traded commodity in the world, cultivated in over seventy countries.

When it comes to talking about drug wars our view is similarly restricted. Again, we think in terms of enforcement agencies taking on murderous foreign drug cartels, and drugs cut with rat poison that cause boy/girl next door drug deaths. But in recent decades, courtrooms around the world, especially in the US, have seen the tobacco companies fighting a war not *against* drugs, but *for* drugs. Their years of skewed science, bribery and corruption have gradually unravelled as the true human cost of smoking has been revealed. Big Tobacco kills around 50 per cent of its customers, more than 6 million deaths a year globally as against around 250,000 that result from illegal drug use.

Alcohol companies are hardly much better, fighting against minimum alcohol pricing and denying allegations that alcopops were introduced in the

UK to lure young people back to drinking after the early years of rave culture that took place in largely alcohol-free venues. Let us not forget also the class actions brought against the pharmaceutical industry for the damage caused by a whole range of psychoactive drugs – most recently opioid painkillers – vehemently denied on their behalf by the same legion of expensive lawyers engaged by the tobacco industry to argue there was no evidence that smoking caused cancer.

However, the war *for* drugs is not a phenomenon of recent history. Consider this. You meet your friends in the local chain of a global coffee brand, one of you has an espresso, another orders tea and a third hot chocolate, all with sugar, while a fourth goes outside for a smoke. Much of the growth of the international trade and the beginnings of globalisation was dedicated to bringing those very drugs to the West. From the fifteenth century onwards, a 400-year-long avaricious and utterly ruthless war *for* drugs was fought across the world, leaving in its wake misery and death for millions.

Prologue

Empires of the Senses

The genesis of international trade as we know it today goes back to the Middle Ages and the growing fashion among wealthy aristocrats for highly seasoned food created by using spices from the East. Spices served three main purposes: to mask the taste of food that might be going off, to add flavour to an otherwise bland and boring diet, but above all, as a demonstration of wealth. The spicier the food, the more prestige for the host. Just like those middle-class after-dinner party moments when the cocaine is supposedly passed around, a selection of cloves, mace, cinnamon, saffron, ginger and pepper would move from guest to guest on a silver platter. Then as now, a compliment that somebody has 'taste' reflects our admiration for their sophistication and appreciation for the finer things in life.

There was another element to the appeal of spices. They came from that mystical foreign land called The East, known to most only through fable and rumour. The smell of spices evoked the exotic and the mysterious. Lovers exchanged spices as gifts. The medieval fascination with these far-off places was an early example of orientalism that would later rise again in a more sinister vein when the British public were lusciously horrified by tales of opium dens, white slavery and the demonic presence of the arch villain Fu Manchu.

Like textiles such as silks, which adorned the bodies of the rich and decorated their castles, the trade in spices relied on Arab traders to bring goods from India and the surrounding regions through Syria and Egypt to sell to Venetian traders, who would resell them into Europe. Inevitably, demand for spices began to filter through society, setting the future pattern for tobacco, coffee, tea, chocolate, sugar and distilled spirits. All these substances began their percolation downwards: initially they were highly acclaimed medicines, universal panaceas in a period of primitive medical knowledge, and then, because of rarity and cost, they were taken up for recreational and domestic purposes by the rich and powerful, before finally being absorbed into popular usage.

Over time, however, the old Eastern trading mechanisms could not keep up with demand; the route was long and arduous, and the transport technology not up to the job. A more powerful symbolic reason was also in play: while nowadays the West would rather not be dependent on Arab oil, back then the main European seaborne powers, Portugal, Spain, Holland and England, wanted to find alternative routes to the East not only for commercial reasons but because of the background of conflict between Christendom and the Islamic states. Political changes too were threatening spice supplies. The Mamelukes took power in Egypt and Turkey and while the spice caravans continued to cross Asia Minor, the new rulers imposed very high taxes on goods en route to Europe and its 'infidel' consumers.

What happened next was akin to the space race of the 1950s and 1960s: the spice race to find a sea route to India. Whoever controlled the spice trade would be a major European political and economic force as demand was vast and growing rapidly. Many tried, but most failed to accomplish this grand obsession of the fifteenth century. It would fall to Christopher Columbus and Vasco de Gama to enter the history books. Columbus got it spectacularly wrong, but his mistake sparked a major development in global commerce. Through de Gama, the Portuguese stole the march on everybody regarding the spice trade but once the Americas opened up to world trade, spices eventually lost their appeal. Markets became saturated and tastes changed. Now it was all about a new exoticism, the New World and El Dorado. The commercial move from east to west marked the break with the Middle Ages and the beginning of early modern history.

Tobacco

Native American and Caribbean tribes were using tobacco for religious and medical purposes long before Columbus turned up. Immediately apparent to the new settlers was the addictive power of nicotine, named after Jean Nicot, a French diplomat who introduced it as snuff to the French court in 1559. A Dominican friar, Bartolome de las Casas, reported that Columbus sent scouts into Cuba who described 'men with half-burned wood in their hands and certain herbs to take their smokes, which are some dry herbs put in a certain leaf, also dry ... These, muskets as we will call them, they call tabacos. I knew Spaniards on this island of Española who were accustomed to take it, and being reprimanded for it, by telling them it was a vice, they replied they were unable to cease using it.'

Sir Walter Raleigh is credited with introducing tobacco to the court of Queen Elizabeth around 1578. Overall, for the first half-century of its European use, tobacco was regarded as a sacred herb with miraculous healing powers. It was suggested by one commentator that tobacco could cure thirty-nine separate maladies. Nothing much changes though; fortunes are still being made with fad diets that do not work, the search for the non-addictive opioid analgesic goes on, we expect a pill for every ill, and the addictions field has been plagued by snake oil merchants peddling 'cures' for decades.

Although tobacco 'drinking' as it was first called (in pipes and as snuff) was tearing through Europe like wildfire, not all were enamoured of this 'Holy Herb', as the naturalist Nicolás Monardes named it in 1571. (Note that Monardes did have significant financial interests in the Spanish colonies.)

James I issued his famous *Counterblaste to Tobacco* in 1604 blaming what he perceived as the moral decline of the nation on the drug and declaring it as a 'custome lothsome to the eye, hatefull to the Nose, harmefull to the braine, dangerous to the Lungs, and in the blacke stinking fume thereof, neerest resembling the horrible Stigian smoke of the pit that is bottomless'.

In 1621, Ben Johnson dubbed the smell of tobacco 'the Devil's fart', while in 1624, a Holy Roman Empire ambassador to the Netherlands reported on the new fashion in 'fog drinking' which 'outdoes all other passions for indulgence in drink, old and new, imbibing and noisily drinking into their bodies the smoke of a plant they call nicotina or tobacco with incredible avidity and inextinguishable zeal'. In 1642 Pope Urban VIII condemned tobacco on the grounds that priests were smoking during Holy Mass. But some regimes went way beyond barbed words of condemnation.

In 1633, Murad IV, ruler of the Ottoman Empire, banned tobacco in Istanbul as well as alcohol and coffee. One strike and you were quite literally out. He would reportedly patrol the streets and taverns of Istanbul in civilian clothes at night and then cast off his disguise before beheading the offender with his own hands. If you fancied being flogged or having your nostrils split, then the officers of the Patriarch of Moscow would oblige. In China, the Chongzhen Emperor tried to shore up his collapsing Ming Dynasty by banning smoking, especially targeting 'the common people'. The Manchu Dynasty took up the fight regarding smoking as an even worse crime than neglecting archery. In perhaps one of the earliest examples of the 'unintended consequence of drug policy', once tobacco was banned, the Chinese people switched to opium smoking.

The story of tobacco also represents the earliest example of the failure of retrospective prohibition. By the time James I was railing against noxious tobacco, there were over 7,000 retail outlets in London and in an oft-repeated sequence of events, prohibition, punishment and condemnation gave way to the temptations of taxation. Earning revenue through the taxes and excise initially on tobacco and then on the whole range of psychoactive substances gripped Europe. Why? The revenues were vital to fund the endless succession of European wars in which the English, Dutch, Spanish, Portuguese and French battled it out in a merry-go-round of alliances to gain control of both foreign lands and international waters and the burgeoning, highly lucrative commodity markets that the land would produce and the sea would deliver.

Realising that as much as he hated tobacco it was a crucial cash cow, James sought to levy a high tax so that tobacco use would be confined to 'the better sort'. This is a familiar trope through the whole history of psychoactive drug use; in the eyes of the authorities, it is not only the drug that is viewed as the problem, rather, as we will see, it is the people who are using it. But James' high taxation policy was a disaster because 'the lesser sort' were already using tobacco on a grand scale. High taxes encouraged rampant smuggling along the lengthy coastline as well as the adulteration of tobacco. The excise men were hated: local residents often protected the smugglers; and the king found himself having to introduce legislation to protect the purity of the very product he had so desperately wanted to ban. Tobacco revenues had the added effect of enabling American colonists, the major suppliers of tobacco to England, to buy huge amounts of English merchandise. By the beginning of the eighteenth century, 80 per cent of tobacco consumed in Europe came from Virginia with overall consumption figures rising from 25,000 tons in the 1720s to more than 60,000 tons by the 1770s.

Coffee

Ethiopia was ground zero for coffee, but according to Dr Ralph Hattacks, interviewed for a BBC World Service documentary in January 2016, 'Yemen is where coffee found its soul.' It was called 'the wine of Islam' and 'the poor man's gold, and like gold it brings a feeling of luxury and nobility'. The usual establishment figures criticised coffee houses rather than the drink itself: there were no inns or taverns in Islamic countries to fulfil the social need for public meeting places so it was thought that men would gather in coffee houses to speak of treason and sedition. Coffee was briefly subjected to failed banning attempts even though in some countries simply visiting a coffee house was a capital offence. Coffee culture reached its peak as a social and cultural force in Constantinople, capital of the Ottoman Empire, and eventually spread to Europe once the Dutch stole bean plants and replanted them in their colonial territories of Indonesia and Brazil.

Because alcohol was banned in Islamic countries in favour of coffee, the Pope weighed in with attacks on the 'beverage of Islam', 'the invention of Satan' and 'the infernal black beverage they call coffee'. But the public would not be denied its first mass market hot drink. The first coffee house opened in London in 1652 and by 1700, the capital had spawned around 3,000 establishments. Although there were plenty of inns and taverns in England, these were deemed to be rowdy and unseemly places where men drank and fought. The coffee houses on the other hand became places where men (and only men) could gather to talk of business, politics, the latest news and other weighty matters, while drinking coffee and smoking tobacco – drug habits that were seen as sober and orderly, a sign of bourgeois respectability. Like any modern coffee chain store, the phenomenon of the coffee house embodied an aspirant business and social lifestyle. In the Middle Ages, spices handed the wealthy a symbol of sophistication and refinement; during the Age of Reason and Enlightenment, their aristocratic counterparts alongside both rising middle classes and the upper tier of respectable working men found it in coffee, tea and chocolate. Eventually the coffee house went out of fashion to be replaced by restaurants and private men's clubs. Some morphed into other businesses; Lloyds Insurance of London started out in 1686 at a coffee house in Tower Street run by Edward Lloyd.

Sugar

Arguably though, coffee (nor tea slightly later) would have made quite the impact it did had it not been for sugar. Sugar had a production history in southern Europe and on the Atlantic islands before Columbus took sugar cane to the New World where the first plantation was established in 1493. Colonial growers in Cuba, Puerto Rico and Jamaica began exporting to Europe, but were outgunned by the Portuguese supplies coming from Brazil. The British seizure of Barbados in 1627 proved a turning point for the British sugar industry. By 1650, England was consuming 500 tons of sugar annually and exporting 1,000 tons to the rest of Europe. A century later, we were importing 55,000 tons and only exporting 300 tons. Sugar had moved from sweetening the drinks of the few to becoming an essential daily product for everybody for its calorific value and taste.

Distilled Spirits

For centuries, weak beer and ale were the only daily drinks for most people, as water was unsafe. Alcohol provided a source of sustenance as well as intoxication. The early days of alcohol distillation were marked by a belief in its beneficial nature. The new drinks were called 'spirits' as they represented the blurred boundaries that existed between the physical and spiritual worlds. The perceived qualities of spirits encouraged belief that they could purify the body and the soul. Spices and distilled alcohol came together in Dr Stevens' Water, recommended for everything from the common cold to dropsy (oedema) and gout.

English distilled spirits became a commercial commodity after the mid-seventeenth century when sugar cane replaced tobacco as the chief crop of the English Caribbean colonies. Distilling a by-product of the sugar production process created a spirit called rumbullion, or rum for short (possibly derived from a slang term for tumult or disorder), which dominated the Atlantic drink trade as it became part of standard rations for English sailors.

Rum, though, was not the cause of alcoholic mayhem on the streets of eighteenth-century London. During the 1650s, Franciscus Sylvius, a professor of medicine at Leyden University in Belgium, developed a new drink through the distillation of grain and flavoured juniper berries: 'Junever', then 'geneva' and finally 'gin'. England's upper crust got the first taste, but then politics intervened to make them even more enthusiastic about the latest drug fashion. Wars against the French had thrown up protectionist barriers against French brandy. At the same time, William III needed increased revenues to pay for these wars. As gin began to make inroads into society, the king not only encouraged landowners to turn over any surplus grain to the making of gin, he offered a level of protection to the distilling industry that made it affordable for everybody.

By the early eighteenth century, London was the largest city in Europe but much of the population was living in dire poverty. The introduction of cheap, strong alcohol saw in excess of 8,500 outlets spring up across the capital (about one for every eleven houses), providing an escape from the miseries of everyday life and an income for otherwise impoverished families. This grim example of what happens when strong drugs are suddenly introduced to an already traumatised society has continued.

Native American communities were devastated by the arrival of colonial whiskey against the backdrop of genocidal policies which saw them butchered and deprived of their land. A similar process played out among Aboriginal tribes in Australia. In the 1980s, crack cocaine ripped through the poor black urban areas of the USA while in the UK, during the same period, heroin might not have insinuated itself across the land but for the wholesale destruction of Britain's heavy industry and manufacturing capacity, leaving millions without either work or hope. History has repeated itself in the USA with a catastrophic wave of opioid painkiller and heroin deaths affecting those poor, white regions of Middle America most hit by economic depression.

Having encouraged and protected gin production, William and his government were now alarmed at the prospect of a gin-sodden labour force, drunken mothers and sickly, malnourished children whose parents spent all their money on gin instead of food. These concerns, best visualised in Hogarth's *Gin Lane* (1751), produced a flurry of anti-gin pamphlets, sermons, parliamentary debates and medical investigations. In the face of what could be called England's first drug scare, the government enacted legislation aimed at curbing gin drinking by taxing retail sales at such a level that in effect, it introduced prohibition. Londoners responded by rioting.

Ultimately, the Gin Act of 1751, which prohibited gin distillers from selling to unlicensed gin merchants and increased fees to sellers, did kill off the small gin businesses. By then, however, the adverse effects of excessive gin drinking were more widely known and accepted, which probably had more to do with curbing gin drinking than any legislation. As the *London Magazine* noted in an editorial published in January 1737 after the most draconian of the Gin Acts targeting the poor had been introduced,

> To inflict a Penalty upon a real Crime, to punish an Action which is generally thought pernicious and scandalous, is not only necessary but popular; but to inflict Penalties upon Actions which are thought neither pernicious nor scandalous will always be thought oppressive; and consequently must alienate the Affections, at least of those who actually suffer by such Regulations.

The eighteenth century was supposed to be the Age of Reason and Enlightenment, a time of civility and control. Doctors therefore could not understand why people would voluntarily get completely out of control through drunkenness. Reason, they argued, was what separated us from all other species, which meant that the drunkard must be a beast, a farm animal, not (yet) a drug fiend, but someone whom the devil could tempt to indulge in the demon drink. This wasn't condemnation of the outcomes of drunkenness such as violence, the inability to work, or a cause of the neglect of family; this was more to do with the very act of intoxication itself – the ingestion of toxins. The religious and moral take was that men were embarking on a vicious and sinful indulgence; but while not at odds with the moral arguments, the doctors of the Enlightenment began as well to think of a voluntary sickness of the mind – some sort of disease.

In Europe during the eighteenth century, with more disposable income around for luxuries, drug consumption exploded; tobacco imports rose from 25,000 tons to 62,000 tons; coffee from 1,000 tons to 60,000 tons; chocolate (mainly for drinking) from 1,000 tons to 7,000 tons. As international trading systems became increasingly more efficient, the gentlemen of the London coffee houses could rest easy that there would be pipe tobacco, coffee, tea and chocolate for both their refreshment and for neural stimulation as they conducted business transactions and engaged in intellectual debate. However, uninterrupted supply rested entirely on one of the horrible paradoxes of the Enlightenment: slavery.

> I do not know if coffee and sugar are essential to the happiness of Europe, but I know well that these two products have accounted for the unhappiness of two great regions of the world. America has been depopulated so as to have the land on which to plant them. Africa has been depopulated so as to have the people to cultivate them.
>
> French writer and botanist J. H. Bernardin de Saint Pierre, 1773

Twelve Million and Counting

Most, if not all, ancient civilisations employed slaves – mainly prisoners of war – to serve in all areas of public life, from the army and the household to the fields and the brothels. Slaves were an integral part of the labour force from as early as 8,000 BC. The term 'slave' was derived from Slavic people sold into slavery to work the early sugar plantations of the Mediterranean. But the new slave trade beginning in the sixteenth century was a very different affair. This became a highly organised and very lucrative business that in itself was global in reach and pivotal in establishing global trading routes between nations and continents on both sides of the Atlantic. The slave trade was dominated by the English, Portuguese and Spanish who not only shipped some 12 million slaves from Africa to work in colonial plantations and mines, but those nations also acted as middlemen slavers, buying slaves to sell on.

The trade began in the West Indies; as the demand for sugar escalated in Europe, so the plantation owners needed to find new sources of labour beyond the indigenous tribal communities who had been pretty much worked to death by the heat and humidity and imported diseases. British plantations had survived not only on local labour, but on criminals who had been given a deportation option, political or religious dissidents on the run, people selling themselves into slavery to pay off debts and straightforward abductions, including children, from where we get the term 'kidnap'. They too succumbed to the harsh conditions and many died.

What began as a trickle of slaves imported from the West African coast became a flood into Spanish and Portuguese-held Caribbean islands. But by the mid-seventeenth century, these colonial powers began to realise they didn't have the trade all to themselves. In 1652, John Hawkins initiated the English slave trade with a first trip to Africa followed by others including

Richard Baker, whose slaving voyage was supposedly the inspiration for Coleridge's *Rime of the Ancient Mariner*.

From the start, the English slave trade was financially backed at the highest level. That very first voyage was funded by the Navy Treasurer and the Lord Mayor of London. Queen Elizabeth endorsed Hawkins' trade so long as slaves were carried off with their consent, which otherwise 'would be detestable and call down the vengeance of Heaven upon the undertakers'.[1] A young Sir Francis Drake accompanied Hawkins on his third trip to sell slaves to Portuguese coffee growers in Brazil. Hawkins was also not above attacking ships to steal their slaves. The huge profits to be earned from the slave trade sparked sea battles, hit and run piracy, smuggling, bribery and corruption. Slave captains would come into their destination harbour declaring fewer slaves than they had on board, selling the undeclared slaves to other slavers at a massive profit. One major slaver, Jorge Fernandez Giamaxo, made frequent trips to the Colombian port of Cartagena de Indias where he would house undeclared slaves prior to selling them on. He owned several large properties in the area, built on the proceeds of previous illegal sales. Centuries later, activities in the same region by drug trafficker Pablo Escobar resulted in him also owning extravagant properties.

England soon established itself as the major slaving nation of Europe: companies were formed as outsourcing contractors to supply slaves to other nations with colonial interests in the Caribbean and the Americas. Following the Treaty of Utrecht in 1713, the Royal Africa Company won a 30-year contract to supply slaves to Spain. There was a torchlight procession through London to celebrate and Queen Ann made a speech. Her successor George I sold the company for £7.5 million to the newly established South Sea Company set up primarily for the business of delivering the contract. Among the many aristocratic and notable investors was the Earl of Halifax, who founded the Bank of England; Sir Joseph Jekyll, the Master of the Rolls; Daniel Defoe; and Sir Isaac Newton, who personally lost £20,000 when the South Sea Bubble famously burst in 1720. The collapse ruined many but not Thomas Guy, whose financial success in this venture led to the building of a hospital in his name.

Slavery wasn't just a London business 'success story'; the development of Bristol and Liverpool owed much to their role as slave ports boosting the demand for shipping. Liverpool was proud enough of its slaving enterprise for the facade of the Exchange to carry reliefs of African heads with elephants. One street was named Negro Row. Having secured contracts to sell slaves to Spain in 1713, success against the French in the Seven Years War gave England the French sugar islands in the Caribbean including Cuba, which became the world's sugar bowl, and access to all France's African slave connections.

Apart from tobacco, coffee, sugar and chocolate, rum too had a vital role to play in the slave trade. There were two triangles to the Atlantic trade: English slaver ships sailed to Africa (via English ports), from there to the Americas, then returned to England with tobacco, coffee, chocolate and cotton. The second triangle was all about rum made from molasses in the

Caribbean and traded to African tribal chiefs in exchange for slaves. So valuable was slavery, that tribes would deliberately start wars with each other in order to take captives for sale to the colonial traders. Slaves would then be transported back across the ocean to work on the sugar plantations and turning molasses into rum for sale to the Americans and the English. African warlords were also partial to 60 per cent proof cane spirit from Brazil, another drug traded for slaves.

Just how aware English investors were of what was being done in their name is unclear, although as Hugh Thomas notes in his magisterial history of slavery, 'The Renaissance in Europe had no humanitarian pretensions ... it reburnished the ideas and practices of antiquity, the institution of slavery among them.'[2]

And institution is the right word; it is doubtful that anybody frequenting a coffee house, hot drink in one hand, pipe in the other or the thousands of ordinary housewives now using sugar in domestic cooking gave a thought as to where these goods came from or how they were produced – and among those who did know, there was either a belief or a rationalisation that however harsh plantation life was, it was still better than life in the 'savage jungle'. Similarly, people nowadays may not want to know the precise circumstances in which their technology, fashion clothes or sporting goods are produced. Occasionally an Asian sweatshop scandal is exposed, the major companies and brands involved deny having full knowledge, instead blaming local outsourced agents.

Back then and until the early rumblings of the abolition movement, little thought was given to the true horrors of the lives and deaths of slaves. They were regarded as no more than beasts of burden, to be used up and disposed of when they could no longer work. Slaves who became ill on the long and arduous voyage caged up in appalling conditions and not fit for sale at journey's end would literally be left to die on the quayside if they hadn't already been thrown overboard.

The best estimate of slaves from Africa who actually made it to North and South America and the West Indies is approximately 12 million. The most potent image of slavery with all its horrors and humiliations is cotton picking in the American south. However, of those 12 million, the American slave states imported about 500,000 Africans to work in the cotton fields, while those transported to the sugar plantations numbered 4 million, with 2 million put to work growing coffee in Brazil. And those figures do not include the countless numbers who committed suicide while still tied up in African harbours, who died or were murdered en route after involvement in slave rebellions, or who were born into slavery far from home.

Addressing the House of Commons in 1792, Prime Minister William Pitt the Younger said, 'No nation in Europe ... has ... plunged so deeply into this guilt as Great Britain.' His comments were increasingly echoed in literary and philosophical commentary which condemned the slave trade (although not necessarily slavery itself). The Church and politicians generally stayed quiet on the subject fearing the political consequences of being seen as 'soft on slavery'.

Although they were themselves implicated in slavery in the early colonial era, the Quakers pushed the Commons to launch an enquiry into the slave trade while John Wesley made the first significant religious intervention with an attack on the very institution of slavery. William Wilberforce, as MP for Hull, is credited with carrying the abolition fight into the political arena, but he was persuaded in this by Thomas Clarkson, a Quaker who in 1787 set up the Committee for Effecting the Abolition of the Slave Trade. Following several parliamentary debates and plenty of opposition from vested interests, the slave trade was abolished in British colonies in 1808 and slavery itself in 1833.

Though the infatuation with spices had long since passed, the East still produced highly valuable commodities to swell the coffers of the British government and its wealthy supporters and business partners. Those commodities would result in Britain engaging in two wars of global significance.

East is East: Tea and Opium

Compared to the rest of Europe, Britain was late to the table when it came to drinking tea. Rare and expensive at first, although stocked by the coffee houses (Samuel Pepys wrote of ordering a takeaway tea), it didn't really become embedded in British culture until the eighteenth century when its domestication outside the coffee house helped change the face of the Great British breakfast to a meal more resembling the tea/bread combination so familiar to us now.

Tea was imported from China to Britain courtesy of the East India Company, founded in 1600 under a royal charter from Queen Elizabeth. It granted them a monopoly on all trade east of Africa and west of the Americas. After Cromwell's time, the charter was renewed by Charles II and it not only reaffirmed the monopoly but gave the company extraordinary powers to make peace or war with any (non-Christian) peoples and erect its own garrisons so long as all enterprises were for the benefit of the British government. With a stroke of the pen, the king created one of the most powerful multi-national corporations the world had yet seen, which would dominate international trade.

Tea imports rose from 13,000 pounds in 1699 rising annually to nearly 5 million pounds or 2½ tons by 1751. However, actual consumption was much higher because tea was still too expensive for most people both because of the company charges and British taxation. As ever, this encouraged wholesale smuggling and adulteration.

The death penalty was regularly meted out to convicted smugglers, so they took enormous risks smuggling tea into the country. Similar to modern-day drug cartels, the risks were so high and the cargo so valuable that smugglers used extreme violence against anybody who threatened their liberty and livelihood. In his book *Tea: Addiction, Exploitation and Empire*, Roy Moxham recounts the story of the Kent-based Hawkhurst gang whose 2-ton tea cargo was seized by customs officers and locked in a Dorset customs house. The gang broke into the warehouse and stole it back only be informed on by somebody known to one of the gang members. A customs officer took the informant with him to identify the smugglers, but the gang got to them first. They were both horsewhipped and dragged for miles under the bellies of two horses with the hooves hitting them in the face. Spikes were driven into their foreheads and their testicles crushed. Having survived that, the customs man was burned alive while the informant was thrown down a well, suffered a botched hanging and was then stoned. Still breathing, he was buried alive. The law caught up with the gang, and eight of its members were tried and hanged.

There were many versions of the Hawkhurst gang throughout Britain and, despite their reputations, they were largely protected by local people who resented the level of taxation, hated the excise men and wanted to enjoy cheap tea. Smuggling and adulteration declined as levels of domestic taxation were reduced – a lesson the government failed to learn when it came to the American colonies; the consequences for the British government far outweighed all the brutalities of smugglers.

Over the course of the eighteenth century, the East India Company fell into financial difficulties; tea smuggling and adulteration had diminished legal exports to Britain to such an extent that the company had a stockpile of 21 million pounds, four years' supply, sitting in warehouses. Their charter prohibited direct trade with the American colonies, which had taken up tea drinking in a big way. However, the company managed to negotiate a deal allowing it direct access to American markets. This was granted by the Tea Act of 1773 with a duty levied at three pence (3*d*) per pound. The colonists were outraged: they already had an existing and long-running dispute with Britain; they argued they should not be taxed at all to fund the British administration of the colonies. Instead taxation should be spent to fund American legislatures. Coming on the heels of new tax impositions in 1765 and 1767 to pay for the war against the French, the new tea tax was the last straw. The East India Company made a bad situation worse by deciding to sell tea in the American colonies through its own agents and not established American merchants. Matters came to a head in December 1773 when four tea ships in Boston Harbour were caught in a stand-off between local protestors who tried to force the Governor to allow the tea to be landed without paying the duty, which would simply be passed on to customers. He refused. Eventually 1,000 people boarded the ships and indulged in the 3-hour Boston Tea Party, hurling more than 100 chests into the sea. Other cities followed suit in attacking tea consignments. Over the next two years, encouraged by their success, local militias regularly engaged with British forces until 1775 and the start of the War of Independence, which killed over 200,000 soldiers and sailors and caused tens of thousands of casualties. As one anonymous poet wrote at the time:

What discontents, what dire events
From trifling things proceed?
A little tea, thrown in the sea
Has thousands caused to bleed.

In 1834, the East India Company lost its trading monopoly with China, but by then, its main trading interests were in India where it was transformed into a virtual arm of the British government, engaged in administration and tax collection. From about this time onwards, various botanical experiments were conducted to see if tea would flourish in India, bringing it under control of Britain and ending the reliance on Chinese imports, which were draining the government's silver reserves. Once successful tea planting was established, London venture capitalists funded development and production so that by 1860, Assam boasted over fifty tea companies. By 1886, the dream of the British Empire was realised: imports of tea from India finally exceeded those from China. But at what cost was tea delivered to the British breakfast table for the humble morning cuppa?

> The mortality among immigrants to the tea districts in the early days of the industry is generally understood to have been very great; but few people I believe realise how appalling it actually was.
>
> J. W. Edgar, Junior Secretary to the Government of Bengal, 1873

The main growing area in India was Assam. Few locals wanted to work on tea plantations or in factories. The population had been decimated by war with Burma and those who survived had their own crops to tend. In order to meet the demand for a growing and very labour-intensive industry, a ready supply of cheap labour needed to be exploited. The East India Company had ceased trading in slaves when the practice was abolished in India in 1843, 10 years after other British-held territories. A way had to be found around this. Desperately poor Indian labourers from regions gripped by famine signed up on a 5-year 'voluntary' contract and found themselves shipped far away. The journey could be hundreds of miles on foot and by boat, and many died on the way. The tea regions were so remote that even those who saw out the contract often never made it home to their families.

As bad as the journeys were, life on the plantations was even worse, especially in Assam. Hardly any thought had been given as to how to feed tens of thousands of immigrant workers; accommodation was primitive and overcrowding caused diseases such as malaria to spread quickly, further weakening an already malnourished and debilitated workforce. Anywhere from a third to a half of the workers on any given plantation died. Powerful tea planter associations managed to block legislation aimed at improving working conditions. The contractors who sold the labourers on to the plantation owners were little more than what we now call human traffickers. Often with a criminal background, they would entice men into signing up with a promise of going to the better paid plantations while girls and women would be promised marriage only to be dumped at river or seaport quaysides and shipped off to the plantations. Others were simply kidnapped and illicitly sold, having signed no contract.

Once there, anybody caught running away or not working hard enough would be routinely flogged, often adding to the death toll. Prosecutions for brutality and murder were rare. Even into the early twentieth century, conditions had hardly improved. As Roy Moxham notes, 'At the end of the nineteenth century, India had produced 200 million pounds of tea (about 100,000 tons). Of this 85 per cent was exported to Britain. Across India about half a million acres were given over to tea plantations. Virtually all this tea had been planted in only 40 years – but at a terrible cost'.[3]

* * *

In 1840, educator and historian Thomas Arnold wrote, 'Surely you will agree with me in deprecating this war with China which really seems to me so wicked as to be a national sin of the greatest possible magnitude... Cannot anything be done by petition or otherwise to awaken men's minds to the dreadful guilt we are incurring?'

The opium poppy was not an indigenous plant in China: opium was probably brought in by Arab traders from the eighth century onwards to be either eaten or drunk, as an important part of the Chinese pharmacopeia. There was no smoking of opium for recreational or any other purpose. The idea of smoking opium took off following the ban on tobacco and quickly spread through the Imperial court, the military, the civil service and wider population.

So alarmed was the emperor about the spread of a habit that seemed to be enervating large sections of his vast empire, that he issued a ban on all imports except under licence for medical purposes. Anybody caught dealing could expect a severe public flogging and time spent in a portable pillory called a cangue.

The East India Company was in a quandary. Historically, the Chinese wanted little Western produce, regarding Western traders with an attitude ranging from condescension to outright hostility. They barely tolerated having them live in a limited enclave in Canton. By contrast, British demand for Chinese tea was seriously draining the silver reserves of the Exchequer: tea exports from China grew from about 46 tons in 1700 to 1,500 tons by 1751. By 1800, the company were buying 11,500 tons of tea a year for export to Britain, costing £3.5 million in silver. The government's commercial arm in the East needed a commodity that would be attractive to the Chinese: opium. But the company's trading rights with China had been hard won. If in the light of the ban, they were caught smuggling opium into China it would be very costly. Yet they urgently needed the income stream that opium would provide. The company's agents in Canton sternly warned against trying to sidestep the ban: Chinese opium smokers carried on relying on opium smuggled in by Portuguese sailors or pirates. Dramatic events in India changed everything.

Following an attack on the company's Calcutta headquarters in 1756 by the new ruler of Bengal and the imprisonment of more than 100 British subjects in 'The Black Hole of Calcutta', the company – led by Robert Clive – went to war. They won the Battle of Plassey in 1757 bringing Bengal, the richest province in India, under company control with a puppet ruler. As the imbalance of trade with China worsened, Clive's successor Warren Hastings, who became Governor General of India, decided that the potential to sell now British-controlled Indian opium to a potential market of 300,000,000 Chinese was too great a chance to be missed. He knew full well what he was doing; he wrote that opium was 'not a necessity of life but a pernicious luxury which ought not to be permitted but for the purpose of foreign commerce only and which the wisdom of government should carefully restrain from internal consumption'. By 'internal' he meant British India but, as we shall see, opium use was not exactly unknown in Britain itself.

The Indian princes of states neighbouring Bengal noted the rising price of opium and began to encourage production in their own provinces. In response, Warren Hastings made them an offer they couldn't refuse – sell only to the company or risk making an enemy of the British government, not dissimilar to the 'silver or lead' deals offered to local and national officials by the Colombian and Mexican drug cartels.

But how to get the drug into China without directly implicating the company and the British government in what was not even a clandestine trading arrangement, but out-and-out drug trafficking? There was a wider purpose at work; yes, to improve cash flow, but also to force the Chinese to join the fold of international trading nations. A first step would be to legalise the opium trade. The answer to the most pressing problem was to sell the opium to Indian merchants who would ship opium to China on so-called 'country ships' flying under their own flag and then offload onto junks to be landed ashore.

Everyone involved of course wanted their nose in the trough; very soon bribery of Chinese officials was so flagrant and widespread that the country ships were blatantly sailing right up the Canton estuary to the port rather than offloading onto junks out at sea. The Chinese ordered all boats to be searched and any opium cargoes confiscated. The smugglers retreated down the estuary to Lintin and continued trading from there, fighting it out if necessary, with the government junks sent to intercept them. The relatively safe haven of Lintin allowed opium imports to rise sharply during the 1820s.

It didn't go unnoticed among MPs that having won the colonial moral high ground by abolishing slavery in 1833, the British government were now overseeing the smuggling of a known dangerous drug (De Quincey's *Confessions of an English Opium-Eater* had been published in 1821) in ever-increasing quantities. But whatever political qualms were voiced back home about the morality of the trade were quickly countered by the company which pointed out that the revenue raised from opium smuggling contributed about half of the money needed to pay for the Crown and the Civil Service.

Under pressure to rein in the trade, Foreign Secretary Lord Palmerston tried again to persuade the Chinese to open up the country to foreign trade and in the process to legalise opium use. He sent Lord Napier to negotiate the deal. It didn't go well. His ship was blockaded and a ban imposed on trade with any British ship. The spurious grounds for the much-documented Opium Wars were laid.

In fact, the Chinese emperor was hearing from some of his advisers that opium had got such a hold that further bans were useless and he should indeed legalise use. In May 1836 one official wrote to the emperor admitting that opium smoking was a 'vile practice', but that prohibition not only failed to deal with all the evils, it created more. This might have appeared a liberal stance: it was anything but. The harsher the penalties, he wrote, 'the more widely do the evils arising therefrom spread'. His point was that prohibition bred violence, greed, blackmail and corruption, affecting many parts of society; the tougher the penalties, the higher the bribe needed to tempt officials. On the other hand, if you legalised opium, went the argument, the only people affected would be the smokers and if they died, it would help an already overpopulated country.

However, after due consideration, the emperor was persuaded that the real culprits were not the addicted smokers, but the foreigners trying to import the drug. In 1839, he sent Lin Tse-hui to Canton. Lin had the full authority of the emperor to do what he could to disrupt the trade.

British officials on the ground knew that morally they didn't have a leg to stand on in what they were trying to protect. Palmerston's view though was that British property had been seized and destroyed, trading in a valuable commodity threatened and so a show of force was required. To the doubters at home, he used the classic arms dealer argument: 'If we don't sell it, somebody else will.' The first Opium War ended in ignominious defeat for the Chinese; Lin lost his job and the Chinese lost Hong Kong, which remained a British colony until 1997.

Debate continued to rage at the emperor's court, most of whom, including the emperor himself, were addicted to opium, about what to do about this situation. The war resolved little; the Chinese authorities continued to act against British traders while Palmerston was looking for a pretext to send in the gunboats again. The emperor provided the excuse for British action in 1856 by arresting the crew of *The Arrow*; the British Navy (aided by the French) responded by taking the Port of Canton and burning the emperor's summer palace in Peking, eventually forcing Chinese capitulation and the signing of the second of what Chinese historians called 'unequal treaties'.

***

The British secured the legalisation they had been pressing for, in exchange for duty payments and the inevitable rise in Chinese use. As Britain was no longer dependant on China for tea, it was the Chinese exchequer that was now feeling the drain on its cash reserves to pay for British opium. In response, given that it was clearly impossible to restrict opium use, the Chinese decided to grow their own opium, although by the end of the century, political and public pressure curtailed Britain's involvement in the opium trade and it became relatively less commercially important.

Through all the political debates about the opium trade, it was taken for granted that opium was indeed a dangerous drug that would enslave all who used it. Outside of Parliament, the Society for the Suppression of the Opium Trade (SSOT) was at the forefront of public opinion, pushing for a ban. Yet there were conflicting opinions about the dangers of opium use. It would be expected that those with a commercial interest in the drug would downplay the dangers; instead it was the doctors and missionaries based in India who were expressing an alternative view.

A Royal Commission on Opium was set up to investigate the issue and concluded that, in the main, opium was not used to excess and in moderation was not that detrimental to health, although the Quaker Joseph Rowntree produced a damming minority report saying that of the fifty-two Chinese missionaries who had submitted evidence, the Commission had only quoted the views of the few who had been less fervent in their condemnation.

Drilling down into the evidence, it would seem there were differences in the Chinese and Indian experience and, over time, within India itself, all of which again demonstrated that the impact of drugs on society is not limited to the chemical interaction of body and drug. True, in China the drug was smoked rather than swallowed as in India. Next to injecting a drug, smoking is the quickest and most effective way of getting a drug into the brain. The experience of swallowing a drug is less intense as it has to travel around the body before entering the brain. This meant the witnesses to the Commission who worked in China were more likely to condemn opium than those who worked in India, but not just because of the more intense effect of smoking. The Chinese missionaries were despised by all strata of Chinese society and when the Chinese refused to embrace Christian teachings, the missionaries blamed opium-induced stupor for the otherwise inexplicable refusal to give in gracefully.

That wasn't the whole story though. What happened in Assam was probably closer to the heart of the issue. When opium was introduced into Assam in 1839 along with the cheap labour for the new tea plantations, the major disruption caused to the community's way of life created a growing body of users. Opium had, in the words of one official, reduced the population from 'a fine race of people to the most abject, crafty and demoralised race in India'. Yet 50 years later when use was higher per head than in any part of India, one British Commissioner reported that opium use was no more of a problem than when 'a good Englishman would take his peg' (an Indian term for a shot of whiskey). Over time, opium had been normalised within that society where informal social controls had, at a whole population level, limited excessive and problematic consumption.

All the Drowsy Syrups

It is hard to imagine these days that not much more than a century ago, you could walk into any British pharmacy or even local grocery store and buy a wide variety of pure opium products including pills, lozenges, powders and sticks, plus an array of patent medicines with gloriously Dickensian-sounding names such as Daffy's Elixir and Mrs Winslow's Soothing Syrup.

The medical use of opium goes back at least 6,000 years to the time of Sumer, one of the earliest urban civilisations located in what is now southern Iraq. Ideograms from the period describe opium as 'the plant of joy', suggesting that perhaps use was not only for medicinal purposes or that, as with many psychoactive drugs through history, the lines between strictly medical use and subsequent reasons for consumption rapidly become blurred. But the early historical record restricts itself to evidence only of medical use throughout the Ancient World.

Opium was known in England by the fourteenth century. An early pioneering surgeon, John Arderne, mixed up various opium-containing concoctions to put his patients to sleep, 'so that he schal fele no kuttyng', while Shakespeare included mention of 'drowsy syrups' in a famous passage from *Othello* knowing his audience would understand the reference.

In the sixteenth century, the influential Swiss doctor, chemist and philosopher Paracelsus (also known as Philippus Aureolus Theophrastus Bombastus von Hohenheim) was supposed to have formulated opium in a pill form he called 'laudanum', meaning praiseworthy. However, it was British doctor Thomas Sydenham who in the 1660s invented the more familiar liquid form of laudanum, a tincture of alcohol and opium. He said that 'medicine would be a cripple without it' and he was right. In the centuries before there was a clearer understanding of the actual causes of diseases, those professing some medical knowledge could only treat symptoms – and the most distressing symptom of all was (and still is) pain. So, when a whole range of pain-killing products appeared on the market from the late seventeenth century onwards, it was literally a huge relief to millions of people, most of whom could not afford a doctor and were simply self-medicating their discomfort.

There was no real concern about opium addiction; Dr John Jones recognised the condition in his *Mysteries of Opium Reveal'd* published in 1700, but he also wrote of the pleasurable aspects of opium use. Right up to the mid-nineteenth century, opium use in all its formulations was universal among all ages and classes, without any moral opprobrium attaching to those who used it. Yet by the end of the century, users were classed as diseased and sick. How did that happen?

The story of opium's journey from universal acclaim and availability to fear and regulation is not straightforward, certainly not simply a case of medical science progressing to the point where dangers were recognised and action taken, although that is part of the story. Professor Virginia Berridge covered the whole saga in exhaustive detail for her peerless study *Opium and the People: Opium Use in England During the 19th and Early 20th Century*, so what follows can only be a brief summary – a knotty twisted skein of medicine, machination, myth and morality.

From the mid-nineteenth century, there was a coming together of middle-class medical, public health, moral and social reforming interests who collectively gave much of their attention to the plight of the poor. The Industrial Revolution had created dreadful squalor and poverty in major cities like London and Manchester. The cholera outbreak of 1831 focused civic minds on improving urban sanitation, manifested in Edwin Chadwick's landmark report of 1842, *Sanitary Conditions of the Labouring Population of Great Britain*, which recommended ambitious civil engineering projects to improve water quality, sewerage and drainage. Several parliamentary reports and publications such as Engels' *The Condition of the Working Class in England* (1844) brought conditions further into the light.

The scope of public health concerns began to ripple out into other areas, including controls on the sales of poisons. The 1844 Manchester Police Act placed the first restrictions on the sale of arsenic and prussic acid. The Act also provided for what was probably the first example of stop-and-search for possession of arsenic or prussic acid that had been bought in violation of the new restrictions. The Arsenic Act of 1851 placed more restrictions on the sale of arsenic while The Bolton Improvement Act 1854 introduced controls on the sale of 'virulent poisons'.

Attention also centred on the rising incidence of children overdosing on opium products. Nowadays we take official statistics for granted; governments enumerate the lives of the population from every possible angle providing the evidence base for State interventions. But this was new in Victorian England; the post of Registrar General was created in 1837 and from then on, the statistics on the state of the nation began to increase, including figures on infant opium deaths. The evidence demanded action.

This tied into another thread – the growing movement encouraging self-help, people taking personal responsibility for their own actions. Heading this movement was Samuel Smiles who believed that a lot of poverty was caused by irresponsible habits. In this climate of moral improvement, working mothers were blamed for irresponsibly dosing their children so they could go out to work, but in fact most women working in factories left in their early twenties specifically to get married and have children. The real causes of infant overdosing were the unhealthy living conditions and poor diet: babies fell ill with stomach complaints and as there was no access to regular health care, mothers used easily available potions. However, the official view was that to tackle infant doping and the adulteration of opium by unscrupulous vendors, there had to be some way of controlling access to the drug. What happened next leads us to the next thread.

Doctors and chemists were starting to organise themselves as legitimate middle-class professions. The British Medical Association, the doctors' trade union which manages the medical register, was formed in 1832, the General Medical Council in 1858, the Pharmaceutical Society in 1841 and for those chemists not in the Pharmaceutical Society, they could belong to the short-lived United Society of Chemists and Druggists while the Society of Apothecaries was founded as long ago as 1617. They all had one common interest: open sale of opium products undermined their business and professional interests. The doctors wanted opium to be only available on medical prescription; they just wanted to restrict sales to their own premises as opium could be bought in a variety of grocery shops and general stores and reportedly from even more unlikely sources such as bakers, basket makers, rent collectors and cobblers.

The 1868 Pharmacy Act was really a victory for the pharmaceutical profession as it simply added further sales restrictions to existing poisons legislation requiring registration of premises, specific labelling of poisons and a register of those purchasing the more lethal products, which did not include opium. The doctors certainly did not achieve the prescribing monopoly they sought. Moreover, the Act did little to inhibit general sales as it did not include opium-based patent medicines, a highly profitable industry at the time. One manufacturer, Thomas Holloway, was a multi-millionaire and one of the richest men in the country, able to spend £50,000 annually just on advertising. His country seat was Tittenhurst Park, a Georgian mansion, later home to both John Lennon and Ringo Starr. The founding of Royal Holloway College, now part of the University of London, was one of Holloway's philanthropic legacies.

But while the Pharmacy Act had little impact on sales, it did, along with the other bits of poisons legislation, establish the principle of State intervention to control access to drugs. Even before the Act was passed, previous poisons legislation had drawn criticism from John Stuart Mill in his treatise *On Liberty*, published in 1859, an attempt to establish standards in the relationship between State authority and individual liberty. On poisons legislation he wrote, 'The sales of poisons open a new question; the proper limits of what may be called the functions of police; how far liberty may be legitimately invaded for the prevention of crime, or of accident.' He went on to suggest that if the only reason for buying poisons was to commit murder, then prohibition would be justified. However, because they can be used 'not only for innocent but useful purposes', restrictions to protect against nefarious use also impinged on those whose intent was perfectly lawful. His view was that it was one thing to warn customers through labelling about the potential dangers of a product so they could make a choice, quite another to make the choice for them by making it difficult or impossible to purchase, for example by giving the doctors the monopoly on prescribing – which would put the product out of the reach of most ordinary people.

Although doctors had failed in their attempt to establish the principle that opium use was potentially dangerous enough for them to have control over public access, the seed had been sown. It took the next step to bring the drug use more firmly within the orbit of medical expertise.

Nobody had any idea how many working-class people were addicted to opium or how many were using it for morally reprehensible 'stimulant' or 'luxurious' purposes (what we would now call recreational use). Controlling working-class opium use was more an issue of availability than treatment. The notion that addiction per se was a pressing problem only emerged after morphine came into general medical practice and with it the perfection of the hypodermic syringe as the most effective delivery system for the new drug.

At the beginning of the nineteenth century, three chemists, two from France and one from Germany, were working independently to isolate the active ingredient, the pain-relieving chemical from the opium poppy. It was the German chemist Friedrich Sertürner who coined the name 'morphium' after Morpheus, the Roman god of sleep, and by 1820, Thomas Morson, who founded the Pharmaceutical Society, was producing morphine in commercial quantities. His main competitor was J. F. MacFarlan Ltd from Edinburgh (which merged with other firms and currently, as MacFarlan Smith, still has the monopoly on diamorphine supplies to the NHS).

Coincidentally, three doctors were also working simultaneously on perfecting the hypodermic syringe so that by the 1860s it was acknowledged in medical circles that a combination of the more powerful morphine in conjunction with the capacity to inject the drug close to the source of pain was not only the most effective form of pain treatment, but gave the medical profession an expertise it could truly call its own.

Given the expense of the new drug and with access to doctors still limited to those who could pay, treatment through morphine injection was only available to wealthier groups in society. Very soon doctors noted that some of their patients, while starting out as medical patients, had become chronic morphine injectors. Doctors wrote up their observations in the medical press, generating concern based on little more than a handful of case studies. When originally published, De Quincey's *Confessions* had made only limited impact save for some literary magazine reviews and interest from the anti-opium lobby. Now it went into several editions and was pored over for insights into the 'addicted' mind. It was well known too in polite society that high-profile public figures William Wilberforce and Robert Clive had been chronic opium users. English doctors were also influenced in their thinking by the writings of their counterparts in Germany and America, where morphine addiction was prevalent. Influential medical works included Levinstein's *Morbid Craving for Morphia* (1878), Kane's *The Hypodermic Injection of Morphia, Its History, Advantages and Dangers* (1880) and Crothers' *Morphinism and Narcomanias from Other Drugs* (1902).

So how was the 'disease' of addiction conceptualised? To quote Professor Berridge, 'Disease was generally defined in terms of deviation from the normal. A hybrid disease theory [of addiction] emerged in which the old moral view of opium eating [use not confined to medical] was reformulated in "scientific" terms, where social factors were ignored in favour of explanations in terms of individual personality and biological determination.'[4] Physical aspects of addiction such as tolerance and withdrawal were recognised, but the strong emphasis was on the psychological. In England, drug addiction came to be regarded as an offshoot of alcohol-related 'inebriety'. There was legislative action for the control and care of 'habitual drunkards', the champions of which formed the Society for the Study of Inebriety in 1887. There were strong links too, between those doctors involved in the development of disease theory, the temperance movement and those campaigning for the abolition of the opium trade.

There was a certain amount of medical pushback about the moral aspect of addiction, but even so, the prevailing view was that addiction was a disease of the will – a disease and a vice. There was talk of 'moral bankruptcy' and 'moral insanity'. Addicts were responsible for the condition in which they found themselves while at the same time addiction increasingly became a condition that was not only in the purview of doctors but those with a special expertise. In effect, a win-win for the medical profession: doctors would be in charge of treatment, but if it failed it was the fault of the addict/patient. Moreover, some of the treatments advocated very much played to the notion that people needed to be punished for their 'vicious indulgence': abrupt withdrawal (cold turkey), emetics, dousing in cold water, head-shaving and electric shocks. The idea that punishment should be an integral part of 'treatment' never went away. For years, cold turkey was the only option for those in prison; the regimes of much later residential rehabilitation houses in the UK and the USA subjected residents to public humiliations and shaming; while even today, 'treatment' meted out to those with drug problems in some countries is as far removed from any conception of human rights and civil liberties as you can imagine.

As mentioned above, running parallel to the developing notion of addiction as the product of a diseased mind was the campaign to end the export of opium from India to China spearheaded by SSOT. Their campaigning had little relevance to the domestic experience of opiate use, but the amount of energy they expended in public speaking, petitioning and parliamentary activity further added to public awareness of the iniquities of opium use including opium smoking, something unknown in Britain until the barbaric practices of far-off lands appeared on our very doorstep with the arrival of the Chinese opium den.

A small Chinese community grew up close to the dock areas of east London and Liverpool to service the needs of itinerant Chinese seaman: lodging houses, shops, restaurants and laundries. Visiting sailors, looking to relax after arduous voyages, brought with them the now long-established Chinese practice of opium smoking. The whole community probably never numbered more than a few hundred and the 'dens' could just be a room in one of the lodging houses, although others might be more elaborate. What turned an innocuous habit among a small isolated community into a growing public scandal were the lurid tales of debauchery and moral depravity found in the fictional presentations of Charles Dickens in *The Mystery of Edwin Drood* (1870) and Oscar Wilde's *The Picture of Dorian Gray* (1890). Depictions of opium dens played on a number of fears and stereotypes that would later be articulated more crudely by the burgeoning tabloid press.

In the early years of the twentieth century, the general landscape of opium use changed. The trade with China reduced in importance as the Chinese were producing their own supplies although, from a British point of view, that story was far from over. There were increasing domestic controls on the patent medicine trade to remove opium and morphine from products or reduce the percentage content while new drugs came onto the market to replace opium, especially for insomnia. So, at the turn of the twentieth century, a British government official would have been pretty smug about drug control mechanisms in the UK. The Americans had other ideas.

The League of Gentlemen

After the American Civil War, the country experienced a period of rapid industrialisation and urbanisation. With it came a rising tide of protest led by rural-based as well as middle-class moral, social and religious reformers who campaigned against a range of issues they saw as signs of a decaying and morally bankrupt society including alcoholism, child labour, prostitution, immigration and, increasingly, drug use among poor urban youth. Concerns about immigration mainly centred on the influx of Chinese labourers who came in the 1840s, primarily to build the railways. However economic depression in the 1890s increased already rampant hostility towards the Chinese whose use of opium provided an easy target. There were local ordinances against opium smoking well before the federal government introduced its first Act aimed at dangerous drugs in 1914.

The combination of economic depression and anti-Chinese sentiments posed a problem for the federal government. To offset the impact of the economic downturn, officials began to look overseas for new markets for American goods. Although they overestimated the actual size of the potential market, China looked very tempting. The Americans were also concerned that in the wake of internal strife in China caused by the Boxer Rebellion (1899–1901), existing colonial powers such as Britain, France, Germany, Russia, Japan and the Netherlands might take advantage and instigate a 'scramble for Asia' as they had in Africa. America did not want to lose out for both economic and strategic reasons; it wanted its own sphere of influence in the western Pacific region.

The USA too had a growing sense of its place in the world; it saw itself as a burgeoning global power, which, alongside any economic or military strength, had a moral duty to bear some of the 'white man's burden' to match the colonial missionaries and their muscular Christianity. As part of this colonial muscle flexing, America had fought a war with Spain, spoils from which saw the Philippines become a US colony. What the Americans hadn't bargained for was a responsibility for extensive opium use among the islands' Chinese population. President Theodore Roosevelt received a letter from Charles Brent, the Episcopal Bishop of the Philippines and an anti-opium hardliner, raising the issue of opium use and lobbying the president for an international meeting to discuss how to curb production and supply in the region.

Supporting China in the fight against opium use was just the diplomatic wedge the US State Department was looking for because Sino–American relations were at a low ebb as the USA had instigated tough immigration laws to stem the flow of Chinese migrants. China responded with a boycott of US goods.

So, in 1906, the US Ambassador to the UK asked Foreign Secretary Sir Edward Grey for the British government's view on having an international commission investigate the opium trade and the opium habit in the Far East. A new Liberal administration had been elected in 1905, which immediately came under pressure from its backbenchers to end the Indo–China opium trade. The MPs were encouraged in their campaign by the appointment of John Morley as the Secretary for India as he had an anti-opium track record. However, once in post, Morley was resistant to anything that might undermine Indian government revenues. The British already had in place a treaty, signed with the Chinese in 1906, whereby the British pledged to reduce exports if the Chinese reduced home production and didn't import from elsewhere. In the very early days this seemed to be working quite well, so the British saw absolutely no need for an international meeting on the subject. However, Morley and senior civil servants at the India Office in Whitehall reasoned that an international commission could play to their advantage. While the trade could be put at risk by subsequent bi-lateral agreements, where several nations were involved all with competing strategic and economic interests in the region, it would be far harder to come to an agreement that would jeopardise the trade. Therefore, both Grey and Morley were minded to accept the proposal from the Americans, because to refuse might accelerate backbench moves to abolish the trade and it offered the chance to kick the idea into the long grass.

The Americans sent out invitations to fourteen countries, all with an interest in the opium situation in the Far East. All agreed to attend a meeting except Turkey, a major producer and exporter of opium. Their excuse was the Young Turk Revolution of 1908 which caused an internal constitutional crisis, but Turkey's absence did not auger well for the outcome of the meeting.

Before it, there was more backstage swordplay over the terms of reference. The American view was that the meeting was to focus on helping the Chinese deal with its opium problem, whether among its own population or in other territories in the region such as the Philippines, declaring opium use as an 'unmitigated evil'. The India Office objected to this description of opium use, citing the conclusions of the Royal Commission on Opium as evidence. In order to deflect attention away from specific consideration of the Indo–Chinese trade, the India Office insisted the delegates should consider opium use in their own countries – not just in China. The British also refused to engage in any discussion about their existing treaty with China. The Americans knew that without the British, the whole enterprise would be pointless, so they agreed.

The British via the India Office had boxed clever. If it was determined that opium was not an 'unmitigated evil', as already concluded for India, then there was no need for international controls. If it was, then the Commission would have to consider global implications, not just those that applied to the Indo–China trade.

The US delegation was led by Bishop Brent. With him was another staunch anti-opiumist, Dr Charles Tenney, an ex-missionary and Secretary of the US Legation in Peking. But its most important member was Hamilton Wright, who was to have a major influence on the development of both US domestic and international drug controls. Wright was not a US Federal employee, but more what we would call these days a consultant to the US State Department. This allowed him more freedom of action. From his investigations into opium use in the USA and the Far East, he concluded that the only option was strict prohibition.

By contrast, the UK delegation was led by Sir Cecil Clementi Smith, a former governor of British territories in the Far East and as equally determined as his colleagues in the India and Colonial Offices and the Indian government to block any attempts at undermining opium revenues. The meeting, which started in Shanghai on 1 February 1909, chaired by Brent, was the first ever international meeting between global powers not to be discussing the provisions of a treaty to end a war. As it turned out, it was the inaugural meeting which started one.

In truth, while all the delegates represented powers with interests in the region, the main players standing toe to toe were the Americans and the British, with everybody else essentially supporting the USA and China to a greater or lesser extent. After some bad-tempered exchanges, the Americans proposed nine resolutions, mostly written by Hamilton Wright. Heading the list was the proposal that opium use should be restricted to medical use only. Clementi Smith objected on the grounds that such a ruling would be impossible to enforce and that as far as India was concerned, opium had a cultural and social role to play that went beyond simple medical use. Every proposition put forward was either rejected or watered down with the inclusion of vague phrases such as 'careful regulation' as opposed to outright prohibition and that the Shanghai Commission 'recognises wide variations between the conditions prevailing in the different countries'. From the American point of view, the outcome of the commission was highly unsatisfactory; it committed the powers to little more than aspirational goals around suppressing production and supply from their own countries and amending any trade agreements with China that might serve to hinder Chinese anti-opium efforts. The Foreign Office regarded the whole meeting as a farce, but there was a sting in the tail.

The problem with vague diplomatic language is that it is open to very wide interpretation. In this case, despite their disappointment, the US delegation came away from Shanghai convinced that there was an appetite for another meeting, but this time one that could actually pass international laws that would bind the attending nations: in other words, the delegates would have plenipotentiary powers. It took Wright about seven months to come up with a list of fourteen propositions that were sent to the Foreign Office, all focused around international restrictions on the production and supply of 'opium, its derivatives and preparations' with penalties for contraventions. The initial reaction of the British was incredulity. A senior clerk in the Far Eastern section of the department wondered mischievously, 'Is it not possible to administer opium in strong doses to the United States Government when they get on the opium warpath?'[5] That said, Edward Grey, thought it would be diplomatically awkward for Britain to stand alone by refusing to go to a second gathering. It was decided to call an interdepartmental meeting to decide how to respond to the American proposals. The Foreign Office was really just the messenger; it tended to defer to colleagues in the Indian and Colonial Offices who in turn pretty much gave the Indian government free reign; in effect, the Indian government had almost as much autonomy to deliver policy on the ground as the East India Company.

It was in the interests of the British government that existing opium revenues were not put in jeopardy. Previously as a deflecting tactic, the British had insisted that all the powers at Shanghai should consider opium use in their own countries not just China and the Far East. Now when they eventually replied to the Americans a year later, in September 1910, they insisted that the conference should consider not just opium, but also morphine, cocaine, and any other drug considered dangerous. One of the four American proposals, which the British rejected outright, was the idea that an international agency should be set up to oversee the implementation of any agreement. After further exchanges of letters, in the end the sole prerequisite for British attendance was assurance that the other nations agreed in advance to place severe restriction on the illegal/unlicensed traffic in morphine and cocaine from their countries. After more delay, the conference finally opened in The Hague in December 1911.

Because the delegates would have plenipotentiary powers, the government did take the Hague conference more seriously. Nevertheless, the view was that like Shanghai, the whole point was to deal with drug use in the Far East. Nobody gave any thought as to what an agreement might mean for the situation in Great Britain. None of the departments responsible for the pharmacy laws had been invited to the interdepartmental meeting called to discuss the strategy for the Hague Conference. Article nine of the final Hague Convention did stipulate that if they hadn't already done so, the contracting powers would enact pharmacy laws and regulations that would 'limit manufacture, sale and use of morphine, cocaine and respective salts to medical and legitimate use only'. But as far as the British government was concerned, it was already in compliance. There was no serious non-medical drug use. A tighter Pharmacy Act was introduced in 1908. All the bases were covered.

As there was no agreement on the opening agenda for Hague, negotiations and compromises meant proceedings ground on as the parties inched their way towards what needed to be an all-or-nothing agreement. Italy wanted cannabis to be controlled in its African possessions, Portugal sought to protect the opium revenues enjoyed by its colony in Macao, Russia refused to contemplate restrictions on poppy cultivation and Germany was unhappy about the implications of control for its cocaine industry. There were concerns that while Hague Convention proposals would apply to the nations that attended, what about the ones that did not – such as Turkey and also Switzerland with its significant pharmaceutical interests?

As the fine details of the Convention were being hammered out through 1912 to 1914, interdepartmental discussions were now underway in Whitehall as to what more needed to be done in the light of the Hague commitment to tighten up on domestic drug control. Initial thinking didn't extend much beyond having a look at existing pharmacy laws and increasing medical supervision of prescriptions. There was no appetite among civil servants or the medical profession for the sort of controls already existing at state level in the USA, further tightened by the passing of the punitive Harrison Narcotics Act in February 1914, copies of which were handed around at a series of meetings of Whitehall civil servants and medical and pharmaceutical interests. The Act did make an impression on the gathering, but in the end, there was not much more than tinkering around the edges. It was agreed retail and wholesale transactions of raw opium would be controlled and that import and export of prepared opium for smoking would be banned. It was also agreed that any preparations containing more than 2 per cent morphine or more than 1 per cent cocaine (way above the 0.2 per cent or 0.1 per cent as stipulated in the Convention) could only be obtained with a doctor's prescription. It would be up to the individual chemist to decide if requests for medicines under these limits were for 'legitimate and medical purposes'.

Then there was the question of which department would take the lead in drug regulation. Nobody was that keen. The police and the Pharmaceutical Society brought individual prosecutions for contraventions of pharmacy and poisons regulations. As it stood, oversight of these regulations came under the loose supervision of the Privy Council Office. Neither the Foreign nor Colonial Office wanted to take it on, nor did the Board of Trade. The Home Office was not even represented at earlier meetings and took the view that the Privy Council Office should deal with domestic control and sale while the Board of Trade should be responsible for import and export issues. There was no Ministry of Health until 1919. Then everything changed. On 15 July 1914, Britain ratified the Hague Convention. Three weeks later, the country went to war against Germany.

1

DORA, Billie and Freda

At the end of August 1915, Britain's ambassador to China Sir John Jordan sent a memo to the Foreign Office raising concerns about the smuggling of opium into China aboard British ships owned by Alfred Holt and Company, sailing from British ports. There does not seem to be a written response to this, presumably because the government was not sure what to do about it other than to ponder the question of trying to prevent the drugs getting aboard in the first place. There were no effective laws in place. The only controls on these drugs was the Pharmacy Act of 1868, as amended in 1908. The idea behind these Acts (and other legislation concerning poisons) was to ensure that only qualified persons dispensed a range of poisons, including opium products, and that there were administrative procedures in place at the point of sale to regulate the actions of pharmacies. There had been no conception of somebody legally buying drugs over the counter and then selling them on the streets. But while this memo was no doubt being moved from one departmental in-tray to another, the press, in particular the new generation of sensation-seeking mass market newspapers, came to the government's aid. Stories began to appear concerning the sale of drugs by prostitutes to soldiers coming home on leave.

Read in Tooth and Claw

The idea of producing newspapers that would play to the less noble instincts of society while making a fortune for the owners and shareholders was born in America, the brainchild of two of the very first media magnates, William Randolph Hearst and his arch-rival Joseph Pulitzer. Hearst was given control of the *San Francisco Chronicle* by his rich father and later moved to New York City and took over *The New York Journal*. He started a bitter circulation war with Pulitzer (who cut his journalistic teeth owning the *St Louis Despatch*) and his *New York World*. The rapid rise of mass-circulation newspapers in the USA was founded on two developments – the spread of the railways across the country and advertising revenue from the patent medicine industry, whose products contained the very drugs that would provide a rich harvest of scandal and outrage for what became known as yellow journalism. The essential features of this style are very familiar to us still, including scary headlines in huge print often relating to minor news stories, bad science, candid photos, misleading information, and unattributable quotes of the 'experts say' or 'critics say' type.

Hearst and Pulitzer went head-to-head to bring their readers the most lurid and sleazy stories about crime, sex and corruption. But their impact went deeper than just some vicarious thrills over the breakfast marmalade. These papers helped shape societal constructs about all sorts of people who were 'not like us', especially on subjects that most readers knew little about, such as drugs and drug users.

During the second-half of the nineteenth century, there was much concern in the USA about growing drug use, especially among urban youth, manifesting itself in pamphlets, speeches, books and articles in the medical press. But just as we talk today about 'echo chambers', so much of the anti-drug (and anti-alcohol) campaigning existed mainly among the members of various religious, social and moral reforming groups and their political allies and those who took the trouble to attend temperance meetings. What Hearst and Pulitzer realised was that the drugs issue ticked all the right boxes for their style of journalism. They became the willing megaphones of anti-drug campaigns claiming they were doing their bit to preserve the moral integrity of the nation.

The actual dangers of the drugs themselves were almost incidental; drug use became a proxy for some very deep-seated fears in American society at a time of social and economic turmoil. There was xenophobia and fear of the threat from outside because opium, morphine, heroin and cocaine originated in the poppy and coca fields of lands far away. Then racism; these foreign drugs were being used by foreigners such as the Chinese who were spreading their evil habits through opium dens enticing white people inside to sample sin and debauchery. Black slaves working in the fields and on the docks were given cocaine to make them work longer for less food. The narrative was now that freed slaves represented a clear and present danger, especially to white women. It was Hamilton Wright, the US international opium control negotiator, who helped promulgate the idea of the 'cocaine-crazed negro', prompting police in some southern states to be issued with higher-calibre guns. Use of drugs by young people became a metaphor for threats, both to the family and to the future of the young country, of a drug-addled generation unable to take the country forward. Maybe the biggest threat of all was miscegenation, the mixing of the races seen as an almost inevitable outcome of white women lounging around with black and Chinese undesirables, or worse, being seduced and drugged into white slavery. At an even deeper level, there was the notion that drugs (as anthropomorphic entities) and the people who sold them were inherently evil in the truly supernatural sense of the word. The belief was that drugs had a hold over their victims and somehow those victims themselves became infected with evil. This is where the mass market press played a particularly pernicious role. Hearst and Pulitzer knew full well a picture told a thousand words. They employed the best graphic artists to illustrate their scurrilous stories. On those pages was born the enduring image of the supernatural drug or dope fiend: the vampire, the walking dead, the outsider who only appeared at night to infect others; the grim reaper just waiting for the next victim. The fiend and the drug user became synonymous, the drug user became the scapegoat, responsible for society's ills and stigmatised with the mark of the beast. While people might be seduced by the demon drink, the implication of the dope fiend was that the evil resided in the person.

Scapegoating has a history that goes back to the Ancient World when a laden goat would be sent out of the city into the desert, its burden representing the sins of the people who saw this as necessary to cleanse their souls and appease the gods. In Ancient Greece, two men – a slave and somebody physically disabled, a criminal or an otherwise 'disposable' person, known interestingly as 'pharmakoi' (derived from the Greek word for poison) would be exiled from the city in times of war, disease or famine as an act of purification. Academics have argued over whether the pharmakoi were sacrificed, thrown from city walls or beaten and stoned but their end was not a happy one.

Stigmatisation occurs when a person possesses an attribute or status making the person less desirable or acceptable in other people's eyes and which then affects their interactions with others. When stigma takes centre stage, the person becomes identifiable only by the label attached to them. This is the lot of the chronic drug user; it becomes their master status. It doesn't matter that they may be many things: a mother, father, brother, sister, bank clerk, nurse, whatever – at best they are only an 'addict' or at worst a 'dope fiend', a 'junkie'. And these labels are readily accepted by those affected. Battered by very low self-esteem, they have bought into the narrative and embraced the stigma. For the sake of selling newspapers, this is the narrative on drug users that quickly became a deeply entrenched trope.

One British publisher of the time, Arthur Harmsworth, was particularly influenced by the example set by Hearst and Pulitzer. Born in Dublin in 1865 but educated in England, Harmsworth (later Viscount Northcliffe) began his newspaper career as a freelance journalist, moving on to publish a series of cheap and very successful periodicals such as *Comic Cuts*. He turned his attention to the national newspaper business, rescuing ailing newspapers such as the *Observer* and *The Times*. From a business point of view, he achieved most success as the founder of the *Daily Mail* in May 1896 (tagline the 'busy man's daily journal') and the *Daily Mirror* in 1903 (originally run by women for women as more of an entertainment 'light relief' paper). These papers along with *The Times* and the *News of the World* (founded as a scandal sheet as early as 1843), the *Daily Express* and the *Sunday People*, would embrace the new phenomenon of the drug scandal.

The drug at the centre of the first wave of British press hysteria about drugs was not morphine, heroin or opium, but cocaine. The cocaine alkaloid was first isolated in Germany in 1855 and became popular as a local anaesthetic in dentistry and an important ingredient in American patent medicines for hay fever, rhinitis and similar conditions, sometimes packaged conveniently with a rubber tube for snorting. Briefly, a coca-infused alcoholic drink called *Vin Mariani* was all the rage in Europe, but coca leaves don't travel well, making long-term production unsustainable. The main European production and export centres for pharmaceutical cocaine were the Netherlands (using coca leaves from their colonies in the East Indies) and central to the war panic over the drug – Germany.

* * *

A mythology has grown up that Britain believed the war would 'all be over by Christmas'. There is little evidence that this was the popular view, much less the official view of the military or government. In May 1915, the Germans sank RMS *Lusitania*, then the world's largest passenger liner, with the loss of 1,198 lives. This heightened hostility towards all foreign UK residents: not only were German shops attacked, accompanied by anti-German riots in London, Manchester and other cities, but also premises belonging to Jewish, Swiss, Russian and Chinese owners. As the war dragged on, fuelled by incidents like the sinking of the *Lusitania*, a feeling grew that perhaps forces were at work at home undermining the war efforts of an empire upon whom the sun was never supposed to set.

Confirmation of dirty deeds done cheap were revealed in February 1916, when the *Daily Mail* and *The Times* reported on the conviction of petty thief Horace Kingsley and prostitute Rose Edwards for selling cocaine to Canadian soldiers based in Folkestone. Apparently, Kingsley had just walked into a Dover chemist willing to sell him the drug without recording Kingsley's details as the Pharmacy Act required. Rose Edwards said she got her supply from a London dealer who, she said, 'sells to all us girls'.[1] The *Daily Mail* reported on 11 February under the headline 'Dopey Soldiers' that the Canadian military had

> for some time past … been trying to find out the source from which Canadian soldiers were getting large quantities of cocaine … The habit of taking cocaine made it useless to try and control the men who were often very unreliable and it very often resulted in insanity.

The Times added weight to the cocaine insanity story with an article by 'Our Medical Correspondent' titled 'The Cocaine Habit – Ruinous Results of a Drug – the Soldiers' Temptation'. Although claiming that cocaine was 'more deadly than bullets' and describing a plethora of debilitating effects, it did acknowledge that cocaine was bound to be a temptation for the soldier 'subjected to nervous strain and hard work' and that 'it will for the hour charm away all his troubles, his fatigue and anxiety; it will give him fictitious strength and vigour'.

Kingsley and Edwards were charged under Regulation 40 of the Defence of the Realm Act 1914 (DORA), which made it an offence to supply 'intoxicants' to members of the Armed Forces in order to make them 'drunk or disabled'.

The main purposes of the DORA were to defend the country and also boost morale at home. It gave sweeping powers to the government to requisition buildings or land, and to impose a whole raft of social control mechanisms. This meant strict censorship of news and information available to the public and permitted in letters passing between soldiers at the front and their families. Many banal everyday actions were banned such as loitering near bridges, whistling for a taxi in case people thought it was an air-raid warning or kite flying for fear of attracting zeppelins. You weren't allowed to buy binoculars, and when food rationing came in, feeding animals at the zoo was also banned. Prime Minister David Lloyd George, a long-time temperance advocate, used DORA to dramatically cut back on pub opening hours, restricting them to 12 p.m.–3 p.m. and 6 p.m.–9.30 p.m. The imposed afternoon break remained until the Licensing Act of 1988 allowed pubs to open from 11 a.m. to 11 p.m. Under DORA, buying a round of drinks was also banned to discourage drinking.

The Act was amended throughout the war, increasing the regulations from 66 to in excess of 200 including the introduction of the death penalty, which claimed the lives of eleven Germans found guilty of acts liable to aid the enemy. In Cardiff, six women were sent to jail for 62 days just for being in a public house, which caused such an outcry that the Home Secretary stepped in and quashed the sentences.

In the case of Kingsley and Edwards, the prosecution failed to prove intent, an important element of the regulation under which they were charged. *The Times* (12 February 1916) reported that, 'the evidence seemed to show that they acted on their own initiative and were actuated only by motives of personal greed'. But the public interest in the case, the fact that soldiers were involved, the defendants were of 'a certain class' and that Germany was a large manufacturer of cocaine, all told against them and they were sentenced to 6 months' hard labour.

The outcome of this case compared starkly with the two separate cases brought against Harrods and the chemist shop Savory & Moore and concluded just a day before the Folkestone convictions. These reputable establishments were accused under the Pharmacy Acts of advertising for sale gelatine sheets impregnated with morphine and cocaine as 'useful presents for our friend at the front'. The prosecution in the Harrods case was led by Sir William Glyn-Jones, Secretary of the Pharmaceutical Society, who declared that 'it might have the effect of making them sleep on duty or other very serious results'.[2] No hard labour for the proprietors, of course; just a token fine.

There was more than a hint of double standards, not just in these cases, but in the whole issue of British military use of cocaine in the First World War. In his book *A Short History of Drugs and War*, Lukasz Kamienski relates that 'the British Army used extensively a medicine available on the market… [named] "Tabloid" or "Forced March"'. The strapline was 'Allays hunger and prolongs the power of endurance'. The drug contained cocaine and cola nut and was manufactured by Burroughs Wellcome, 'a well-known London pharmaceutical company and also the first to launch cocaine in tablet form'. And the company address in London? Snow Hill Buildings EC1. According to this account, the drug was used by the polar expeditions of Ernest Shackleton and Captain Scott, and by Ronald Amundsen, who beat Scott to the South Pole. 'Because Forced March worked so well during these extremely wearying expeditions, it is hardly surprising that the command of the British Army decided to try it out on the soldiers of the expeditionary force in Europe.'[3]

As if to underline the vagaries of the law, very shortly after the two Pharmacy Act cases, another cocaine possession charge came before Bow Street Police Court. In April 1916, police had information about a gang selling cocaine to prostitutes, chorus girls and others. Police were told where sales were taking place in and around Soho and apprehended one of the gang, Willy Johnson, whose escape was probably hampered by his artificial leg. However, when the case came to court it was dismissed because there was no evidence that the cocaine had been acquired illegally, possession was not an offence and Johnson wasn't caught selling any drugs. The frustrated magistrate declared that he 'sincerely hoped that the result of this case would lead to a speedy and drastic alteration in the law with regard to the sale of poisons'. The prosecution added that the use of cocaine constituted 'a grave social evil which the authorities did not have in their minds when the Defence of the Realm Act was passed'. This was an interesting comment, the implication being that drugs did not just pose a threat to the efficiency of the army but was a general threat to the nation in time of war.

Yet while it appeared that Canadian soldiers were being targeted and so portrayed as victims of evil pushers, they also came under attack themselves for supplying cocaine for drug-fuelled West End 'orgies'. One publication, *Umpire*, made the *Daily Mail* look positively restrained: 'Vicious Drug Powder – Cocaine Driving Hundreds Mad'; 'Women and Aliens Prey On Soldiers'; 'London In The Grip Of Drug Craze'; 'Secret Parties Of Snow Snifters'. Americans over here as visitors (soldiers didn't arrive until 1917) set up opium dens in and around the West End patronised by the whole panoply of Soho *demi-monde* night people.[4] Generally, though, it was easier to blame prostitutes and petty criminals for undermining the war effort than the brave lads come to save us from the ravages of the Hunnish hordes.

Meanwhile, the shipping firm Arthur Holt and Company sent a lengthy memo of its own to the Foreign Office explaining that it employed many Chinese sailors and firemen; it was these men who were taking opium on board and selling it once the ships had docked anywhere where there was a Chinese community. The company said it was impossible to police this as the drug was so readily available in Britain and thus it felt the only option (because the unlicensed export of opium and cocaine from Britain was banned in November 1914) was for the government to tackle the problem upstream and deal with internal supply and possession.

Cognisant of the pressure to act, an Army Order in Council was issued in May 1916 (under Regulations in the DORA Consolidation 1914) which went further than simply banning 'intoxicant' sales to members of the Armed Forces. 'Intoxicant' had been very generally defined and could have included any of the drugs that the new Order specified, but presumably for the purposes of a legal instrument with penalties attached, a level of specificity was required. The drugs listed were not just cocaine, but barbiturate (a sleeping pill first synthesised in Germany in 1903 and marketed as Veronal by Bayer from 1904), and other sedative and hypnotic drugs such as Sulphinol and chloral hydrate; Indian hemp, opium, morphine, codeine, and diamorphine.

These could not be supplied, sold or procured for and on behalf of a member of the Armed Forces unless ordered by a doctor on a written prescription dated and signed by him and marked 'not to be repeated'. The chemist continued to be obliged to note all the relevant details in a register.

The medical press was very supportive: doctors had fought for years for this level of control over the supply of what were now known as 'narcotic drugs'[5] rather than poisons only to be knocked back by the retailers and their professional organisations. *The Lancet* observed that the order was 'yet another instance of an innovation, long advocated in years of peace being secured without controversy under the stimulus of a great war'. The article went on to suggest that the new drug law should apply to society as a whole and not just the Armed Forces and it should be done in wartime to prevent more resistance from vested interests once the war was over.[6]

The government now had two memos on the problems of smuggling from UK ports, a growing body of evidence that drugs were being supplied to soldiers as well as the medical, judicial and mainstream press pushing for further action. But the Army Order of itself wouldn't deal with the general smuggling issue, only supply to the military. The question arose as to which existing regulations could deal with largely unrestricted retail (and wholesale) supplies of the listed drugs.

A government interdepartmental meeting was convened in June 1916 at the suggestion of the Colonial Office to consider how best to deal with this wider issue of drug supply. Rather than engage in more battles with pharmaceutical interests by more amendments to the Pharmacy Act, it made more bureaucratic and political sense simply to add a new regulation to the DORA. There were existing regulations concerning the importance of 'war materials' and certainly opiate-based drugs were valuable war materials crucial in dealing with injuries sustained in battle. Ordinarily it would have been harder to argue for cocaine's inclusion as a vital war material, but the scandal over sales to soldiers was justification enough to include cocaine in the DORA drug regulations.

The Home Office did not even attend previous interdepartmental meetings concerning international drug control, but now the issue focused on domestic controls. The police were already charged with street-level enforcement of such drug regulations that did exist, but under the umbrella of war and protecting the nation, wider powers would clearly fall under the overarching jurisdiction of the Home Office. The department now moved centre stage, driven by the civil servant who would become the lead official on UK drug control, Sir Malcolm Delevingne.

Delevingne was born in London in October 1868, to Ernest and Helen Delevingne. Ernest was a wine merchant, born in Paris to British parents, but of Huguenot descent. His son won a scholarship to Trinity College, Oxford, in 1887 gaining a double first in classical moderations and *Literae Humaniores* in 1891. In 1892, Delevingne passed the civil service examination, starting off in the Local Government Board, then transferred to the Home Office. He was knighted in 1919, eventually rising to the rank of Permanent Under Secretary in 1922, a post he held until his retirement in 1932.

Once at the Home Office, his privately held religious views and his sense of social responsibility came to the fore. He was instrumental in pushing through landmark factory and mines legislation to significantly improve the safety and general working conditions for employees. He was also involved with the children's charity Barnardo's from 1903 and joined its board on his retirement.

According to his entry in the *Oxford Dictionary of National Biography* and his *Times* obituary published on 1 December 1950, he was variously described by colleagues as imaginative, innovative, 'clever and able' and was imbued with drive, determination, and a 'remorseless quest for precision'. Senior colleagues also regarded him as courteous, kind, loyal, and even lovable.

Even so, while his personal views on some important departmental issues were undoubtedly humanitarian, he was also a man of his times. And as the suspect and troublesome supply of drugs appeared to be located within an equally suspect and troublesome segment of society, Delevingne had no compunction but to act and has gone down in history as the architect of UK drug prohibition.

His methods sometimes attracted criticism. This was partly because he was something of an autocrat who preferred to deal with a matter personally rather than to delegate, and partly because he 'sometimes gave the impression of being too much the bureaucrat who thought that to settle a matter you had only to tie it up in a bundle of regulations, preferably of his own drafting'.

This was nicely demonstrated in 1931 at an international conference that tried to hammer out further international controls on opium production. As well as being at the helm of UK domestic drug policy, Delevingne not only represented Britain at the international level, but also played a key role in the development of international drug policy in the interwar years. The conference of 1931 rejected proposals largely drawn up by Delevingne, that the raw opium-producing countries should have a world monopoly under a quota system to try to limit international distribution. He was so annoyed at this rejection that he publicly withdrew his cooperation but stayed in the meeting reading *The Times*. As the meeting stuttered to a halt over yet more drafting problems, the chairman asked Delevingne for his help, a request abruptly refused. At this, the Canadian delegate sitting behind Delevingne piped up that the British official's attitude would have been more convincing, 'if you did not read the London *Times* upside down'.[7]

Back to the summer of 1916. If Delevingne and his fellow civil servants needed any further ammunition at least about cocaine, it was provided by *The Times* on 13 July which in a leading article demanded that unauthorised possession and sale of cocaine be 'punishable with a substantial term of imprisonment without the option of a fine' because the 'moral and physical effects of its abuse are inevitable and disastrous'.

Five days later, on 18 July 1916, Regulation 40B of the Defence of the Realm Act (known as DORA 40B) came into force. The Army Order of May remained in place, banning the supply, sale and procurement of a long list of drugs to military personnel. This new regulation introduced a general ban but focused on cocaine (because of all the concerns and pressures) and opium (to deal primarily with the export smuggling issue). To demonstrate that opium controls were not just about smuggling, the already ingrained suspicions about opium dens were underpinned by further restrictions in October 1917 specifically aimed at the Chinese community where the preparing of opium for smoking, allowing premises to be used for opium smoking and being in possession of the necessary paraphernalia were all outlawed.

The introduction of the word 'procurement' in the new drug regulations was a recognition of a signal moment in the development of the embryonic drug scene. Such as it was, the scene was very small, located mainly in premises in and around the streets of Soho whose patrons would have been primarily actors, actresses, chorus girls, dancers, small-time crooks and the more louche, playboy elements of the upper classes. But small as it was, the group represented a new market for psychoactive drugs and one that would not mainly be serviced by doctors, but by third parties who either bought supplies legitimately or courtesy of a bent chemist or dentist, and then sold them or even gave them away as gifts, favours or bribes.

In the months following the introduction of the new drug laws, the Home Office seemed well pleased that it was successfully dealing with a problem which, it admitted in a memo, didn't really amount to much in the first place:

The reports (from police forces) ... show that the Regulation is working smoothly ... in a number of cases it is reported the effect has been negligible as cocaine and opium were so little used before ... Attempted infringements are few in number and in most cases are not, perhaps, intentional ... References to persons known or suspected to be victims of the cocaine habit, or opium takers, are exceedingly few.[8]

This complete lack of a cocaine 'epidemic' was confirmed in February 1917 when a committee convened to investigate cocaine use in dentistry concluded that there was 'no evidence of any kind to show that there is a serious or perhaps even noticeable prevalence of the cocaine habit amongst the civilian or military population of Great Britain'.[9]

Regarding opium, another Home Office memo of the time recorded with some satisfaction that the new regulation resulted in twelve Chinese men being deported from Liverpool causing 'a holy panic throughout [the city] and cast feeling of terrible insecurity among the Chinese population'.

In the main though, in the two-and-a-half years between the introduction of general prohibition against cocaine and opium and the end of the war in November 1918, there were very few prosecutions, mainly involving the Chinese community where the sentence was usually a fine or sometimes a short term of imprisonment. On 21 December 1918, a case came before the Thames Police Court involving Lau Ping You charged with being in possession of opium smoking equipment. The magistrate, Mr Rooth, admitted that he had a 'difficulty here to contend with' that opium smoking was 'universal' in China, but regarded as a 'national vice' in this country for which the man could go to prison for 6 months and fined £100 or, as a foreign national, be deported. Rooth went on to say that whatever happened in other courts was not his business, and he was also mindful that the police were satisfied the equipment was for personal use and the defendant was addicted to opium, a habit he was trying his best to overcome. Lau Ping You was fined £10. His Scottish wife Ada was not so lucky and found herself at the centre of Britain's first celebrity drug story.

* * *

The illegitimate daughter of a chorus singer, Florence Leonora Stewart was born in London in September 1896 and brought up by her aunt. Despite her unpromising start in life, she became well read, fluent in French and German, and an excellent pianist. Changing her name to Billie Carleton, she left home aged 15 for a life on the stage. Lacking a father, she gravitated towards 'father figures', but being a very attractive teenager, no doubt older men were also attracted to her and as she progressed in her chosen profession, she gathered a triumvirate of sugar daddies around her. The first such figure in her life was John Marsh, a playboy with private means and reputation for throwing his money around. Billie lapped up the lavish lifestyle: the flat in Savile Row, trips in the Rolls-Royce, champagne and a personal bank balance at one point of £5,000 when the most she ever earned was £25 a week. The second older man was her doctor, Frederick Stuart, who became her friend and took on the role of managing the money generously supplied by Marsh. The third member of this trio was Raoul 'Reggie' de Veulle, the son of a British consul, one-time actor now a theatrical dress designer. He was already a cocaine user and introduced Billie into the West End's tight drug-using circle. As she moved rapidly up the theatrical hierarchy, Billie's use of opium and cocaine became an open secret. Dr Stuart's concern about his young charge's drug use (he once confiscated her cocaine) was mitigated somewhat by giving her morphine injections for wisdom tooth pain and a supply of Veronal barbiturate sleeping pills.

Like Marilyn Monroe, she was a rising star, a very attractive young actress able to keep powerful men at her beck and call through a combination of sexual allure and apparent innocence. She was working in a cut-throat, stressful profession and using various drugs probably to self-medicate against loneliness and depression. One of her escapes from reality was a trip to Limehouse, in the company of an actor, Lionel Belcher, to the opium den run by Ada Lau Ping who also supplied some low-grade cocaine. Billie herself hosted opium parties when she was staying at Reggie's flat in Dover Street, much to the annoyance of Reggie's wife, Pauline. Billie had her whole life ahead of her and with the end of war in November 1918 came the promise of a role in a production in Paris and maybe even America.

Billie did become a household name, but in the most unfortunate circumstances. On 27 November 1918, she attended a Victory Ball at the Royal Albert Hall. She returned to her flat in the early hours of the next morning with Lionel Belcher and Pauline de Veulle. They had breakfast together and the guests left the flat around 5 a.m. with Billie sitting up in bed. About 10 a.m. Billie made a call to friend. Housekeeper May Booker arrived for work at approximately 11.30 a.m. to hear loud snoring coming from the bedroom. By 3.30 p.m., the snoring had stopped. May went in, tried unsuccessfully to wake Billie and called Dr Stuart. His attempts at resuscitation failed; Billie Carleton was declared dead.

Billie's death opened up the London drug scene to very public scrutiny. The case received widespread coverage in all the major newspapers and magazines. Reporting on the inquest, the *News of the World* (5 January 1919) revelled in faux outrage: 'Young women and men have frankly confessed to being drug takers – the drugs indulged in being cocaine and heroin. So far as it has gone, the inquiry into the death of Billie Carleton has shown that in the West End of London, in the quiet seclusion of luxurious flats, the most disgusting orgies take place.'

Billie's death resulted in the arrest and trial of Ada Lau Ping accused of supplying opium and smoking equipment. *The Times* (21 December 1918) reported,

> After dinner, the party adjourned to the drawing room of the flat and having provided themselves with cushions and pillows placed them on the floor and sat thereon in a circle. The men divested themselves of their clothing and got into pyjamas and the women into chiffon nightdresses. In that manner, they seemed to prepare themselves for the orgy. There were about five or six of them. Miss Carleton arrived later at the flat from the theatre, and she, after disrobing, took her place in this circle of degenerates. In the centre of it, Mrs Ping officiated. She had an opium tin and the lamp, the opium needle and all the accessories. She prepared the opium ... The party remained apparently in a comatose state until about 3 o'clock on the following afternoon.

Albeit that the charges against Ada Ping were more serious that those faced by her husband, she had the misfortune to be in front of very different magistrate. Francis Mead (who would later fine a man for sunbathing without his shirt on) accused Ada of being 'the high priestess of unholy rites' and sentenced her to 5 months' hard labour.

The inquest itself attracted much attention: the court was packed for the five days of the proceedings and among the crowds were some well-known actors and actresses, keen to hear what was going on but perhaps fearful too of an unwelcome mention. So intense was the interest that after the third day, the coroner barred the public to allow room for the witnesses, lawyers and the large press contingent. Lionel Belcher and Alfred Toose were called as witnesses but were also in the firing line for supplying cocaine. In his defence, Toose said that he had simply been given the cocaine by Belcher to destroy after Billie died and he didn't want to drop his friend in it, a plea to honour that clearly impressed the coroner; neither men subsequently faced any charges. The case needed a fall guy: the spotlight fell on Reggie. He admitted supplying cocaine to Billie but not on the day of her death. With no evidence presented, counsel representing the others instead launched a character assassination of Reggie, even calling his sexuality into question as Reggie was not only a dress designer but also exhibited 'effeminate' ways. The inquest jury concluded that Billie had died of an accidental self-administered dose of cocaine, but that it had been supplied in a 'culpable and negligent manner'.

The jury didn't name Reggie: following the verdict, the coroner declared that 'somebody supplied her – that is certain and it is an unlawful thing to supply anyone with cocaine'. He went on to say that if one person supplies another and it leads to a death, the supplier is guilty of manslaughter and on that basis, Reggie de Veulle was charged with the manslaughter of Billie Carleton and conspiracy to supply cocaine.

The Old Bailey trial went over all the same ground as before, yet on 5 April 1919, after three days of proceedings, the jury took only 50 minutes to find Reggie not guilty of manslaughter. He was subsequently sentenced to 8 months, without hard labour, after pleading guilty to the conspiracy charge. Despite the inquest verdict, the coroner's statement and Judge Salter's unequivocal direction in his summing up at the Old Bailey, the jury were not convinced that cocaine alone was responsible for Billie's death, thus Reggie could not be convicted of manslaughter. Nor was there any evidence that Reggie had supplied the fatal dose. Expert witnesses at the trial disagreed as to whether or not Billie's state of health could have been a contributory factor. There was a suggestion the sleeping pill Veronal could have been the cause. None were found in her system, but that didn't mean, admitted the Public Analyst Percy Richards, that she hadn't taken any, betraying the embryonic state of forensic science at the time. Billie had had some Veronal in the room, which Dr Stuart, who had given her the drugs, apparently managed to pocket at the scene and they were never produced in evidence. Given the way she died – she just went to sleep and never woke up – it does seem more like a sleeping pill than cocaine overdose, although equally she could have had a cocaine-induced heart attack. We will never know. Nor do we know what became of Reggie de Veulle after his spell in Wormwood Scrubs, save for a solitary credit as a costume designer in a 1926 West End musical.

* * *

It was always the intention of Home Office officials to continue the controls on drugs once the war was over. The Billie Carleton case made it clear that despite initial official optimism, DORA 40B had not shut down the drug scene. The *News of the World* (5 January 1919) reported that rather than a handful of entertainers taking drugs, 'hundreds of others were in the same situation', ensnared in 'a drug cult'. Readers were led to believe that drugs were readily available in every Soho café and on every street corner; anybody

> who knows the ropes can buy heroin, cocaine, morphia or any of the preparations of opium … Hashish, the drug of the Assassins[10] – is available in cigarette form, in compressed tablet or in the dark green treacly liquid' to the extent that 'hundreds' of young men and women 'were indulging in the vicious habits of the drug slave, taking part in indescribable orgies and courting the dangers so painfully exemplified by Billie Carleton's fate.

And despite the regulations in place, there were still cryptic newspaper headlines blaring 'Limehouse Secrets/Barred Doors/Trap Flaps and Hidden

Bell in Opium Raid' and 'Opium Den Raid/Chinaman's Three Savage Guardians/Drug Heavy Air'.

If more robust legislative justification was needed, it was provided by the outcome of the Paris Peace Conference, which opened in January 1919. Despite two more Hague Conferences on international drug control which took place before the outbreak of war, the Hague Convention was still not formally in operation. Although not directly a concern of those negotiating the Versailles Treaty, it was thought that it would be convenient to deliberate on the Convention as all the major powers were in the room. The Treaty was signed on 28 June 1919; Article 295 obliged the contracting powers to introduce such legislation as was necessary to bring into force the International Opium Convention not later than a year after the signing. In May 1920 the Liberal Home Secretary Edward Shortt duly introduced the Dangerous Drugs Bill.

Apart from the usual difficulties from pharmaceutical interests, the Home Office now had a new adversary to deal with from within its own civil service ranks. A Ministry of Health had been created in 1919 and attempted to define control of 'narcotics' as part of its responsibility. Malcolm Delevingne gave the idea short shrift and won the day by sheer weight of obstinacy, although he agreed that the two ministries would have joint responsibility for the detailed regulations that would attach to the Bill.

The Bill went beyond both DORA 40B and the Opium Convention by empowering the authorities not only to regulate, in any way necessary, morphine, cocaine and opium and all current and future salts and other alkaloids, but any drug that might have similar effects to either morphine or cocaine with the potential to cause harm if 'improperly used'. The only organisation with concerns was of course the Pharmaceutical Society keen to protect the interests of its members now that the Home Office could no longer point to the imperatives of the war effort and national security. But such technical issues as existed were quickly resolved.

The Bill itself was so uncontroversial and generated so little parliamentary interest that when it was scheduled for committee discussion, the meeting failed four times to convene a quorum, eventually romping through the business in 20 minutes. The only debate in Parliament was the continuing disquiet among the remaining anti-opium lobby about the British manufacturing involvement in morphine addiction in the Far East. The Dangerous Drugs Act (DDA) passed its third reading in July 1920.

While the passage of the Act was smooth, agreeing the 1921 Dangerous Drugs Regulations and subsequent amendments to the DDA in 1923 was a different matter. The Home Office turned its attention to opiate-based proprietary medicines proposing that any such medicine should only be available on prescription, which in those pre-NHS days would mean that everyday medicines would become far more expensive. Such was the furore that it reached the newspapers: the *Sunday Post* (6 February 1921) declared. 'Would you believe it? Every man, woman and child in this country today is either a dope fiend or heading that way. You may smile and say the idea is ridiculous. In that case, I simply refer you to the intellectual giants of the Home Office.' Pharmacists were also appalled at what they saw as unacceptable increases in the level of record keeping now expected of them. Any oversight could lead to fines or even imprisonment for the most minor slip-ups. But the Ministry of Health was not sympathetic to complaints, believing that pharmacists were just out to undermine the DDA in their own interests. Dismissing medical protests was a different matter.

Because the law since 1916 had put 'narcotic' drug prescribing in their hands, doctors voiced little criticism. But amendments put forward for the DDA in early 1923 included a proposal that doctors would no longer be allowed to prescribe narcotic drugs for themselves. The medical press condemned this as unenforceable and an insult to the profession when the problem resided only in a few 'degenerates'. So strong was their objection that even Delevingne had to back down. While pharmacists had no political clout, the medical profession had influential political and social connections, a reality that would shape Delevingne's future *modus operandi* over drug control.

***

Due to their rarity, true life cases like Billie Carleton's attracted much attention. However, since the turn of the century, the public had been drip-fed a steady stream of fictionalised accounts that added heft to the mythology of the dope fiend. From its earliest days, the film industry in Europe and America brought to life stories ripped off from the newspaper headlines. *Chinese Opium Den* was made as early as 1894, *Rube in an Opium Joint* (1905), *Dream of an Opium Fiend* (1906), the Danish film *Opiumsdroemmen* (1914), *The Secret Sin* (1914) and one of the most famous drug films of the era, D.W. Griffiths' *Broken Blossoms* (1919), which actually depicted the Chinese opium smoker in an unusually sympathetic light. Some of these films used the vehicle of the opium dream to try out new ideas in special effects.[11]

Sax Rohmer (born Arthur Henry Ward, pseudonym Arthur Sarsfield Ward) based his novel *Dope* on the life of Billie Carleton. In the casual and unremarked upon racism of the period, he gave us the archetypal oriental evil genius, the ever-inscrutable and eternally diabolical Dr Fu Manchu. Starting in 1912, Rohmer managed to squeeze out thirteen books, with numerous film adaptations, based on this character, probably doing more than any press magnate to daub the entire Chinese community with the paint of infamy. Then, in 1922, real life kicked in again and set the British press off on another exploration of London's vice-ridden streets.

Freda Kempton was a wannabe actress who was very much part of West End nightlife, dancing until the early hours, having breakfast and finally arriving home as the sun came up. Freda was noted for her energetic cocaine-fuelled dancing style. Having spent the night of Sunday 5 March partying and clubbing, she spent most of the next day in bed. Around 8 p.m., her flatmate arrived home to find Freda crying out in pain, banging her head against the wall, whereupon she collapsed, foaming at the mouth, and died. Because Freda had left the burnt remains of what read like a suicide note, the coroner recorded death by suicide due to drugs supplied by person or persons unknown. But the press was in no doubt who supplied the drug; a well-known 'dope king' of London, Dr Fu Manchu in the flesh: 'Brilliant' Billy Chang. Yet Brilliant Chang looked nothing like the evil pigtailed doctor dressed in traditional Chinese garb, hands clasped in sleeves, lurking in the shadows, plotting his devious schemes of ensnaring innocent young women. Sporting Savile Row suits and fur-trimmed overcoats, Chang came from a wealthy family with business interests in Shanghai and Hong Kong. He had a smart office in the City of London from where he conducted family business, including contract work for the Admiralty, and had part-ownership of a Chinese restaurant in Regent Street. He was a charismatic, attractive playboy, a central and highly visible figure of West End nightlife, an exotic and erotic Svengali character as far as women were concerned, and an alleged supplier of cocaine to Freda, an accusation he denied at the inquest.

This new round of investigative reporting about Soho's seedy underbelly focused not on doped soldier war paranoia, but on the wider issues of young women and their cocaine indulgences. Only six weeks after Freda's death, a film simply called *Cocaine* was banned by the Board of Film Censors (BFC). Delevingne saw the film and denounced it, perhaps surprisingly, as too over the top and an unscientific portrait of the effects of cocaine, showing as it does a girl becoming 'an abandoned hussy' after a single dose. The members of the BFC itself thought the film might encourage rather than discourage use.

But even allowing for press hyperbole, while geographically circumscribed, there was a healthy traffic in cocaine – easily the most popular recreational drug of the times. The Metropolitan Police upped their game in trying to clamp down on cocaine trafficking with women officers (now allowed to undertake police duties under the Police Act 1916) posing as prostitutes. Penalties for dealing were increased under the Dangerous Drugs Act 1923, especially for repeat offenders and the Metropolitan Police did manage to sweep up quite low-level operators in the period 1922–23 to the extent that by Christmas 1923, *The Times* was reporting a significant reduction in cocaine trafficking.

So where had all the cocaine been coming from? An amount was in circulation from corrupt chemists and dentists, but with the end of the war and a resumption of normal European travel, the drug was also being smuggled into Britain in small parcels, mainly from Germany. There were occasional large seizures: in 1922, an Australian passenger from Germany was arrested coming into Britain with 3½ pounds of cocaine hidden in a false-bottomed suitcase.

Back in December 1918, the *Daily Express* claimed that drug supply in London was in the hands of a criminal organisation called 'The Vice Trust', who had interests in prostitution, gambling and nightclubs and who used women as drug dealers selling primarily to women on the club scene. The term 'Trust' came from the American white slavery scare of the period and was perhaps another example of how the British press took their cue for sensationalism from their American cousins. The US press often used the word 'Trust' to imply some form of coordinated conspiracy or corruption in the financial world. As the recent BBC TV series *Peaky Blinders* portrayed, there were some very violent gangs operating in London at the time, mainly connected to gambling and protection, but perhaps apart from Brilliant

Chang's operation (he made a brief appearance in one episode) – there was no evidence of gangs being involved in high-end drug supply.

The police really wanted Brilliant Chang who, despite seeing some of his restaurant staff arrested on dealing charges, remained out of reach. Having paid two fruitless visits to his house in search of drugs, they finally claimed success in April 1924 when police paid another visit to his home and 'found' a small packet of cocaine in a cupboard. Would as sharp an operator as Chang have made such a stupid mistake, especially as he had already been visited by the police? In court, the police said that many of those arrested over the past couple of years claimed Chang was their supplier. The police knew what Chang was up to, but just couldn't get him for what he did. In any event, he was sentenced to 11 months in prison and deported.

But from a press point of view, the Soho scene just kept giving, not just a real-life Fu Manchu, but another figure exemplifying the exotic, erotic and dangerous world of drugs: Edgar Manning, a black jazz musician. Born in Jamaica, Manning was another well-dressed magnet for young women, seducing one Doreen Taylor and then living off her immoral earnings as a prostitute. His first documented run-in with the law though came after shooting three men in the legs following an altercation in the West End. But despite a shooting in broad daylight in the middle of usually crowded streets, a stylish display of civility and remorse defended by Huntly Jenkins, who had defended Reggie de Veulle, saw Manning get off with a charge of unlawful wounding instead of attempted murder, earning him the relatively light sentence of 16 months' hard labour.

Manning was now on the police radar and when a former soldier addicted to heroin died of an overdose in Manning's flat, although Manning was out at the time, he became a 'person of interest' implicated in the supply of cocaine (including to Freda Kempton) but with no evidence to substantiate the allegations. He set up a flat with a Greek woman, Zenovia Iassonides, where a more discreet clientele would come and use drugs on the premises. Police received a tip-off that Manning had a whopping 2 pounds of cocaine in his room. They rushed round but found nothing. Manning wrote in aggrieved tones to the Metropolitan Police Commissioner.

Only a week later, however, Manning was caught red-handed. The full inventory of the police haul was 15 tablets of morphine, a bottle of cocaine, opium smoking kit, needles and syringes, a set of pornographic photographs, 13 ounces of opium and a gun, scales, a price list of injectable drugs and a hollowed-out silver can for transporting drugs. Manning got a month for the gun and 6 months for the drugs, but by the time he was inevitably arrested again with a similar array of drugs plus a gun in his possession, the stakes were much higher. An amendment to the DDA in 1923 meant he now faced a maximum sentence of 10 years' penal servitude in the toughest prisons, although in the end the sentence was 3 years in Parkhurst on the Isle of Wight.

He was released in November 1925 and in February 1926 sold his story to the *World Pictorial News*. In an overcooked, breathless article, he claimed that he came to Britain to fulfil his parents' dream to see him become a respectable member of society until he was seduced by a white woman and introduced to the mad excitement of Soho. He went on to describe wild coke parties and sex orgies driven by pulsating jazz rhythms, claiming that not only was he the 'dope king of London' but introduced Brilliant Chang to the scene. As far the press was concerned, he was not somebody who had taken the wrong path, but simply 'The Evil Negro' and 'The Black Devil'. He was a portent of a new threat to white girls; the suave, well-dressed, predatory, black drug dealer whose easy charm tinged with danger made impressionable young white girls putty in his hands as they swayed to the throb of jazz's intoxicating beat, the soundtrack to a life wrecked by 'reefer madness'. For Manning, though, he was broken in health and spirit by a succession of jail terms and died in Parkhurst prison hospital in February 1931.

***

In *Dope Girls*, Marek Kohn's study of the early years of the British drug scene which forms the basis of this chapter, his central point was that the subtext of all the hyperbole about illicit drug use was less about drugs and more to do with the fact that those who seemed most attracted to them, especially cocaine, were young women who became the poster girls for post-war 'modernity'.

The tenor of the press reporting portrayed these users as immature, highly strung 'flappers', of a nervous disposition, fragile butterflies in need of protection from the predatory foreign and older men. This was really a Victorian view of womanhood, delicate flowers best left at home to do womanly things. But the war had changed much.

Women had emerged from behind the curtains of Victorian respectability and submissive compliance to replace a workforce lying dead in the trenches. Women were seen smoking in public, going out together to restaurants, dancing the night away in clubs and cocaine 'warehouse parties', early forerunners of the ecstasy-driven rave venues of the 1990s. The women's suffrage movement, on hold during the war, picked up with new vigour and in November 1918, the Representation of the People's Act gave the vote to all men over 21 and women over the age of 30 so long as they met various property criteria. It took another 10 years for women to be on an equal electoral footing with men, but the 1918 Act was a recognition that the war was a watershed between the old world and the new.

This was exemplified by the contrasting presentations about Billie Carleton at the trial of Reggie de Veulle. Judge Salter took that Victorian view of young women being led astray and taken advantage of recalling those comedy images of the villain in the frock coat and top hat, twirling his moustache, plotting the downfall of the innocent. In defence of his client, de Veulle's counsel Huntly Jenkins presented a contrasting view. Billie was no hapless victim, but Reggie's peer, totally responsible for her own actions and as free to follow her life choices as anybody else.

2

A Very British System

The notion of somebody becoming addicted to opium, morphine or laudanum was a recognised phenomenon in the late nineteenth century even if the scale was unknown, especially among the working class. Such documentary evidence as there was, appeared as case studies written up in the medical press concerning middle-class individuals who had succumbed to some kind of disease of the will. There was no public concept of recreational, hedonistic drug use in Britain until the early years of the First World War. Legislation enacted from then on focused on controlling import and export of 'narcotics' and clamping down on domestic supply and possession, first in the national interest, and when war was over, in the interests of national moral probity. DORA 40B and the DDA aimed to tackle drug use for pleasure on the night scene. However, what about those people who simply could not give up, whose regular use had reached a point where they needed drugs to feel normal, receiving legal prescriptions from doctors in support of their addiction? How did they fit into the new scheme of things?

The primary aim of the Hague Convention was to deal with the drug problem in the Far East, obliging the signatories to enact domestic legislation to limit as far as possible the export of raw and prepared opium, morphine and cocaine and all their analogues. But Hamilton Wright, the American driving force behind the international negotiations, wanted more than that. He had been thwarted at home in 1910 when his legislative proposals for a tough prohibitionist drug law (the Foster Bill) had been defeated by the pharmaceutical industry. Yet Article 20 of the Convention required signatories to consider introducing laws making possession of these drugs illegal as well as all the stipulations around manufacture, production, supply, distribution, import and export.

Wright went home and using America's treaty obligations as leverage, fended off the objections of medical and pharmaceutical interests and saw his drug prohibition proposals adopted as the Harrison Narcotics Tax Act in December 1914. The Act was formulated as a tax and revenue measure, so anybody involved in 'narcotic drugs' had to be registered, pay relevant stamp duties and keep several detailed records. To formulate the legislation in this way was really a ruse to mask its intent as an instrument of social and moral control. As a tax measure, enforcement fell under the jurisdiction of the Inland Revenue Bureau's treasury agents. The detailed regulations that followed stated that a consumer could not be registered and could only obtain supplies from a registered doctor. This meant somebody with a drug addiction could not register and even if they had a prescription, the doctor could still be in violation of the Act if the amount prescribed to a user was not a 'normal dose'. There was no definition of a 'normal dose', nor was there any guidance for chemists who received instructions from the Bureau to watch out for prescriptions involving 'unusually large' doses of drugs.

It soon became clear that the Bureau was running into legal problems: its interpretation of the Act as prohibiting doctors from prescribing morphine to those addicted to the drug, was not shared by district court judges around the country. The matter was settled (for the time being) by a Supreme Court judgement in June 1916, in favour of maintenance prescribing. However, in a rerun of the cocaine scare in Britain, other factors came to the aid of the Federal government in turning the climate of opinion around.

The temperance movement scored a historical success with the passing of the Volstead Act in 1918 ushering in alcohol prohibition, while in 1919, the country was gripped by perceived threats to the nation as a result of entering the war and also by radical labour groups inspired and allegedly orchestrated by Bolshevik revolutionaries. This in turn heightened fear and loathing of any activity that might lead to antisocial behaviour and general undermining of national strength. High on the list was drug use under any circumstances. In this febrile atmosphere, the previous Supreme Court ruling was overturned and maintenance prescribing outlawed. However, it was accepted that there were those who could not immediately give up their drugs so it was proposed that instead, medical facilities would be established but in the expectation that patients would be on reducing doses of drugs. Several clinics were set up around the country, but strictly enforced time-limited treatment was never going to work. Few clinics could report any cures and by around 1925 all the clinics had been forced to close. Those with a drug problem caught in possession of drugs and the doctors prescribing for them were now criminals. In Britain, Malcolm Delevingne faced the same issue, albeit it on a much smaller scale.

In requiring signatories to ensure that the drugs listed were only available for 'medical and legitimate purposes', the Hague Convention left it up to the individual powers to define exactly what that meant. In Britain, the validity or otherwise of maintenance prescribing was never considered during the deliberations over DORA 40B. Neither did the precise wording of the Dangerous Drugs Act 1920 or the Regulations 1921 settle the matter. The relevant Regulation 11 did not directly interfere with the clinical independence of a doctor as he was 'authorised so far as it is necessary for the practice of his profession … to be in possession and supply the drugs'. But in relation to 'dangerous drugs', again what did this mean? What exactly was legitimate medical practice and who would determine this?

Henry Bryan 'Bing' Spear joined the Home Office Drugs Inspectorate in 1952, rising to Chief Inspector in 1977 until his retirement in 1986.

As we shall see, he was a unique and central figure in the history of UK drug treatment policy, but his importance at this point in the narrative is the book he wrote, an insider account of government drug treatment policy, *Heroin addiction care and control: the British System 1914–1986*, which I had the privilege of publishing in 2002 while working for DrugScope. In his usual trenchant style, Spear took to task academics and commentators for characterising Delevingne as an unreconstructed prohibitionist who wanted to outlaw addiction maintenance but who was ultimately frustrated in his ambition by the medical profession. Although Delevingne was never interviewed on the matter nor did he leave a record of his personal views, he did believe that the key to eliminating use was cutting off the supply. As Britain had such a small problem to deal with, given total free rein, he may well have opted for a ban on maintenance prescribing. Then again, he had already seen some of his Dangerous Drug Regulation proposals knocked back by the medical profession, which might have made him more cautious about taking on the doctors. Does this mean that his intentions were frustrated by the powerful medical profession? To a degree: as he set out in a memo to the committee eventually charged with coming to a conclusion on this, his view was that while the DDA and the Regulations did not inhibit freedom of medical practice, nevertheless 'the supply of drugs by a doctor to enable him to indulge in his addiction would be an offence punishable under the Acts'. But then somebody would have to determine the meaning of the word 'indulge'. Did this mean that such prescribing would only be allowed in reducing doses to affect a cure over a limited time period, as was originally allowed in the USA?

Whatever his own views or interpretations, Delevingne was also a British civil servant and there has always been a tradition of interdepartmental collaboration and consultation where policy issues overlap. And as far as drug control was concerned, there was certainly a cross-departmental interest where it overlapped with health, foreign and colonial policy. Delevingne had refused to allow the new Ministry of Health jurisdiction over the DDA, saying it was a police matter. But at the suggestion of the Chief Medical Officer, he had agreed to active cooperation which saw health ministry official Dr George McCleary appointed as liaison officer to the Home Office.

Delevingne wanted what he called 'an authoritative statement' from medical experts about the legitimacy or otherwise of maintenance prescribing. In his book Bing Spear denied that Delevingne had a hidden agenda or that he was deliberately looking to expert medical opinion to validate what he thought should happen. But while there is no evidence of a hidden agenda as such, it does seem that in his dealings with health colleagues, he was certainly hinting as to how he thought policy should play out. In May 1922, at his suggestion, a pamphlet produced by the Canadian Department of Health was sent to the Health Minister with a covering letter asking for his 'observations upon the criticisms therein contained of the treatment of addiction by diminishing doses' going on to point out that the pamphlet contained 'the strongest criticism of the system which the Home Office has come across'. However, his request for 'some pronouncement [from the Ministry] on the subject for the guidance of the medical profession' was rejected in words that do suggest Delevingne's starting position:

> The Minister is advised that the question of the immediate withdrawal of the drug in the treatment of drug addicts is one upon which there is considerable diversity of medical opinion in this country. In these circumstances, the Minister does not feel that at the present time he could usefully issue any pronouncement on the matter.[1]

Delevingne wrote again in November 1922, this time quoting officials from New York who, he said, were against gradual withdrawal, but still asking for some 'authoritative pronouncement...on the subject'. The Ministry's response was to commission a report from Dr Adams, one of their medical staff, to examine the question. Meanwhile Delevingne wrote yet again in December 1922, but this time acknowledging another angle that needed official clarification – the possibility that there were individuals so far down the road of their addiction that they couldn't give up drugs 'without suffering greatly and possibly without a complete breakdown of health'.

While trying to get a definitive statement from the Ministry, Delevingne persisted in sending through examples of cases brought to his attention of doctors he regarded as acting like glorified chemists and just dispensing drugs without trying to affect a cure, backing this up with information about South African legislation banning the prescribing of any habit-forming drug for other than a 'medicinal purpose'.

There was the case of Dr Donald Grant, a GP from Glasgow who had earned a reputation for being a rather shambolic drinker and known locally as 'the daft doctor' who came to the attention of the authorities for suspect levels of morphine and cocaine prescribing to one individual. Then there was Dr Conor, based in Soho and known for prescribing cocaine to 'men and women of the underworld' who admitted to dispensing the drug simply to 'satisfy' an addiction and other procedural irregularities. But the options for criminal prosecution or even General Medical Council sanction evaporated while the whole issue of addiction prescribing was unresolved.

Another difficult category was doctors prescribing for themselves. Doctors H. W. and J. A. Boddy, a father and son general practice based in Manchester, were prescribing morphine and using it daily. The drugs were dispensed by a wholesaler who reported his suspicions to the Home Office while at the same time the doctors received a visit from the Regional Medical Officer to explain themselves.

Why Boddy senior was taking morphine every night is not recorded but his son claimed his own daily injections were to deal with diarrhoea. All the Home Office could do was recommend to wholesalers not to supply any more morphine. And in lieu of any regulations specifically banning doctors from prescribing controlled drugs for themselves, all that could be done was for the Home Office to write to both doctors to obtain written undertakings that in the case of the son (who was using most of the morphine) he would not order any more morphine and would seek help while the father would undertake not to order any more morphine 'beyond the amount strictly required for the purposes of your profession'.

There was an irony in Delevingne insisting that drug control was a police matter because he was faced with cases regarding the actions of prescribing doctors where the police seemed powerless to act.

Dr Adams reported back in February 1923 that it was impossible simply to withdraw drugs of addiction (with the possible exception of cocaine) unless it was done under proper medical and nursing care in an appropriate institution, which hardly existed in Britain. He goes on to say, 'drug addiction can only be regarded as a disease ... the best opinion is unanimous on this point' although he conceded that there were those who took drugs for 'purely vicious motives' – in other words for immoral non-medical purposes and so a police matter.

Delevingne replied in March 1923 in a slightly different vein, apparently accepting Adams' view that there might be instances when continued prescribing was medically justified, so long as the person put themselves under close medical supervision 'until the cure is effected'. He was still, though, looking for a statement allowing him to ban prescribing of drugs in support of an addiction when there was no attempt at a cure. Internal memos between the medical staff of the Ministry of Health reveal they too thought doctors prescribing drugs for the 'mere satisfying of a craving' were no different to a street-corner dealer. However, they resisted making the definitive official statement themselves because they felt unqualified to do so. As civil servants, they could no more come up with solutions for the difficulties Delevingne faced than he could. After more memos flew between the departments throughout 1923–24, it was eventually decided the only way forward was to set up an independent committee to examine all the evidence and make recommendations to the Ministry of Health. In September 1924, two years after Delevingne first raised the need for clarity on addiction prescribing, Health Minister John Wheatley announced the setting up of the Departmental Committee on Morphine and Heroin Addiction to be chaired by Sir Humphrey Rolleston, whose landmark findings became known as the Rolleston Report.

The Rolleston Committee was made up of six members, all medical men. The two most distinguished were Rolleston himself, holder of several prestigious medical posts, doctor to George V and knighted in 1918, and Sir William Willcox, an eminent pathologist and forensic adviser to the Home Office who gave evidence in famous trials including Dr Crippen's. But not only did they all have medical backgrounds, but the group was heavily weighted towards those who had experience in treating, writing and lecturing about addiction with ties to the Society for the Study and Cure of Inebriety. Given their composition and experience, it was always likely the committee would take a softer rather than a punitive view of the issues placed before them, not only because they were doctors and not policemen but also as a means of protecting the clinical independence of their profession.

From October 1924 and for the next year, they conducted twenty-three sessions taking views from over thirty witnesses including Delevingne and the Director of Public Prosecutions. Their final report published in January 1926 was a very thoughtful and in modern parlance 'evidence-based' piece of work.

Steeped in the disease model of addiction as they were, the committee set their stall out early by defining an 'addict' not as some deranged and evil dope fiend, but 'a person who, not requiring the continued use of the drug for relief of the symptoms of organic disease, has acquired, as a result of repeated administration, an overpowering desire for its continuance, and in whom withdrawal of the drug leads to definite symptoms of mental or physical distress or disorder'. And in their discussion about the nature of addiction, 'there was general agreement that in most well-established cases, the condition must be regarded as a manifestation of disease and not as a mere form of vicious indulgence'.

They began with some scene-setting. On the question of the prevalence of morphine or heroin addiction, their overwhelming conclusion was that this was 'rare'. 'Some experienced general practitioners have stated that they had never been called upon to treat such cases; others that they have only seen two or three cases in the course of twenty to thirty years' practice'. They also concluded that this was by and large an urban phenomenon and restricted to those who either had access to the drugs such as medical professionals or, as was generally thought, those of an academic or intellectual disposition and so more prone to mental fragility and nervousness, and presumably more likely to be able to afford medical consultations. One witness, Sir James Purves-Stewart, put flesh on this by presenting a breakdown of the 62 patients to whom he was mainly prescribing morphine, but also heroin, chlorodyne and cocaine. Of the 36 men, nearly half were medical practitioners; the rest were military men, businessmen, barristers, politicians, professors and an explorer. Of the 26 women, 17 were married (12 of whom were categorised as 'society women') and 9 were unmarried, 5 of whom were '*demi-mondaines*'.

The committee also concluded that the addiction was in decline largely as a result of the Dangerous Drugs Act which had reduced supplies on the streets for those unable to afford to see doctors. They considered at length and in some detail what treatment options were available, making the Rolleston Report almost a blueprint for the Department of Health addiction treatment clinical guidance, the first edition of which didn't appear until 1984. Despite evidence from prison doctors, they dismissed abrupt or rapid withdrawal options on similar grounds to Dr Adams, that there just wasn't the care structure available to safely manage this otherwise 'barbaric and inhumane' intervention. Most of the treatment focus centred on the reducing dose option, which the committee clearly favoured, emphasising the need to take every precaution that doctors were not simply 'satisfying a craving'. On the basis of evidence presented, they recommended that the patients should gradually have the dosage withdrawn over three months, acknowledging that the last few grains were always the hardest – a grain being 60 milligrams. They thought the doctor should see the patient at least once a week, never prescribe more than would be used between visits and that if the patient was away for an extended period, he or she should seek the help of another doctor who should in turn contact the first doctor to coordinate care. And if they saw an addicted patient for the first time, they should check out the case history with the patient's previous doctor.

The committee even asserted that simply getting people off drugs wasn't enough to prevent relapse and recommended what is now called 'multi-agency working', although of course it wasn't expressed in those terms. They stated there should be psychosocial support both during and after treatment and 'scarcely less important than psychotherapy and education of the will is the improvement of the social conditions of the patient, and one physician informed us that he made it a practice, wherever possible, to supplement his treatment by referring the case to some Social Service Agency'. They also considered the more enforcement-specific proposals of the Home Office which wanted some way of controlling the actions of the Grants and Conors of the drug world. Two proposals were rejected; one was that a doctor would be forced to get a second opinion every time he saw a new addiction case and second that doctors should be compelled to notify the Home Office of every new addiction case to prevent people seeing a number of doctors concurrently. Also rejected was the idea of circulating a blacklist of doctors to wholesalers. The Home Office still lacked a mechanism for bringing irresponsible doctors to book; but rather than have doctors dragged through police courts to face fines or even prison and publicly stain the reputation of the whole profession, the committee concluded (on a recommendation from the British Medical Association) that the Home Office should establish a Medical Tribunal composed entirely of doctors who would sit in judgement on their suspect colleagues to deal with those doctors who seemed to prescribing irresponsibly either to themselves or others.

The key statement from the committee was the acceptance that prescribing morphine or heroin in support of an addiction was legitimate medical practice for two groups of people – those subject to a gradually reducing dose whose care the committee had set out in some detail, and also:

Persons for whom, after every effort had been made for the cure of the addiction, the drug cannot be completely withdrawn either because complete withdrawal produces serious symptoms which cannot be satisfactorily treated under the ordinary conditions of private practice or where a patient, who while capable of leading a useful and fairly normal life so long as he takes a certain non-progressive quantity, usually small, of the drug of addiction, ceases to be able to do so when the regular allowance is withdrawn.[2]

The idea that a doctor could prescribe morphine, heroin, cocaine or any controlled drug in support of an addiction, even on a reducing dose, let alone potentially on a lifelong basis was unprecedented medical practice anywhere in the world and would come to be known by American medical writers and journalists as 'The British System'.

Even so, the Rolleston Committee's conclusion could hardly be said to be a ringing endorsement of opiate maintenance; it was a measure of last resort, the dosage should remain small and not be increased, although of course, there were no specifics which would have seen to be interfering in clinical judgement. Their view should be regarded in the wider context of the time. Evidence showed that addiction was rare and reducing and those few who did suffer were usually the 'better sort' who could afford discreet visits to private doctors posing no threat to wider society.

To what degree then was Sir Malcolm Delevingne thwarted in his ambitions? He got the authoritative statement he was looking for, although his memos to the Ministry of Health do suggest he would have preferred a more prohibitive outcome. Most of his proposals were rejected, but he did get a Medical Tribunal. In a memo to Sir John Anderson, Permanent Under-Secretary of State at the Home Office, Delevingne declared that he thought the Rolleston Report 'admirable and important' and believed that the Medical Tribunal would provide him with the mechanism to deal with 'doctors who cannot safely be trusted with possession or use of the drugs or the treatment of persons addicted to the drugs'.[3]

Any politician or civil servant looking at what evidence existed, would have every reason to believe that the tough provisions of the Dangerous Drugs Act had done the job. But not everybody was convinced. Arguments about the details of the Act had been played out between the Home Office and various professional and commercial interests, but nobody at the time publicly called into question the need for the Act itself or suggested what might be the unintended consequences, save perhaps for a few lone voices such as Aleister Crowley's. Author of the semi-autobiographical novel *Diary of a Drug Fiend* published in 1922, writer, mountaineer, 'mystic' and general con artist with a great facility for beguiling the gullible, Crowley was an unabashed user of heroin and cocaine. Writing in the June and July 1922 issues of *The English Review* he decried in his typically overblown, bombastic style, attempts to deprive doctors of the right to prescribe to those who could lead normal lives as long as they received prescriptions for their drug of addiction. He also wrote more generally that

> despite repressive legislation, there is an international industry making its many thousands per cent on an enormous turnover and occasionally throwing some peddling Jonah overboard when some brainless dancing girl happens to kill herself ... if the people of England want to see their cities in the hands of petty tyranny patting the paunch of corruption, well and good, strengthen the Act! ... There has been so much delirious nonsense written about drugs ... But it ought to be obvious that if England reverted to pre-war conditions, when any responsible person ... could buy drugs at a fair profit on cost price ... the whole underground traffic would disappear like a bad dream.

He predicted that under such a scheme that it was 'probable' that initially a number of people would kill themselves, but it would be nothing compared to the loss of life in the war so that 'we should not miss a few score wasters too stupid to know when to stop. Besides we see ... that the people who want the drugs manage to get them one way or the other at the cost of time, trouble and money which might be used more wisely'. His view was that restrictions on alcohol in the USA and to a lesser extent in Britain had contributed to increasing drug use but thought the main culprit in generating interest was the press. He slammed the coverage he called 'nauseating'. 'Indulgence in drugs is described with an unholy leer. It is connected lewdly with sexual aberrations; and the reprobation with which the writers smear their nastiness is obviously hypocrisy of the most oily and venal type' – a view of media reporting (and also on the efficacy of drug laws) that would be shared by many down the years.

***

After 1923, prosecutions for all drug offences fell dramatically. Britain's drug scene until that point was small, which made it relatively easy for concerted police action backed by tougher penalties under the DDA to close down illicit drug operations. Prosecutions for the most popular drug, cocaine, fell from an average 65 cases a year in 1921–1923 down to just 5 in 1927–1929. Across Europe (especially in Germany) and the USA, cocaine had become regarded as a social menace meaning tighter controls around the world. Drug laws and cocaine's negative reputation saw other alkaloids such as novocaine gain precedence in dentistry, while the appearance of amphetamine in the 1930s diminished the legal market for cocaine still further. Amphetamine was a much cheaper stimulant which the pharmaceutical industry could produce in its own laboratories and factories. There was no illicitly produced cocaine coming out of the main producer country Peru at that time, so as the medical market for cocaine largely dried up, recreational use almost (but not quite) disappeared until it re-emerged under very different circumstances in late sixties America.

In discussing the early years of Britain's drug scene, the American drug historian Terry Parssinen noted that 'perhaps only in the 1920s, when the nation enjoyed a short period of peace and prosperity, sandwiched between the two world wars and a major depression, that Britons could indulge themselves in the luxury of worrying about a social problem, like narcotic drugs, that touched so few of their lives'.[4]

No less than today, though, people did enjoy reading about the lives of others and for many people, nothing provides more relish than reading about somebody in a privileged position falling from grace. The deaths of Billie Carleton and Freda Kempton shone a light on the London drug scene and the nefarious deeds of Brilliant Chang and Edgar Manning. There wasn't too much attention paid to the women themselves, who were just regarded as hapless and naïve victims of evil men. The story of Brenda Dean Paul, arguably Britain's first publicly exposed high-society drug user, was very different.

Brenda Isabell Francis Theresa Dean Paul was born in London in May 1907, the daughter of Sir Aubrey Dean Paul, Baronet of Rodborough, and a descendant of the first Duke of Marlborough and Irene Regina, an accomplished musician and composer. Aubrey was establishment, his wife more wedded to the bohemian life of an artist and they eventually separated in 1922. Home life was not happy; Brenda was educated in convent schools while her parents drifted apart. Brenda aspired to a stage career and played minor theatrical roles before trying her luck in the Berlin film industry. However, she was quickly drawn into the interwar decadence of Berlin's hectic nightlife where morphine and cocaine were freely available. Although there is no direct evidence that she was using drugs then, when she later witnessed heroin sniffing at the home of a Parisian playboy, she said in her ghost-written autobiography published in 1935, that this white powder did not have the 'bright glitter' of cocaine.

Having failed a screen test in Berlin she returned to London in 1927 to become a notable presence among that group known as the Bright Young People. Described by D. J. Taylor in his book of the same name, as 'one of the most extraordinary youth cults in British history', they were essentially from well-to-do families, often landed aristocracy, with too much money and too much time on their hands. Among their number were some who became household names such as Cecil Beaton, John Betjeman, Nancy Mitford, Cyril Connolly, William Walton, Lytton Strachey and Evelyn Waugh who satirised their antics in *Vile Bodies*. By and large though they were a shallow, feckless and talentless bunch who loved to drive around drunk in fast cars and throw endless fancy dress parties. They were Britain's first celebrities: craving publicity and creating a whole new genre of journalism – the gossip columnist. Their American contemporaries were the Hollywood stars of the silent screen whose scandalous private lives became very public under the watchful gaze of tabloid reporters and Hollywood's own insiders. There was a crossover; the gloriously outrageous Tallulah Bankhead, famed for her promiscuity and drug use, had a successful stage career in London during the twenties and was a regular on the party scene.

But beneath the paper-thin gaiety and the glitter that could be as short-lived and illusory as the sparkling cocaine which fuelled the night, often lay stories of fractured, dysfunctional families. As the twenties rolled into the thirties, where fortunes were wiped out by the Crash of 1929, fun and laughter gave way to drink, drugs, disappointment and in some cases early death.

Brenda's problems appeared to start in Paris following a car crash; she was admitted to hospital and given morphine. Then she either had a miscarriage or an abortion, probably the latter because she was dumped by her lover once he found out she was pregnant, and generally she was in poor health, a misery compounded by concerns about her beloved mother whose health was also failing (she died in 1932). With all the unhappiness in her life, her drug use, relieving mental as well as physical distress, understandably escalated.

In her autobiography, she was at pains to describe herself as a 'drug victim' rather than a 'drug addict' or 'dope fiend', 'Individuals like myself have contracted the habit while ill. It has never been a game, never was a pleasure or dissipation. I never enjoyed real happiness of the senses from them, though it has been a relief and godsend and vital necessity.'[5] She also claimed that once hooked, society victims were blackmailed by their dealers into introducing more users via their privileged networks. This didn't seem to apply to her as she stated she was legitimately receiving morphine on prescription, and using about 10 mg or one-sixth of a grain a day, which clearly helped: 'From my emptiness and misery, I would be filled with a warm stream of contentment as if any icy driving blizzard had ceased and I had found shelter in a warm sunny place.' But that warm sunny place would eventually be replaced by the cold reality of Holloway prison.

The exact circumstances of the mess she got into are unclear but in December 1931 she was convicted at Marlborough Street Police Court on seven counts of 'unauthorised possession of dangerous drugs' as she had been obtaining prescriptions from more than one doctor. The police became involved after her father went to Scotland Yard to implore them to stop his daughter obtaining any more drugs.

Detective Sergeant Griffey of Scotland Yard was tasked with arresting Brenda but discovered that she had vanished from London. Enquiries traced her to Devon, where she had spent her childhood. On a cold November night, as Brenda waited in her car outside the local doctor's surgery while her maid collected her morphine script, a torch flashed in Brenda's face and so began a period of fame far different from that she had craved as a teenager. She was bound over for 3 years on condition she went into a nursing home for the first of several attempts at a 'cure'.

The Rolleston Report had recommended that any withdrawal procedure should only be undertaken under careful medical supervision in an appropriate institution. The end of the process for Brenda was to be given injections of hyoscine, also known as scopolamine, with a range of medical uses, but also found in one of Dr Crippen's victims and tested as a truth drug during the 1950s. Side effects include hallucinations, nightmares and seizures, a brutal endgame in addiction treatment. Any such cure was bound to fail of course, because none of Brenda's psychological and emotional pain was ever dealt with. She was the classic Rolleston patient for whom a regular prescription would help her to lead something like a normal life.

She was convicted of illegal possession after a friend sent some of her prescription through the post and she picked up various convictions for minor fraud and deception offences. Eventually she was sent to Holloway where she had to endure cold turkey. On leaving prison, she weighed just 5 stone.

Accompanying her court appearances through the 1930s and 1940s were headlines such as 'Drug addict's fate: Brenda Dean Paul said to be incurable'; 'Doctors give up on Brenda Dean Paul'; 'Society girl lives five weeks without dope, but would die without it in luxury nursing home'; 'Unless she receives ever-increasing doses of drugs, Brenda Deal Paul will go mad and die'.

Although at times she was her own worst enemy, once she was on the police radar, there was a certain cachet to be earned by dogging her tracks. Prosecutions brought under the Dangerous Drugs Act had been what we might call these days 'the low-hanging fruit': itinerant seamen, prostitutes and anybody likely to be found lurking around the Soho streets. In that age of deference, the Bright Young Things were pretty much untouchable. I am reminded that back in 2005, the new Commissioner of the Metropolitan Police, Sir Iain Blair, committed the service to targeting middle-class cocaine users. He said he was determined to make 'a few examples' of this group (*Daily Telegraph* 2 February 2005). In 2018, Home Secretary Sajid Javid made a party conference declaration along similar lines, as did Metropolitan Police Commissioner Cressida Dick. Nothing happened any more than the

Hooray Henrys of the 1920s were herded into court by way of example. This left Brenda Dean Paul as the fall girl for all her peers who got away with it.

At one point in the 1940s, she changed her name to Isolla Hampton – her grandmother's maiden name – and was charged under that name on drug possession charges in 1949 and 1950. She worked as a waitress and shop worker, but interviewed by the *Sunday Dispatch* in 1951, she claimed she was off to America to warn teenagers about the dangers of drugs. She also claimed in the interview that she had found a cure: 'I am keeping that to myself for the moment because on my return to this country, I want to open a clinic.' She never did of course. Worn down by addiction, she finally realised her ambition to act when she won the leading role in Ronald Firbank's 1920 comedy play *The Princess Zoubaroff*. Actor and writer Neville Phillips wrote rather snidely at the time,

> The role of the Princess was played by the always newsworthy, once ravishing now ravaged, oft arrested society blonde lesbian drug addict, Brenda Dean Paul, who, owing to her addiction, was not able to do all the performances, giving the ones she could manage the extra frisson of wondering if the police might burst in at any moment and make an on-stage arrest.

She continued to receive regular prescriptions of morphine with a daily cocaine script of 4.2 grams. In 1957, she was admitted to a psychiatric hospital in Rome with a parcel of cocaine in her possession. She died in London in July 1959 officially of natural causes, although there was a suspicion of an overdose. She was 52.

A view of Brenda as victim rather than villain was expressed by the Resident Medical Superintendent of one of the nursing homes Brenda was sent to as a condition of being bound over. He wrote to the court,

> I must express the opinion that Miss Paul has been harshly treated at the hands of the law and I think it is high time the legal and medical authorities took council together to save the soul of this young woman who is more sinned against than sinning.

According to Bing Spear, Brenda's Home Office file 'ran to 97 sub-numbers'.[6] By the time Brenda passed away, the country had long forgotten about opium dens and Fu Manchu. Instead, the press was on to a new scourge of which Edgar Manning was a harbinger; the seductive black drug dealer beguiling his young white female victims in a haze of bebop riffs and cannabis smoke.

3

The Light of the Charge Brigade

As a result of cannabis being added to the Dangerous Drugs legislation in 1925, a black seaman, Abraham Jones, 40, and Elizabeth Cocklin, 29, became the first people to be arrested in the UK on a charge of unauthorised cannabis possession. The arrest took place on 7 March 1929 at a Chinese restaurant in Limehouse. The arresting officers testified that they had been keeping the pair under observation and had seen Jones pass Cocklin a paper packet which she concealed inside one of her shoes. When questioned she produced the packet from her shoe and it was found to contain herbal cannabis. They appeared at Thames Police Court where Jones was sentenced to 3 months' imprisonment with hard labour while Cocklin was given the choice of a 40 shilling (£2) fine or a month's imprisonment.

In 1929, cannabis use was virtually unknown in the UK. There were no public, medical or scientific concerns about the drug, and outlawing cannabis possession and supply was never debated in Parliament. In order to save parliamentary time, the new law governing cannabis (and coca leaves) was simply added to the DDA under rules allowing additions and amendments to existing legislation as secondary rather than primary legislation. Under these circumstances, how did cannabis possession and supply become a crime in the UK?

Across North Africa, the Middle East, China and India, cannabis had a very long history of medicinal, recreational and religious use going back centuries. The plant was not grown in the West until the seafaring powers realised the value of hemp in the manufacture of ropes. Western interest in the medicinal use of cannabis grew during the nineteenth century, largely on the basis of anecdotal reporting from British-ruled India. But one doctor, William O'Shaughnessy, Professor of Medicine and Chemistry at the Medical College of Calcutta, became the first clinician to conduct primary trials into the therapeutic potential of cannabis. His results were remarkably prescient as he described the benefits of cannabis for 'spasmodic diseases', as much later research and personal testimony credit cannabis with relieving some symptoms of multiple sclerosis and Parkinson's disease and similar musculoskeletal disorders. O'Shaughnessy also identified the value of cannabis in general pain relief, in particular, to relieve period and childbirth pain. Inspired by

O'Shaughnessy's findings, it was claimed that Sir Russell Reynolds, Queen Victoria's doctor, prescribed tincture of cannabis for her menstrual cramps. According to Virginia Berridge, this is a myth, although Reynolds did write, 'when pure and administered carefully, [cannabis] is one of the most useful medicines we possess'. The advent of the hypodermic syringe allowing drugs to travel more quickly to the site of pain saw medicinal cannabis fall out of favour in Europe.

Cannabis had economic value too; the British ruled over the largest cannabis market in the world. When the East India Company relinquished its trading monopoly, most of its revenue was derived from the profits of administering taxation on the behalf of the government. Given the widespread use of the drug right through Indian society, there was money to be made from cannabis. Retailers needed a licence from the Colonial Office before approaching producers and there was a proliferation of licences and regulations right along the supply chain to extract as much revenue as possible. In Bengal, the government was earning more revenue from cannabis than opium. However, in another classic case of unintended consequences of drug policy, prohibitive taxation led to the growth of an illicit trade and as British officialdom was already suspicious of cannabis' intoxicating properties, the drug became increasingly associated not only with criminality but also madness. A highly flawed survey conducted by the government in India in 1872 concluded that Indian asylums were awash with inmates who had been incarcerated through cannabis-induced insanity. However, as James Mills explains in the first volume of his two-part history of cannabis in Britain, the numbers produced by British medical officers 'were ... based on bad information, administrative expedience and colonial misunderstandings of a complex society'.[1]

Even at the time, it was realised that the data was unreliable. It was nevertheless seized upon by those MPs concerned about the British involvement in the drugs trade or who had a dislike of imperialism in general and they pushed the government to investigate the issue. In response, the government established the Indian Hemp Commission to conduct a review similar to that carried out for opium. The final report, published in 1894, ran to more than 3,000 pages in eight volumes, including interviews with 1,200 individuals from doctors and the asylum bosses to smugglers, growers and users. The main conclusion was that,

> Viewing the subject generally, it may be added that the moderate use of these drugs is the rule, and that the excessive use is comparatively exceptional. The moderate use practically produces no ill effects. In all but the most exceptional cases, the injury from habitual moderate use is not appreciable. The excessive use may certainly be accepted as very injurious, though it must be admitted that in many excessive consumers the injury is not clearly marked. The injury done by the excessive use is, however, confined almost exclusively to the consumer himself; the effect on society is rarely appreciable. It has been the most striking feature in this inquiry to find how little the effects of hemp drugs have obtruded themselves on observation. The large number of witnesses of all classes who professed

never to have seen these effects, the vague statements made by many who professed to have observed them, the very few witnesses who could so recall a case as to give any definite account of it, and the manner in which a large proportion of these cases broke down on the first attempt to examine them, are facts which combine to show most clearly how little injury society has hitherto sustained from hemp drugs.[2]

Admittedly, as with opium, it was in the interests of the government to minimise the harms of cannabis. Even so, the weight of evidence was impressive, gained by first-hand interviewing, not second-hand anecdote, covering every aspect of the drug's use in India and representing one of the most thorough enquiries into cannabis ever undertaken. It was certainly enough to quash political disquiet, following which cannabis dropped off the UK political radar altogether until the 1920s when it became the subject of scrutiny at an international level.

At this point, the battle lines in international diplomacy on drug control were quite sharply drawn. The American view was that to stop consumption of any dangerous drug, all you had to do was stop production. The British view was, as this position related to opium, if production was decreased in India, somebody else would step in to fill the breach. Instead, the main plank of British policy was to moderate demand rather than stifle production.

In the continuing saga of trying to reach consensus on international drug control against a backdrop of diplomatic power games, the International Opium Conference was called for 1924 to be held in Geneva. Any League of Nations member could attend, not just those with immediate interests in opiate and cocaine production and this gave an opportunity for other countries to raise their own drug-related issues. Malcolm Delevingne, now retired from the Home Office but still a key figure on the international stage, had his carefully drawn-up agenda, which majored on opiate and cocaine control, sideswiped by the Egyptian delegate Dr Mohamed El Guindy. He unexpectedly stood up and launched an impassioned attack on hashish, claiming it was more harmful than opium and causing havoc in his country. He tabled a proposal for the international control of cannabis not only restricting use of hemp to scientific and medical purpose only, but an outright ban on hashish for any purpose whatsoever. In presenting his proposal, Dr El Guindy gave a detailed account of the harms of the drug adding that the Egyptian customs had recently seized in excess of 3 million kilos of illegally imported hashish in a single year. His audience sat stunned as he described the 'terrible menace to the whole world' posed by cannabis and sat down to prolonged applause. What was behind his sudden intervention?

Since medieval times, successive Egyptian rulers had failed to control endemic use of hashish with penalties ranging from heavy taxation to death. The impetus for control gained new strength in the early nineteenth century, when the new Ottoman ruler, Muhammed Ali Pasha, began a process of modernising the country. Hashish was symbolic of old, outmoded customs, but was also seen as a threat to improving the health of the workforce and the military. In 1882, Egypt became a British Protectorate.

While the country was not formally annexed by Britain, it was the British government that pretty much ruled Egypt until independence was granted in 1922, although the British remained involved in Egyptian affairs until the early 1950s. The presence of a foreign power in a country wishing for self-determination saw the growth of a nationalist movement aimed at throwing off the yoke of imperial control. Hashish came to symbolise not only the old Egypt, but also a British imperialism trying to undermine the nation's ambitions by allowing rampant export of Indian cannabis.

Egypt has long, uncontrollable borders and hashish smugglers were every bit as inventive as modern-day traffickers. A report compiled by the Egyptian Interior Ministry was sent to the Foreign Office by the High Commissioner for Egypt and the Sudan, Lord Allenby. The report detailed how the drug arrived in Egypt wrapped up in cotton goods, bundles of newspapers, tins of petrol, and concealed in bricks, marble columns, barrels of olives, hollow bedsteads, and fashioned into inner soles for boots so smugglers would just walk hash into the country. In a rerun of opium smuggling in Chinese waters, consignments would be dumped offshore and brought in by small boats to be loaded onto camels and transported across the desert by Bedouin tribesmen.

Delevingne saw this report, but his view was that British reputation was tarnished enough over opium, the government in India knew that tough hashish controls would never work, and anyway, there was disquiet among some countries concerning British presence in Egypt such that it was best to keep quiet about all this.

In fact, the British head of Egypt's Central Narcotics Intelligence Bureau, Thomas Wentworth Russell, became so exasperated at the failure of his efforts to keep hashish out of the country that he proposed to the Egyptian government that they legalise hashish and run it as a government monopoly, earning valuable revenue instead of spending vast sums on prohibition while Egyptian money flowed out of the country and into the pockets of foreign smugglers. His bosses disagreed; instead El Guindy used Allenby's report to press the case that the only way to deal with hashish use in his country was to impose strict international controls. Relating to the medical evidence, he used the report of another British official, John Warnock, the man who had oversight of Egypt's asylum system.

Warnock had been appointed to reform one asylum, but ended up expanding all the existing institutions, writing new laws on mental health and essentially running the whole administration of the Egyptian asylum system. He was in post for nearly 30 years but in all that time, he never learnt to read or write Arabic, could hardly communicate with his staff and was generally dismissive of Egyptian culture and political ambitions, describing the push for self-determination as 'an infectious mental disorder'. Yet despite admitting a total lack of interest in Egyptian society and cultural traditions, or perhaps because of that attitude, he was more than happy to blame hashish for filling his asylums with mentally ill patients. Simply put, his methodology was to ignore the views of everybody connected to the patients and instead keep questioning them until the poor individuals gave the answers he was looking for. His report was suspect on at least two levels:

the degree to which mental health problems could really be blamed even among the asylum population on the drug and even if there were some legitimate cases, how representative were they of the much larger population of hashish users?

Armed with these reports on smuggling and insanity, Dr El Guindy convinced conference delegates that cannabis needed to be controlled. In calling for extreme measures, he deployed the classic negotiating tactic demanding something he knew he could not achieve in order to be able to compromise. Therefore, while the wording of his proposal was much watered down, mainly due to British objections, El Guindy (who archly commented that this was the first such conference where Egypt was represented by a wholly Egyptian delegation) succeeded in a quite remarkable fashion in having cannabis included in the list of drugs subject to international control. Mills points out the rich irony that objections to cannabis control from one part of the British Empire were totally undermined by reports written by British officials from another hub of British imperial power.

***

In Britain, through the early 1920s, there had been flurries of interest in cannabis. One of the earliest and very brief media references to recreational use was the item in the *News of the World* in January 1919 reporting on the Billie Carleton case. It casually referred to Indian hemp as the drug 'of the Assassins' without any other context as if its readers would know what the reporter meant.

In the wake of the passing of the Dangerous Drugs Act, the Metropolitan Police seemed especially keen to see cannabis included in the Act and wrote to the Home Office claiming that cannabis drove users mad and was equally as bad as cocaine and morphine. The Home Office demurred, while the police had egg on their face when in August 1923 they arrested two foreign waiters working in Soho for allegedly offering to sell a detective some opium, which turned out to be still-legal cannabis. Though the case was dropped, the police's solicitors used the media to stoke up concerns about the drug. The *Daily Chronicle* reported that the case revealed there was a large traffic in a drug that caused madness and other newspapers used the case to run stories that the government was about to include the drug in the DDA and how it had slipped under the radar. The evidence for anything approaching widespread supply and use was entirely lacking yet press reporting and a couple of items in the medical press concerning individuals not from immigrant communities did prompt some parliamentary interest. Even when the Pharmaceutical Society took fright and classed the drug as a poison in 1924, the British government saw no need to control cannabis under dangerous drug laws until forced to do so by the unexpected outcome of the Geneva Conference.

Once it was controlled, the police seemed to lose interest with just a handful of prosecutions of itinerant African and Asian seamen from 1929 through to 1945, but this didn't stop the *Daily Mirror* publishing a full-page shock/horror story about cannabis on 24 July 1939, the first of many to appear in the British press, not only revisiting all the tropes of cocaine and opium reporting, but rehearsing all the standard myths about the drug – addiction, madness, violence and sex. The headline screamed:

Just a cigarette, you'd think, but it was made from a sinister weed and an innocent girl falls victim to this TERROR!

In London there are thousands of them. Young girls, once beautiful, whose thin faces show the ravages of the weed they started smoking for a thrill. Young men, who in the throes of a hangover from the drug, find their only relief in dragging on yet another marihuana cigarette.

One girl, just over twenty, known among her friends for her quietness and modesty, suddenly threw all cautions to the winds. She began staying out at nights. Her parents became anxious when she began to walk about the house without clothes. They stopped her when she attempted to go into the street like that. At times she became violent and showed abnormal strength. Then she would flop down in a corner, weeping and crouching like an animal.

A young and lovely woman, her clothes in shreds, stood perilously perched on a window ledge. Behind her was a man. He too, was wild-looking and dishevelled. Several times the girl made an effort to jump and the man feebly held her back. Soon a third man appeared, coloured and strong, and hauled them both back. They were both marihuana addicts.

And what was the source of this 'terror'? 'Not only nightclubs, respectable hotels and cafés frequented by 'agents' but also 'milliner's shops, hairdressers and antique shops ... in Soho, in little lodging houses run by coloured men and women, the cigarette can be had for a secret password and a very small sum of money.'

With the lure of the drug came the lure of sex: 'For women, the menace of the cigarette is greater than for men. A girl of 21 was persuaded by a coloured man to elope with him.'

Either there was a massive pre-war trade in cannabis going completely unnoticed by the Home Office and the police, or this was just a farrago of made-up nonsense. One pointer to the real source of this story was the reference to 'marihuana', a term not used in Britain. To government officials, the police and others it was 'Indian Hemp'. To users, it was initially 'reefers', but that soon became passé, to be replaced in the 1950s by 'charge', possibly derived from the Indian word 'charas' or the charge or buzz from smoking. In fact, both the word marihuana and the spelling ('h' rather than 'j') are American, suggesting that the reporter cited only as ES just reworked some reefer madness tales from the United States.

The article was published two years after the Marihuana Tax Act was passed in America which effectively outlawed possession and sale of cannabis. In 1930, the Federal Bureau of Narcotics was established, headed by Harry Anslinger, fresh from a failed career trying to enforce prohibition. Part of the problem with prohibition enforcement was the lack of agents in the field, something Anslinger was determined to avoid when it came to drugs. Cannabis smoking had come into the US from Mexico, following a flood of refugees on the run from war and revolution. Despite border states banning the drug, it had become very popular among working people across the southern states and there was pressure for Federal control. Anslinger initially resisted due to resource constraints, but then realised that the best way to secure more Congressional funds was to start a national drug scare over cannabis.

One has to be careful about attributing significant policy changes to one person, but it is probably no exaggeration to suggest that Anslinger, ably assisted by all the usual suspects among the press and faith-based campaigning groups, created the myths of cannabis, promoting its links with the medieval cult of Assassins and all the violence and psychosis that came from that link. He chose to highlight specific cases involving Mexican or black crimes of violence alleging a connection with cannabis and produced the classic film *Reefer Madness* which ironically because of strict US film censorship laws, couldn't be shown in the large, metropolitan cinemas. His plan worked until the 1950s when Congress became increasingly unconvinced about the direct evils of cannabis. In response, Anslinger switched tack and instead promulgated the idea of cannabis as the 'gateway' drug to heroin, cocaine and other more dangerous drugs, a flawed assumption still alive today.

* * *

During the Second World War British families at home lost much: loved ones dead and injured abroad, and for those caught in the Blitz, death and destruction all around. Yet strangely it could also be a time of liberation, particularly for children and young people. Without realising the full horror of what might happen, children were excited by air-raid warnings, rushing for shelters, hearing planes overhead and playing in the ruins the next day. Concerns were raised about bands of feral kids roaming the streets largely free of parental control. Sexual freedom was unprecedented, especially if you were hunkered down in a dark shelter wondering if this night might be your last. And with so much of the male workforce away fighting, women became crucially important in the war effort. But what about afterwards?

Successive post-war governments introduced an impressive array of reforms starting with the Conservative 1944 Education Act and then under Labour, the establishment of the NHS and the Welfare State, all of which significantly improved the lives of ordinary people. To lift morale came the Olympic Games in London in 1948, the Festival of Britain in 1951 and Queen Elizabeth's coronation in 1953.

Nonetheless, Britain was a dingy, dusty and colourless place in the early post-war years; the war had nearly bankrupted the country, meaning more years of grinding austerity with rationing extended to include bread. The weather symbolised the drabness: 1946–48 saw London hit by harsh winters and the killer London smog of 1952 prompted the eventual passing of the Clean Air Act in 1956. For London and its visitors, the West End did offer some relief: the vibrant neon of Piccadilly Circus was relit and bars, cafés, clubs and restaurants came back to life. On a day-to-day basis, though, adults who lived through the war understandably wanted nothing more than safety, stability and certainty, now that the Cold War was offering up new threats to keep people awake at night.

Their offspring, however, were in search of something more exciting. Some might have daydreamed of emulating great sporting achievements; Stanley Matthews winning the FA Cup for Blackpool in 1953 or Roger Bannister breaking the 4-minute mile in 1954. To break the monotony, however, most British youth had to be content with trips to the pub if they could get in, the youth club dance and a quick fumble in the back row of the local cinema.

There was a sub-group of bored young people who were in search of something deliberately outside the mainstream, something daring and a bit dangerous, something their parents and society would hate. For those living in and around London came the chance for such an adventure: the invasion of American GIs during the war and the arrival of immigrants from the West Indies soon after it. The Americans with their smart, pressed uniforms carried the aura of Hollywood glamour, bringing luxuries like nylons and cigarettes and the promise of sex with no strings for young women, although many did end up as GI brides. The men coming in from the West Indies brought similarly exotic promise, colourful clothes and an outlook on life totally at odds with the narrow-minded conservatism of their new hosts. Black and white mingled together in smoky Soho dives to the complex yet compelling sounds of Charlie Parker and Dizzy Gillespie and the smell of cannabis. And for young white people, it all represented one thing – freedom.

The drug scene of the 1950s was still confined to London's West End and those areas in the East End which housed small communities of Chinese and African seamen. Following the 1948 Nationality Act, working-class West Indians were the first wave of Commonwealth citizens encouraged to come to bolster a workforce decimated by war. Once here, they established their own communities in areas such as Brixton, Notting Hill and Ladbroke Grove. And like the Chinese before them, West Indians brought with them their own long-standing tradition of recreational drug use – ganja – introduced into the Caribbean during the nineteenth century by indentured workers from India sent to labour on British-owned sugar plantations. Although the Jamaican white elite and the Church forced through a ban in 1913, use was already ubiquitous among the working class and adopted as a religious sacrament by Rastafarians.

Little has been written about the London drug scene of the fifties, but one long-forgotten source offers up some insights. Born in 1930, Raymond Thorp found his way onto the Soho scene in his late teens. His descent from wide-eyed innocence to convicted drug dealer was charted in an autobiography, co-authored with *Daily Express* reporter Derek Agnew, and published in 1956. *Viper: The Confessions of a Drug Addict* had all the hallmarks of a sensationalised tabloid tale – addiction, sex, crime and betrayal – but it is possible to glean a sense of what the scene was like, suggesting it was rather more widespread than official sources indicated at the time.

In the late 1940s, Thorp, who had a solid but dull suburban family background and a grammar school education, found himself with a dead-end office job in central London. Contemptuous of the 'squares' around him, he sought refuge in the West End jazz scene, initially at a dive called The Boogie Club – one of those here today, gone tomorrow basement holes that didn't even warrant a footnote in the music histories of Soho. Thorp was no less dismissive of the clientele here than his workmates or the people pushing past him on the streets as they scuttled back to suburbia: '[The club] was haunted by musicians on the dole, musicians wasting time and musicians smoking hemp, artists in blue jeans who never painted, writers who couldn't write, philosophers who had never thought, jazz-hungry girls begging life to kick them.'[3]

Initially he spurns an offer of 'charge', but wary of being thought a 'drag' in the cool company of musicians, West Indians, American soldiers and their girlfriends, he accepts a joint from the club barmaid having been assured that it wasn't the asthma cure powder sometimes passed off onto the unwary. In short order, Ray was 'raving high', he was 'above everything. Above it and beyond it. Yet somehow right inside it as well, swimming in a crystal-clear world. The jazz seeped into my body. I felt the notes running through my veins, slipping through my tapping fingers into the air around me.'

Getting deeper into jazz, he gravitates to the Feldman Swing Club in the basement of 100 Oxford Street (which later became 100 Club, still there today). Like The Boogie Club, it didn't matter who you were, what you did, how you were dressed, where you came from or the colour of your skin. Jazz, cigarettes and charge were the social glues that held the scene together. Eventually, Feldman's became the home of New Orleans-style revivalist 'trad' jazz sending some of the crowd, including Thorp, to seek out the new sounds of bebop. The music was played on records in the clubs, but nobody was playing it live until Ronnie Scott, nine other musicians and a manager opened Club Eleven at 44 Great Windmill Street in 1948.

From its earliest beginnings in the red-light districts of New Orleans, there was always a deep suspicion about jazz among the press, religious groups and moral reformers because of its strong ties to the black community. The outlaw musicians, operating on the fringes of society, were accused of being Pied Pipers of 'jungle music', driving young white women into a frenzy of sexual abandon fuelled by booze and drugs.

In 1926, the respected Scottish artist John Souter submitted a painting to the Royal Academy for the Spring show called *The Breakdown* depicting a naked white girl dancing to the sounds of a black saxophonist. Souter had exhibited at the Academy before and was well-known for portrait commissions of the high and mighty and had also painted and exhibited other female nude portraits. The Academy originally hung the picture, but then, incredibly, came under pressure from the Colonial Office to remove the painting as it was felt that 'it would make ruling our natives difficult'; a question of 'state, not art'. The Academy replaced the offending artwork with a portrait of leading London socialite (and David Cameron's great aunt) Lady Diana Manners, which was hugely ironic because her Ladyship was a confirmed and unapologetic injector of morphine who in 1915 wrote enthusiastically about her drug experiences she described as 'orgies' in the company of Katharine Asquith, wife of the Prime Minister's son.[4]

The year 1926, also saw the first edition of *Melody Maker*, whose editor, Edgar Cohen, might have been expected to take a more liberal view of the painting. Instead, he wrote that 'we jazz musicians protest against and repudiate the juxtaposition of an undraped white girl and a black man' and demanded the painting be burnt.[5]

However, the appeal of vibrant, loose-limbed and exciting jazz for young people was not to be denied. Bebop took the coolness of jazz to another level and in a totally different direction. Starting in the early 1940s, it was a reaction of young, black musicians against those they regarded as 'Uncle Toms'. Pianist Hampton Hawes put it like this: 'Our rebellion was a form of survival. If we didn't do that, what else could we do? Get your hair gassed, put on your bow ties, and a funny smile and play pretty for the rich whiter folks?'[6] The music was complex, hard to dance to, the musicians distant and aloof. Black bebop musicians in America were throwing up a wall to insulate themselves from racism, segregation and discrimination. In the UK, it was probably no coincidence that several of the original pre-war Club Eleven musicians were Jewish. White musicians on both sides of the Atlantic flocked to the new sounds, on the run from the narrowness and bigotry of white society. The Club Eleven crew were Norman Mailer's 'White Negroes', exploring an exclusive, underground music in the depths of Soho basements.

For Thorp, Club Eleven was a revelation: 'The clientele was crazy, really gone. From the Bohemian lunatic fringe, to small-time crooks and Americans on furlough. From musicians dropping by for the fun of the ride to teenage girls following the pack.'[7] But life was also getting expensive, stretching his junior clerk wages beyond breaking point. He wanted to dress for the occasion in a style that reads like early Teddy Boy: 'I bought drape-style suits, crepe shoes, bright ties and coloured shirts.' Now booted and suited, hip to the slang and drifting further away from straight life, the more Thorp went to the club, the more he became aware of a serious drug scene beyond the odd joint passed around at Feldman's.

'Now that I had broken through the crust,' he wrote, 'I could see the black-market deals and a little of the drug trade that went on behind its doors.' People he had known for months 'were regular hemp smokers, some were even injecting or sniffing cocaine or heroin'. The scene was getting quite heavy, which sent Thorp back to Feldman's for a while, but the intoxicating atmosphere of Club Eleven proved too much of a draw. As well as the clothes, Thorp was now regularly downing pints of cider, the fashionable club drink, and smoking increasing amounts of dope. He needed money: first he was selling black-market cigarettes and nylons on behalf of American soldiers and from there was introduced to the far more lucrative world of drug dealing.

Apart from Club Eleven, there were other dealing hubs close by. Archer Street ran behind Great Windmill Street and was home to the Musician's Union offices. On Monday mornings in the fifties and sixties all manner of musicians would gather there to find work in dance bands, jazz groups and even classical orchestras. And right in the middle of Archer Street was a greasy spoon café selling terrible food and worse coffee called the *Harmony Inn*.

One of the few late-night places to go to once the clubs and pubs had closed, the *Harmony Inn* attracted trad jazz revellers, all the Club Eleven musicians and representations of some of London's most notorious villains including Billy Hill (mentor to The Krays), Tony Muller (shot dead by the barman at the Zodiac Bar as Muller tried to kill him) and Jack 'Spot' Comer who survived an attack by Mad Frankie Fraser.

Thorp notes that just after the war, 'drug convictions were few and far between. They were such a rarity, in fact, that it was almost hard to realise that selling or using drugs was an offence. No one gave the law a second thought. Pushers did their work almost with the spotlight on them. In a crowded place, hemp was handed over on the spot. If there were not so many people around and it was easy to see what was happening, then the business was conducted in a toilet.'

This was hardly surprising. When Detective Sergeant George Lyle was seconded to Scotland Yard in 1947, he was the first-ever specialist drug policeman. His work came under the auspices of the Vice Squad, whose main activities were policing the porn trade and trying to catch gay men having sex in public toilets. There was a synergy with the Home Office Drugs Branch, which included pornography in its early remit. It also had a role to educate police forces about drugs, yet Thorp claimed that he and his friends took much delight in going up to some rookie constable and asking for a light for their joints. There was no separately established Metropolitan Police Drug Squad until the mid-fifties, but prosecutions for cannabis did begin to rise once the war was over; between 1942 and 1946, there were 17 prosecutions, but then a total of 113 between 1947 and 1950. This reflected not just the influx of cannabis-smoking West Indians, but also the beginnings of use among white teenagers. In August 1951, the first white teenager, a plumber's mate, was arrested for dealing.

Thorp made his first drug buy, spending £5 on cannabis and dividing it up into 80 wraps, from which he hoped to double his money. As plain clothes police were out and about in the West End, using a public toilet to sort out the goods seemed particularly risky, especially as it took him an hour, emerging under the suspicious gaze of the toilet attendant. He went off to the Club Eleven in search of vipers, the slang name for cannabis smokers supposedly derived from the hissing sound heard when a joint was lit. He soon learnt the first rule of drug dealing – if you are new to the game, make sure you are not trespassing on somebody else's turf. Under threat of having his facial features permanently rearranged, Thorp got the message about dealing at Club Eleven, although he did carry on surreptitiously.

He soon built up a clientele of his own though and was looking forward to the time when he could tell his boss at the office what he could do with his job. It was now 1950 and all was going well, until two visitors turned up at work, Detectives Lyle and Carpenter from the Vice Squad. Two weeks before at the office, some cannabis had fallen out of Thorp's pocket in front of a co-worker who assumed it was dog worming powder. Instead of agreeing, Thorp boasted it was cannabis and in consequence received a visit.

The police had begun to move into gear on drugs; a ship's steward caught with cannabis said he bought it at Club Eleven. On 15 April 1950,

40 officers led by Lyle and Carpenter stormed the club in one of the first drug busts of its kind. Ronnie Scott was into a Charlie Parker song when a large policeman appeared at the end of his saxophone. Drummer Laurie Morgan recalled, 'The police came in and stopped everything and searched everybody. They put on all the lights and found all sorts of packets on the floor.'[8]

Three years later in January 1953, George Lyle gave a talk to the Society for the Study of Addiction entitled 'Dangerous Drug Traffic in London' in which he described the raid:

> There were on the premises between 200 and 250 persons, coloured and white, of both sexes, the majority being between 17 and 30. All these people were searched. Ten men [mainly musicians] were found to be in possession of Indian Hemp. Two also had a small quantity of cocaine [including Ronnie Scott] and another man had a small quantity of morphine. In addition, 23 packets of Indian Hemp, a number of hemp cigarettes, a small packet of cocaine, a small quantity of prepared opium and an empty morphine ampoule were found on the floor of the club. All the cocaine had been adulterated with boric acid. All were later convicted and fined. The Indian Hemp cigarettes were being sold at 5/- (25p) and the adulterated cocaine at 10/- a grain (50p for 60 mg).[9]

Three months later on 1 July 1950, an even larger force of 80 officers raided the Paramount Dance Hall in Tottenham Court Road and searched about 500 people, only finding 'eight coloured men' in possession of cannabis. One of the men bit two policemen and another club-goer. Quietly in court, the accused declared that he had only done this because they bit him first. The floor yielded 20 more packets of cannabis and several knives, while as if to underline the vice of white girls mixing with black men, Lyle felt it necessary to mention to the gathered medics that, 'In the ladies' toilet, a large number of contraceptives were found.'

Lyle told of another incident when he and other officers went to a house in Gerrard Street in the Chinatown district of the West End, accompanied by the Chinese representative of a shipping company who employed Chinese seamen. The official gave a password in Chinese, the door opened to reveal a group of men who continued smoking opium as if nothing was happening. Subsequently DS Lyle tried the same trick again, learning the password phonetically, to enter a house in Maple Street. Only this time, there was chaos behind the door and everyone fled, leaving Lyle wondering if his broad Scottish accent was a bit of a giveaway.

Thorp was remanded for a week in September 1951 to Wormwood Scrubs for a psychiatric report followed by a probation order, which stipulated that he lived with his sister and stayed out of the West End. While Thorp was awaiting his fate, the newspapers were picking up where the *Daily Mirror* left off in 1939, but this time suggesting that female smokers were far from young innocents. Under the headline 'Young Girls Who Smoke Doped Cigarettes', the *Daily Telegraph* reported in August 1951,

Home Office inspectors ... are satisfied ... that for the moment the smoking of these 'reefer' cigarettes is confined mainly to young girls of the type who became camp followers when American troops in large numbers were stationed here during the war... The danger, of course, is that they may become confirmed addicts and spread the habit among girls and boys in their own district.

John Ralph wrote a series of articles on cannabis use and dealing for the *Sunday Graphic*. He said he had done 'several weeks ... of exhaustive enquiries into the most insidious vice Scotland Yard has ever been called up to tackle – dope peddling ... As a result I share the fear of detectives that there is the greatest danger of the reefer craze becoming the greatest social menace the country has known.' It was in his last article, published in September 1951, that Ralph got to the heart of the matter claiming that 'the country will all be mixtures ... There will only be half-castes.' However, the idea that cannabis smoking was a nationwide threat was not born out by Thorp's account of his trips to other cities where business was minimal.

The threat of cannabis was the theme of a book published in 1952 by Dr Donald McIntosh Johnson called *Indian Hemp: A Social Menace*, which excited much press interest. Johnson was called as an expert witness in one of the rare UK trials where the alleged link between cannabis and violence was raised.

In 1952, a Nigerian, Joseph Aaku, was stabbed to death in his flat. A bloodstained packet of cannabis was found on the floor, leading the police to assume that drugs were the subject of the heated argument neighbours heard shortly before the attack. The police eventually arrested Backary Manneh who was caught selling the watch that Aaku had been wearing and worked in the restaurant from which the murder weapon had been stolen. It came out in evidence that the men knew each other, both men smoked cannabis, while Manneh already had convictions for possession and violence. The police view was that they met in the flat for a drug deal where Manneh simply attacked and robbed Aaku. But Manneh's defence team decided to try to prove that a cannabis-induced frenzy was entirely to blame for their client's murderous behaviour.

Donald Johnson was their star expert witness who stated categorically that there was a link between cannabis smoking and violence. His evidence was not challenged by the prosecution who may well have believed him about the evils of cannabis, but as the judge reminded the jury, in this particular case, there was no evidence that cannabis had been smoked on the evening of the murder which could account for what took place. The jury convicted Manneh, who lost on appeal, and he was executed on 27 May 1952.

Because of the lack of evidence of cannabis smoking, the judge queried why Johnson was called in the first place. He might have been even more mystified had he known the background to Johnson's alleged expertise. He came with impeccable credentials as a medical man, barrister, hotelier and publisher, except that he never actually practised law, had sold his medical practice in the 1930s following a dispute with an insurance company, his publishing business was always on the verge of going bust and he had to sell his hotel when he was admitted to a psychiatric hospital. Once there, he somehow got it into his head that his mental illness was the result of cannabis poisoning by Russian agents searching for a truth drug, although how this was actually administered was unclear. This set him off on his quest for the 'truth' about dope. On publication, the book sparked a brief bidding war among the press who revelled in the lurid tales that Johnson revealed, many of which could have come from the desk of Harry Anslinger, suggested again by the American spelling of 'marihuana'.

Summing up Johnson and his book, James Mills observes that 'writing about cannabis can often be writing about many other things... [Johnson] seized upon the drug as a topic through which he could articulate the Cold War anxieties and racial fears that he shared with many others in the UK in this decade'.[10] But because of his medical and legal credentials, and because he was confirming beliefs about the drug (even though few in the UK had any experience of cannabis or knew anybody who used it), his 'garbled fantasies' had sufficient credence for the press to give them fulsome coverage and add (however briefly) to the weight of established opinion that condemned cannabis as the 'devil's weed'.

Meanwhile what of the enterprising Mr Thorp? He quickly broke his conditions of probation and was soon back in his Soho haunts. Christmas came early, when he met a petty criminal who knew how to get his hands on 2 ounces of pharmaceutical-grade cocaine, stolen from a wholesaler. The contact knew nothing about the value of cocaine; Thorp said he bought £200's worth of cocaine for £15. Most of their clients were Archer Street musicians except one very special client who lived in a luxury apartment in Park Lane and was clearly somebody quite high up in the Establishment who bought £30's worth of cocaine from Thorp and his partner for 'fantastic all-male parties in this flat and his country house'. No names were mentioned, but this appears to be an early example of the kind of notorious parties which allegedly involved a predatory London clique of the rich and powerful who sexually abused or maybe even murdered teenage boys and young men.

The total haul for Thorp and his partner from sales was £220 (equating to around £6,000 today) when the average weekly wage was around £7. Police records of the time show that most of those apprehended for possession and supply of cannabis were of African and increasingly West Indian descent. This would be another example of apprehending that low-hanging fruit because Thorp's account reveals that several white dealers were also active at all levels. He refers to the mysterious 'Mr Smith' who he met at Lyons tea shop in Covent Garden: '[He] looked like a caricature drawing of a civil servant. He was a cat somewhere in his late thirties, wore glasses, white cutaway collars, dark suit and just the right length of shirt sleeves showing from his jacket.' In his search for 'Mr Smith', Thorp had mentioned his name all around the West End including inadvertently to a plain clothes policeman. Mr Smith's message to Thorp was, 'If you want to do business with me, a little more discretion please.' He never met Mr Smith again; all future business was done through a third party. But he did learn that Mr Smith had connections in Ceylon (modern day Sri Lanka), where cannabis was stashed for export in cases of shredded coconut and other foods, earning Mr Smith around £500 a week. Mr Smith would soon retire on his smuggling proceeds to teach in a country prep school and given the money Thorp says he was earning from cannabis dealing, he too should have been on easy street.

However, he was on the police radar, and London was still a small town as far as drug dealing was concerned. He says he blew all the money and was imprisoned variously for possession, supply and theft. His convictions made him an unreliable dealer and he lost his drug connections, turning in the end to injecting heroin. When Derek Agnew came across him in 1955, Thorp was living in a shabby Paddington bedsit. In his conclusion to the story, Agnew reverts to type, gravely intoning about the impending crisis of cannabis smoking and laying the blame firmly in the lap of West Indian migrants who have not only 'brought their vice with them', but worse still, 'take perverted satisfaction from "lighting up" a white girl. I know. I have watched it happen. And it is a horrible sight!'[11]

As for Raymond Thorp, he continued using heroin and appeared on the Home Office Addicts Index in the early 1960s as being in receipt of the drug from a doctor. What happened in between is unknown, but he was living in Brixton where he died on 12 September 1990.

Coming at the decade from the other end and also offering some insights into the London drug scene of the 1950s was an obscure novel by Terry Taylor called *Baron's Court: All Change,* the story of an unnamed 16-year-old who narrates his adventures of sex, drug use and dealing in Soho. Taylor was more on the inside track of bohemian Soho than Thorp and there are many autobiographical touchpoints in the novel.

In 1956, then aged 23 and working in a Soho amusement arcade taking passport photos, Taylor met the author Colin MacInnes at a drinking club in Berwick Street. Tony Gould wrote a biography of MacInnes, and in it Gould describes Taylor as interested in 'jazz, soft drugs and hustling'. Taylor had no real interest in photography but MacInnes introduced him to the photographer Ida Kar. Despite being nearly twice Taylor's age, she and Taylor became lovers. He moved in with her and her husband in a very typical Soho *ménage a trois.* The protagonist of Taylor's book also gets involved with an older woman. Like Thorp's account, however, the driving force of the novel is the determination to escape dreary suburbia. He spends his days working in a hat shop in Wimbledon, but when night falls, he is on the District line train changing at Baron's Court for the journey into Piccadilly and the heart of the bad lands.

Between the publication of Thorp's book in 1956 and Taylor's in 1961, the London music scene and its audience had expanded and with it came more opportunities for selling cannabis. Initially, there was great hostility between fans of traditional New Orleans jazz of the type personified by Louis Armstrong, often called 'Revivalists' and those fans of the new modern jazz, who became known as 'modernists' or 'Mods'. As revivalist singer George Melly explained, 'The Revivalists were studiously scruffy, so Modernists were sharp. Modernists were cool, so Revivalists were extrovert. Modernists were known to smoke dope, so Revivalists confined themselves to alcoholic excess.'[12]

On the surface this was odd because the twenties and thirties saw a slew of coded drug songs played and sung by the very musicians that the Revivalists revered such as Louis Armstrong's 'Muggles' or Fats Waller's 'Vipers Song' with the lyric, 'Dreamed about a reefer five foot long'.

However, these records never found their way to Britain. Melly also pointed out that many of the bebop musicians were professional, had travelled and met some of their heroes, whereas most of the British New Orleans-style musicians were semi-pros and never had that chance. There was also an awareness that the law was cracking down and dishing out hefty fines and prison sentences. Some of these old hostilities broke down during the 1950s and at least among the musicians, if not the fans, dope smoking seeped into New Orleans jazz circles.

Underground folk and blues clubs opened up to welcome visiting black musicians, who while mainly spirit drinkers were certainly not averse to the odd spliff. More generally, the West Indian community was growing and there was still a sizeable US military presence in the country.

So like Raymond Thorp, Taylor's character sees a chance to make some serious money and break away from the hat-selling business. The moment comes when a white dealer friend of his, Danny, who already had drug convictions, gets 'fitted up' by the police, leaving a dealing vacuum that the narrator is persuaded to help fill by his more streetwise friend Dusty. Danny claims that while he had form for possession and dealing, this time the cannabis had been planted on him. This may refer to a real incident in 1955, when Colin MacInnes was arrested at a black East End gambling club and beaten up by the police. Only later was he accused of drug possession. His lawyer picked enough holes in the police case for MacInnes to be acquitted, but it wasn't the last time that the stink of corruption and racism would stick to some officers of the Metropolitan Police Drug Squad.

Both in fact and fiction, some of the best cannabis in London at the time was Congo Matadi. Matadi is the main seaport of the Belgian Congo (now the Democratic Republic of Congo). The narrator goes into business with Dusty, spending his £50 savings on Congo, which they thoughtfully hide in the flat of a girl (Miss Roach!) they both know without telling her. The narrator's cut from their first sale is more than two months' wages selling hats. They mop up the musician trade, selling ounces at a time, taking £20 a week profit each, but eventually run foul of a white dealer, the big-shot supplier in the area. Somehow the police get to hear of the stash in Miss Roach's flat. Although she knew nothing about it, she, like Danny, has form and is arrested. While Dusty doesn't care, the narrator is guilt-stricken and walks into a police station to confess, changes his mind at the last minute and walks away.

Between the twenties and the early sixties, concerns about cannabis waxed and waned between the police and the Home Office Drugs Branch. Initially, the police had agitated for control in the face of government indifference. Then it was the turn of the Home Office Drugs Branch to collect piles of data and alerting customs officials to a drug they had never seen. Most of the official and press concerns in the fifties centred more on the presence of a growing West Indian community as a baleful influence on young white people than anything to do with the actual effects of cannabis. Policing cannabis became a proxy for policing the new immigrants. From the works of Thorp and Taylor, it was clear that there had to be an international dimension to cannabis trafficking with connections between the UK and source countries, but not on a scale that caused undue official anxiety.

In 1957, the Home Office sent a paper to a conference of Chief Constables expressing a worry that there were no corresponding increases in convictions for cannabis dealing to match the increasing amounts of drugs being seized. Their response was to reject both the proposition that increased seizures equated with more use and that fewer prosecutions meant the police weren't doing their job. But by 1960, the situation was changing. In May that year, Bing Spear at the Home Office was preparing a review paper on the rise of cannabis use in the UK suggesting that the trade was becoming well-organised, a point underlined when in the same month, customs officials made their biggest seizure to date of 169 kilos of cannabis from a ship anchored in Liverpool docks. The seizure prompted Spear to suggest to his boss, Mr Burley, that a special conference should be convened to discuss the evidence of a growing cannabis trade. The implication was that the police were not on top of the situation. Burley's response, perhaps for political reasons, was to deny there was any need for such a meeting. When the Chief Constables met again on 22 November 1962, they had to acknowledge a new landscape of cannabis trafficking although by then, they were excised by evidence of another potentially more serious youthful drug problem and one already a hidden issue for a much wider sector of society – the misuse of amphetamines.[13]

4

Talkin' 'Bout My Generation

As medical science progressed through the nineteenth century, so chemists increasingly looked to traditional plant-based medicines as a source for new treatments. The opium poppy and coca plant gave up morphine, heroin and cocaine, while the Ma Huang or Ephedra plant used in Chinese medicine to treat asthma and as a stimulant would, via the constituent chemical ephedrine, yield amphetamine and methamphetamine.

Lazăr Edeleanu, a Romanian chemist working at the University of Berlin, first synthesised amphetamine, a contraction of alpha-methylphenethylamine, in 1877. Between 1898 and 1919 two Japanese chemists, working separately with similar compounds, synthesised methamphetamine. Not until 1927 though, when American chemist Gordon Alles, who took the drug himself and documented the subjective physical and psychological effects of amphetamine, was the drug formulated into a pharmaceutical product. The American company Smith, Kline & French (SKF) launched Benzedrine decongestant inhaler for asthma in 1933 followed by the pre-war marketing of amphetamine pills and tablets for the treatment of narcolepsy, lethargy and, paradoxically, as a stimulant drug as treatment for what we now know as Attention Deficit Disorder in children.

A drug to fight fatigue, reduce appetite and promote a sense of well-being, confidence and aggression became a valuable addition to the field rations of both the Allied and Axis powers during the war. Use by German troops, Adolf Hitler and other members of the Nazi high command is well documented. But in June 1940, unknown pills were found with Luftwaffe pilots shot down over Britain. The RAF commissioned research to find out what they were. The pills turned out to be methamphetamine and were recommended for British forces, especially for pilots undertaking long, boring flights tracking submarines across the Atlantic. These pilots were already unofficially taking Benzedrine pills, so the RAF was playing catch-up and eventually bought in amphetamine from SKF and methamphetamine from the British firm Burroughs Wellcome. By the end of the war, British service personnel had consumed 72 million Benzedrine tablets[1] while in medical circles, amphetamine was now being recommended for a wide range of conditions from obesity and low blood pressure to depression and reduced libido.

However, medical concerns were raised about adverse effects of the drug as early as June 1936 when the *Pharmaceutical Journal* quoted a report saying Benzedrine caused hypertension. In June 1939, Benzedrine was placed in the Poisons List so that the packet had to carry a label to warn that the drug should only be used under medical supervision and could only be sold by a registered pharmacist to a known customer. It seems most unlikely there was much medical supervision in the heat of battle; tank crews given amphetamine at the battle of El Alamein, for example, complained of numbness and hallucinations.

The hallucinations experienced by tank crews exemplified the aspect of most concern in regular amphetamine use: amphetamine psychosis, which could be so acute as to resemble paranoid schizophrenia. Given the commercial value of the drug to SKF, pre-war alarms were dismissed as just an association rather than a cause. Then in 1956, Dr Philip Connell, a psychiatrist working at the Maudsley Hospital in south London, wrote his doctoral thesis on amphetamine psychosis, which became the standard work on the subject when it was published two years later. Dr Connell went on to become a highly influential and often controversial figure in heroin addiction treatment during the 1970s and 1980s and for some years was chair of ISDD. In March 1957, a year before his book appeared, the *British Medical Journal* published this letter from Dr Connell, the first substantial notice on the subject:

It is the purpose of this letter to draw attention to the widespread abuse of amphetamine in this country, which has not previously been demonstrated, and to mention that a common result of amphetamine intoxication is the development of a paranoid psychosis indistinguishable from schizophrenia, during which the patient may be a serious social danger. A further point of general social importance is that many of the patients studied obtained the drug from inhalers freely available to the general public ... The anomaly of the law which permits the free sale of such inhalers while restricting the sale of tablets has been pointed out on a number of occasions, but there has been a lack of evidence demonstrating the real need for such a restriction. This evidence is now available. It is of interest to note that some drug firms withdrew their amphetamine inhalers from the market because of the considerable increase in the sale of inhalers which took place after amphetamine had been placed on schedule 4 of the poisons rules – meaning that amphetamines except the inhalers, were now prescription only drugs.

His thesis and book identified nineteen different amphetamine-containing drugs on the market and examined the case studies of 42 patients, a mixture of white- and blue-collar workers, some taking up to 1,000mg of amphetamine daily. While admitting his sample was small, Connell wrote:

The medical profession as a whole and psychiatrists in particular who were enthusiastic about the amphetamine group of drugs when they were first used therapeutically and recommended their use on a scale not tempered by caution, must bear responsibility for the number of cases of amphetamine abuse and amphetamine psychosis.[2]

The drug was made a prescription-only medication following reports that pharmacies were being overwhelmed by customer demand, primarily from housewives, although in Connell's study there were more men than women patients. Other forms of amphetamine came on the market, such as dextroamphetamine developed to try and offset what were now the acknowledged risks of 'pure' amphetamine. In 1950, SKF launched Drinamyl, a drug combining dextroamphetamine and amobarbitol for depression, anxiety and slimming. The amobarbitol was a barbiturate included to take the edge off the amphetamine. Despite being triangular and blue, they would later gain notoriety as 'purple hearts'. Preludin was developed in Germany as a slimming pill and another attempt to enhance the claimed benefits of amphetamine without some of the side effects. In reality it was a fantasy to imagine a drug with all the effects of amphetamine would not be used for non-medical purposes. Amphetamines became very popular among long-distance lorry drivers while Preludin tablets would become field rations for bands like The Beatles playing the Hamburg club scene for hours on end.

In October 1957, there was a press report of a wide-scale 'black market' in Drinamyl among women living in the Rhondda Valley in Wales. They 'wait outside chemist shops to buy them from boys collecting the drugs for their mothers. They scrub floors – even steal – to get money for the pills.'

Another newspaper report from February 1959 claimed that five years of amphetamine use had wrecked a woman's marriage and driven her into a mental home. She was originally prescribed the drug for post-natal depression after the birth of her third child. As her dependence grew, she could remain awake all night, only to collapse afterwards from exhaustion. She was going from doctor to doctor to obtain prescriptions, ending up on nearly 20 Drinamyl a day and forging prescriptions as she went along. Her husband left with the children. She collapsed in her husband's office and was taken to hospital in an incoherent state but was released as 'cured' after an eight-month stay.[3]

Similar stories of overprescribing, illicit sales, forged prescriptions and addiction appeared in the press throughout the fifties and sixties without any response from either the medical profession or government. By the early sixties, the NHS was dishing out approximately 5 million amphetamine prescriptions a year, but as the decade progressed, substantial quantities of the drug stolen from wholesale warehouses and pharmacies found their way onto the streets and into the pockets of Britain's first truly visible drug subculture: the new generation Mods and their love affair with speed.

* * *

Back in May 1937 came the first reports that Benzedrine inhalers were being taken apart, the amphetamine-impregnated wadding inside removed and then dunked in coffee or alcohol to release more than 400 mg of amphetamine when the normal Benzedrine tablet contained only 5–10mg. In the fifties, Soho bohemians and black-draped beatniks huddled in dives and coffee bars engaged in intense, speed-driven arguments about poetry, art, philosophy, life, the universe and everything. In *On the Road*, their Beat guru Jack Kerouac wrote the classic description of the speed freak as embodied by the character Dean Moriarty; in real life, Neal Cassady: 'He was absolutely mad. It was a shaking of the head, up and down, sideways, jerky, vigorous hands; quick walking, sitting, crossing his legs, uncrossing; getting up, rubbing his hands, rubbing his fly, hitching his pants, looking up ... sudden slitting of the eye to see everywhere and all the time he was grabbing me by the ribs and talking, talking.'

But the inhalers were gradually withdrawn (although some brands such as Nosaline remained on the market), leaving an array of pills whose new consumers were not into debating existentialism. The generation gap which first appeared as Robert Thorp and Terry Taylor entered their teenage years began to widen. The opportunities for Thorp and his contemporaries to create a world in their own image hardly existed as German bombs rained down on Britain's major cities. In the years immediately following the end of the war, little had changed: those aged 13–18 were adults-in-waiting. By 1957, post-war austerity had receded: Britain was enjoying full employment and a relative consumer boom as Prime Minister Harold Macmillan famously declared that in the face of rising living standards, 'most of our people have never had it so good'. Young people wanted to make the most of the opportunities that increasing disposable income allowed them. They finally had cash of their own and the teenager was born as a unique commercial entity with consumer demands for clothes and records. New music venues and coffee bars fulfilled the demand of young people for places to meet – outside of pubs where they weren't allowed and away from the dreary church-based youth clubs complete with the caretaker who pulled the plug on the record player when it was time for his cocoa and slippers.

Unlike the Beatniks with their studied shabbiness and the black leather, grease monkey bike freak Rockers, Mods – who had nothing to do with their predecessor modern jazz lovers – turned neatness into an art form. They didn't express rebellion through a subversive 'uniform' – quite the opposite – the new Mods had a post-war British working-class attitude to smartness, best described as flash. The wartime and early 1950s spivs (James Beck as Private Walker in *Dad's Army* and George Cole as Flash Harry in the St Trinian's films) were followed by Teddy Boys who hijacked a failed attempt by Savile Row to revive Edwardian elegance with the aristocracy by adding string ties and slick hairdos to a taste for American rock 'n' roll and the Mississippi steamboat gambler. Mods also took some inspiration from the States in their attempt to recreate the sartorial coolness of the black hipster. However, they looked to the Continent, particularly Italy, for the clothes themselves.

The relentless pursuit of fashion eclipsed almost everything else. Neither food, drink nor women mattered because their love affair with amphetamine – really the first youth culture where drugs played a defining role – killed the appetite for all three. Most of the earnings from work went on clothes and pills. Mod fashion was a microcosm of an industrial society which paid homage to the sacred cow of built-in obsolescence. Mods would spend a substantial part of their wages having vents put in or taken out of jackets, the pockets widened or narrowed, knowing that three weeks later they would be out of date. Mods would rather stay home than be seen out in last week's fashion. Probably no teenagers since have paid such meticulous attention to the minutiae of their attire – an obsession which had its counterpart in the way amphetamine users can get totally absorbed in mindless and trivial occupations like washing a plate.

Mods looked normal, but they weren't: they made wearing a suit and tie seem aggressive and threatening. Somehow *too* smart and *too* neat, they caused consternation among upright citizens who saw their own conservative dress sense mocked. The worst thing that could happen to a Mod was to have his parents understand him.

This (and the auto-destruction on stage) explains the appeal of The Who as they morphed into the minstrels of Mod even though they weren't really Mods (unlike the Small Faces). As Pete Townsend said later, their Mod image was dishonest. To keep their credibility intact the band would watch the dance steps Mod audiences were doing and recreate them on stage so that another audience would think the band had invented them. Whether intentional or not, The Who wrote the anthems of the Mod generation including the amphetamine stutter of 'My Generation' (which Roger Daltrey initially didn't want to sing); 'Anyway, Anyhow, Anywhere' with the line 'Nothing gets in my way not even locked doors'; and 'Substitute', about all the insecurities beneath the desperate need to keep up appearances and stand behind the image.

The critical parts of the image – the barely controlled aggression, the threatening, garrulous demeanour and general wired 'up-tightness' of it all – was provided by amphetamines, especially purple hearts. As depicted in *Quadrophenia*, getting blocked on pills at weekends was what separated 'them' from 'us'. The bikers got their speed by racing around at 100 mph. The Mods with their scooters, laughed at by Rockers, favoured instead speed of a very different kind.

For Mods, speed performed another useful function: the Dutch courage needed to take on Rockers. The early Mods had no time for violence but hysterical press reporting after the first major Mod/Rocker clash at Clacton on Easter Monday 1964 became a self-fulfilling prophecy. That well-publicised fracas was the first time most people heard about Mods and Rockers and the press instantly created a new breed of folk devils to rival the Teddy Boys of the 1950s and the Glaswegian razor gangs. Press reports were littered with words and phrases like 'battle', 'attack',' siege', 'screaming mob' and 'orgy of destruction'. The press exaggerated and distorted every aspect of the confrontation, conveying the impression that the conflict was strictly polarised on Mod and Rocker lines. Initially the clashes were more between rival gangs in London and the Home Counties. Only later, in some of the more bloody disturbances, when it became fashionable to be either Mod or Rocker, did these battles take on the lines of a subcultural clash. At that point, the Mod underground, a cool understated bunch of natty dressers, became media darlings.

Nothing really subversive was ever featured in the *Sunday Times* colour supplement, but in the hunt for the ideal Mod to interview, the intrepid journalists came up with Denzil who said, 'pills make you edgy and argumentable (*sic*)'. The pills made Mods hypersensitive to the possibilities of action and generated the desire to go looking for trouble.

Powerful stimulants like amphetamine and cocaine release adrenaline, the fight or flight hormone. If that response isn't satisfied, the brain is all dressed up with nowhere to go, and the user becomes restless and agitated and eventually quite paranoid. In the context of Mod culture, having a rumble with a bunch of greasers was the obvious biochemical response. After the way the press handled the Easter and subsequent Whitsun 1964 incidents, it was obvious that any right-thinking Mod or Rocker out for some free publicity to shock the nation, would get together at appointed times and places predicted by the press in the sure knowledge that the cameras would be ready and waiting.

Denzil had more to say, about an 'average week' in the life of the ideal London Mod:

Monday: dancing at the Mecca, the Hammersmith Palais, the Purley Orchard or the Streatham Locarno

Tuesday: Soho at The Scene Club

Wednesday: Marquee night

Thursday: Washing hair (which had to be dried using a dryer with a hood)

Friday: Back at The Scene

Saturday afternoon: Clothes and record buying

Saturday night: The all-nighter at The Flamingo[4]

It is unlikely that anybody ever kept up a regime like that for long, however much speed they took. It all cost money and although Mods were the most affluent teenagers to date, the money had to run out sometime. Nevertheless, the diary does demonstrate the importance of music in the club scene to all Mods whether hard-core or weekenders.

The West End clubs were also the main centres of retail amphetamine dealing where the dealing networks appeared quite complex. A major hub of speed distribution was one of Denzil's favoured haunts, The Scene Club in Ham Yard at 41 Great Windmill Street. Originally the site of Club Eleven, the club was run by Ronan O'Rahilly, pioneer of pirate radio with the offshore Radio Caroline. O'Rahilly had the walls padded and cushions strewn everywhere so that those who speeded to exhaustion could crash out. Two cousins who manned the door had a habit of relieving patrons of their pills as they entered, pretending to flush them down the toilet and then recycling them. The dealing went on in the club where purple hearts were sold at 3*d* each (around 6p) but were normally bought in tens, twenties, fifties and 100s.

Another venue for speed dealing in the early sixties was La Discotheque in Wardour Street. It was originally called El Condor and from 1957 to 1961 operated as an exclusive nightspot frequented by British royalty. The club was owned by Raymond Nash (who also owned The Scene Club)

and the notorious slum landlord Peter Rachman, who sold the club to former film stuntman and co-founder of the Vidal Sassoon empire Tommy Yeardye and one of Rachman's own protégés Peter Davies for £10,000. However, the new club went bankrupt and reopened as a far more downmarket discotheque. Hordes of young people replaced the upper-middle-class and the smattering of aristocrats. Rachman and Nash resumed control as joint shareholders. They installed a powerful light and sound system. Drinks were 5s (25p) but the place was awash with cheap amphetamines. One of the major dealers on the scene was one of Rachman's loyal soldiers, the aptly named 'Peter the Pill'. Later, he became a road manager for The Animals and Eric Burdon's band War and was involved with the Jimi Hendrix business set-up overseen by the ever-slippery manager Mike Jeffrey.

The amphetamines in circulation invariably had the manufacturer's name SKF stamped on them. The handful of people working with chronic amphetamine users in Soho came to the not unreasonable conclusion that the drugs were finding their way directly to dealers via SKF employees pilfering them from the factory and warehouses. At a meeting of the Society for the Study of Addiction in September 1966, Judith Piepe, a German woman who for many years acted as a freelance social worker trying to help young people on the streets, got up and said so in public:

> Extensive security precautions in a factory cost a great deal of money, it is easy for anybody on the production line quietly to take a handful and augment their wages by selling them. The production cost of drugs like Drinamyl are very low and the cost in money to ensure better security arrangements is considered too high by the manufacturers. They do not consider the cost in suffering to young people.

Replying for SKF, a Mr Schreiner said, 'In regard to the accusation that tablets had been stolen from the manufacturing companies, I regard this as nonsense. Tablets are manufactured under stringent supervision and is highly improbable that any quantities could be stolen from the factories in these circumstances.'[5]

Around this time, the press reported a Gloucestershire doctor saying the amphetamines could be made by teenagers with O-level chemistry. He offered no evidence for this, so the *Daily Mirror* rang various experts to check the story. GP Ian Pearce James agreed anyone with O-level chemistry could make amphetamine pills but wondered how they managed to make the little moulds and stamp SKF on them.

In truth, it is impossible to imagine with so many pills in circulation in West End clubs, mostly owned by London crime bosses like the Krays, that they weren't the source of the drugs bought from crooked SKF employees and corrupt chemists and taking a hefty slice of the retail action. It has always been assumed that British gangsters didn't really get involved in the drug scene until the late seventies, but they were active on the scene well before that even if most of the profits earned in the sixties came from prostitution, pornography and protection. And it wasn't just in London; there was a healthy pill scene in other major cities like Liverpool, Manchester, Glasgow and Birmingham.

But behind the hysterical headlines, the Italian suits and the shiny scooters lay a darker reality, one hinted at by Judith Piepe in her attack on Big Pharma; concerns about the plight of young people coming to the capital, entranced by reporting about 'Swinging London' and expecting the streets to be paved with shiny stuff. These fears came to public notice when a white South African political activist on the run from the apartheid regime had a conversation with a journalist from the London *Evening Standard*.

Lee Harris settled in London as a playwright and actor and was a regular visitor to all the Soho dives. Although by the time the Mods were out and about Harris was in his late twenties, he embraced the culture and had friends running the clubs where drug dealing was going on until he saw what was happening on the streets: 'There were all these young kids wandering about at five in the morning with dilated pupils and chewing their gums. I found out they were taking purple heart pills, sometimes taking 80 or 90 in a weekend at *6d* a time and had comedowns and amphetamine psychosis afterwards, seeing insects and spiders on the walls.' He mentioned this to the Labour MP for Paddington, Ben Parkin, who had recently exposed Rachman, but who knew nothing about amphetamine.

'He told me he would raise it in Parliament, but that if anybody wanted to know more about what was happening, he would give them my phone number. I got a call from Ann Sharpley who was a top investigative reporter on the London *Evening Standard*. She said, "would you like to show me around the West End?". I took her on a tour of the dives and introduced her to this young speed addict I knew called Johnny. She saw all these young people and the dealers passing the pills. That Monday at the beginning of 1964, there was a headline in *Evening Standard*, "I see Soho pep pill craze". In the evening, Soho was deserted. There was a terrific hue and cry: at that point the general view was that the only people took pep pills were housewives in the Rhondda Valley.'[6]

But Harris did more than just give a journalist a guided tour of Soho. Lee and his brother Mervyn, a social worker, began to interview some of the young people Lee had encountered and put together a book called *Living for Kicks*, which remains unpublished. One of those interviewed was 'Gerry', a low-level amphetamine dealer whom Lee met in August 1963. Gerry would regularly get high on his own supply, taking anything up to thirty pills at any one time. Supplies for himself and his customers came, not through pharmacy thefts or factory knock-offs, but by conning doctors about the need for slimming pills: 'A friend of mine gets them from a doctor who lets him have as much as he wants. Some people get them from chemist's assistants who take handfuls from bottles.'

Lee called him 'essentially a product of today, he is the prototype of a new movement, the kicksters'. Gerry was not part of any protest or subcultural movement, but more like Robert Thorp and Teddy Taylor's semi-fictional character, intelligent and aware but simply bored, with little sense of purpose about where he wanted to go. All he knew was that he didn't want to live like his parents and railed against anybody who tried to tell him what to do. As Pete Townsend wrote, 'People try to put us down/Just because we get around'. Gerry was a working-class boy who got by on speed dealing, street begging and bits of petty larceny.

In some biographical notes that Gerry wrote, and Lee kept, Gerry said he came from a large loving family and laid no blame on them for how things turned out for him: 'My life is my own. I chose my pathway.'

He clearly struggled with depression brought about both by a crushing sense of futility and shame about being dependent on drugs which he dealt with either by being blocked on pills or laid out on cannabis. He also found solace in the blues: 'I like listening to music, especially the blues. It's impossible to describe it. When you listen to the blues, you don't want to think, you just want to listen.' Eric Clapton, who himself had a loving but difficult childhood, described the blues as one man and a guitar alone with his back to the wall. Although Clapton later used drugs and alcohol to deal with his own demons, in the early days, he was able to sublimate his anguish in music. Few other young people were that fortunate.

Gerry also had to deal with the comedown from excessive amphetamine use and talked about an exhausted body, swollen legs, nausea and classic speed delusions, hallucinations and formication – the feeling of insects crawling under the skin. Gerry had no illusions about London glamour; not so the young people who found their way there in the early to mid-sixties, often on the run from broken and abusive homes or struggling with a crisis of sexual identity which they self-medicated with amphetamine. Ending up in Soho, many found themselves preyed upon by predatory men whose promises evaporated, leaving boys and girls facing a seedy and dangerous descent into male and female prostitution.

There were few avenues of help for these young people or indeed anybody living on the streets; such help as existed was often Christian in orientation. The Reverend Vic Ramsey, a fire and brimstone evangelical, would preach to homeless alcohol and drug users in the basement of Soho's Orange Street Chapel and in 1964 founded one of the first drug residential rehabilitation facilities, the New Life Foundation Trust. Sally Trench, who came from a well-to-do middle-class family but was a rebellious and troubled teenager, found her faith helping and living with London's street homeless. She was involved at one time with The Simon Community set up in 1963 to support the homeless, which still operates today. Burnt out by her life on the streets, Trench wrote a memoir, *Bury Me in My Boots* – a 1968 bestseller. However, the individual who had most influence at the time in bringing the plight of drug users to wider public and political attention was the Reverend Ken Leech. When he died in 2015, Anglican priest and peace and human rights activist Paul Ostreicher wrote Ken's obituary published in *The Guardian* on 22 September 2015:

Ken Leech ... stood firmly in the proud tradition of radical prophetic priests in the English Catholic, rather than Roman Catholic, tradition – one that comes closest to Latin America's liberation theology. His commitment to allying prayer with political action led him to create the Centrepoint charity for young homeless people in central London, to work tirelessly on promoting good race relations, and to become an influential writer exploring the relationship between intimacy with God and compassionate political commitment to a more just and peaceful world.

Ken was a prolific author whose first book, *Keep the Faith Baby*, was published in 1973 and told of his early days on the Soho drug scene. The title was inspired by the Free Church of Berkeley in California led by Reverend Lyle Grosjean, an Episcopal priest dubbed a 'hippie pastor' in San Francisco's Haight-Ashbury district whose church motto was 'The liberated zone is here' and used The Beatles' 'Yellow Submarine' as its symbol. Ken was no buttoned-up cleric.

His earliest encounter with the London drug scene came in the late fifties when he was living and working in Cable Street in the East End, scene of the famous anti-fascist battles of the thirties. Ken was helping out at a Franciscan mission, taught English to Somalis and help set up a club for African seamen and a hostel for new immigrants. He became involved in the burgeoning heroin scene, but here we consider his account of moving to the West End and the Parish of St Anne's in Soho and his first encounters with young amphetamine users. Speaking to Ken some years ago, he told me that as early as 1961,

> As you walked up Wardour Street and turned into D'Arblay Street, there was a very small area which you could walk around in 10 minutes where there was a very heavy concentration of amphetamine clubs. Within yards of each of other you had ... Le Duce, a gay club, directly opposite you had a club which changed its name several times but was most famous as the Subway. Then you had the Coffee Pot which never closed (and where according to Richard Neville's *Playpower* I'm always to be found!). Underneath was the Huntsman and then opposite, in a smelly cul-de-sac between Wardour Street and Berwick Street, was Wardour Mews with the Limbo Club, the Granada and the Take Five.

True to his word, MP Ben Parkin did raise the issue in Parliament. The resulting legislation, the Drugs (Prevention of Misuse) Act 1964 made it an offence to possess amphetamines without a prescription, but as Ken noted, 'The Act was not particularly effective because it included no controls on manufacture, distribution or record of sales and the traffic continued unabated.'[7]

Just how ineffective the legislation was can be judged by this interview from March 1967 when the underground magazine *Oz* spoke to two 21-year-old dealers called Paul and Cliff. They claimed a joint income of up to £400 a week and both owned smart 1966 Ford Zephyrs. A third of the money was passed up the chain to somebody they called 'Big Sid' and they in turn employed two West Indian minders with whom they shared a 20 guinea (£21) a week flat in Chelmsford, Essex. One interesting point was that they said much of their supply came not from factory or shop thefts, but imports from overseas. The magazine reported:

> Starting their work at the Marquee Club, they sell to a market of 13-year-old Mods. After a meal they move into the clubs around Greek Street and then onto a stand just outside Tiffany's about one in the morning. When necessary, they work a pitch in the Lyons Cafés around Trafalgar Square

and if on Sunday morning they have any pills remaining, move to Chelsea were apparently tired debs are always a ready market. In conversation with one reporter as to the origin of the amphetamines, they say that some of their pills were knocked off, but most came from a regular supply through London docks – they weren't sure where they came from, but apparently that was Big Sid's business. In one weekend they said they never sold less than 3,000 pills and sometimes in excess of 6,000 undercutting other dealers by selling at one shilling each.[8]

During that summer of 1967, 'the summer of love', Ken moved from the East to the West End and into the Parish of St Anne's in Soho where he helped set up the Soho Project and began his outreach work in the clubs and cafés just listening to young people talk about their problems without ramming God down their throats, and he became a trusted figure on the scene. Eventually the Soho Project became a small agency with offices in the Charing Cross Road. From his own account, many of the young people he came across in the clubs were gay or lesbian and living very precarious and often dangerous street lives where 'use of amphetamines by kids in the club was closely related to the confusion about sexual identity. There was as much boasting about the number of pills consumed as about the number of sexual acts.' So important was the idea of being blocked on pills, that there was an expectation you would act high even if you weren't. It is noticeable in speaking to those around the club scene at the time, there was a sense of a highly febrile, narcissistic, self-regarding atmosphere of drama, paranoia and anxious gossip where everybody was either 'mad' or 'outrageous'.

As problematic as chronic amphetamine use could be, with a recovery period sometimes lasting months, an even more serious problem emerged from the scene. Towards the end of 1967 and into 1968 around the West End, there was a sudden surge in the availability of injectable methamphetamine marketed as Methedrine. As we shall see in Chapter Seven, if there was ever a gateway drug to heroin, it certainly wasn't cannabis.

In 2004, the BBC broadcast a London 1960s crime series *The Long Firm* adapted from Jake Arnott's novel of the same name featuring a Kray-type gangster called Harry Stark. Stark's driver and right-hand man is a small-time amphetamine dealer in his forties called Jimmy who knocks around with a much younger speed freak guy, Beardsley. It's 1967, and while Jimmy's at a party doing business, Beardsley turns up, scores some pills from Jimmy and then says to him:

'Can you get me some acid?'
'Acid? Who are you threatening to burn?'
'No, LSD. It's a drug. Everybody's ravin' about it.'

And so they were.

5

Long Strange Trips

On 16 April 1943, Albert Hofmann, a research chemist working for the Swiss pharmaceutical company Sandoz decided to leave work early as he was feeling decidedly peculiar. As he later wrote to a Sandoz colleague Professor Arthur Stoll,

> At home, I lay down and sank into a not unpleasant intoxicated-like condition, characterised by an extremely stimulated imagination. In a dreamlike state, with eyes closed (I found the daylight to be unpleasantly glaring), I perceived an uninterrupted stream of fantastic pictures, extraordinary shapes of intense kaleidoscopic play of colours. After some two hours, the condition faded away.[1]

Hofmann had been working on a chemical called lysergic acid, found in ergot, a parasitic fungus which grows on wheat and rye. Ergotism is poisoning produced by eating food affected by the fungus, typically resulting in headache, vomiting, diarrhoea, and gangrene of the fingers and toes. The fungus was reputedly responsible for causing epidemics of hallucinations and strange burning sensations in charred gangrenous limbs known in the Middle Ages as 'St Anthony's Fire' after Anthony of Padua, who died of ergotism in 1231. The strange and 'unholy' symptoms forged a link between ergotism and accusations of witchcraft and the general outbreaks of uncontrolled hysteria among populations who had eaten bread from ergot-infected grain.

Because it constricts the blood vessels, ergot also appeared in late sixteenth-century herbal remedy texts as a drug to stimulate childbirth and prevent post-partum bleeding. It was this potential for medical use that encouraged chemists at Sandoz to attempt extracting the active chemicals from the fungus for further study, examining too the potential for relieving other conditions such as migraine. Hofmann had been working on the main active chemical in ergot, lysergic acid, with little success. In 1938, he was studying the twenty-fifth iteration of the chemical, but then abandoned the project. He later wrote that he had a feeling there was more to LSD-25 than simply a straightforward medical treatment for physical conditions. He went back to the substance in 1943, and inadvertently stumbled upon one of the most powerful hallucinogenic drugs on the planet.

Believing that LSD-25 was responsible for his strange experience, he took the drug again, dissolved in water and became so disoriented and overwhelmed, he needed help getting home. Not only had he confirmed the power of the drug, but also its extreme potency in minute quantities, just 250 micrograms or 250 millionths of a gram.

To further grasp what he had unleashed, Hofmann continued to experiment on himself, quickly concluding that because of the inexplicable nature of the experience, this might be akin to psychosis and so might help unlock some of the conundrums of mental illness. The personal insights Hofmann says he gleaned from taking LSD led him to think that maybe the drug might help in the still new and controversial practice of psychotherapy. The LSD story travelled along four intersecting pathways – the first being medical.

In 1947, Sandoz marketed LSD as Delysid, sending free samples to researchers who promised they would reciprocate with any research findings. In 1952, Hofmann was visited by Ronald Sandison, a British psychiatrist on a study tour of Swiss mental health clinics in his new role as Consultant Psychiatrist at Powick Mental Hospital in Worcester. Sandison was intrigued to hear about LSD and agreed with Hofmann that the drug might very well have an application in psychotherapy, which he had been trying out at Powick. He had been frustrated by the lengthy and expensive process of generating the necessary trust with the patient for them to open up to the therapist, without which little progress could be made. After a subsequent visit to Sandoz, Sandison returned home with a consignment of LSD ampoules to try on a selected group of patients. Interviewed by Andy Roberts for his history of LSD use in Britain, *Albion Dreaming*, Sandison admitted that the notion of having these trials approved by an ethics committee or seeking informed patient consent was unheard of in the 1950s: 'One was left to get on with it, if one felt the treatment was right.'[2]

Sandison published the first fruits of his research in 1954 in the *Journal of Mental Science*. He concluded that there was sufficient improvement across the patient group to believe that LSD had a future as a psychotherapeutic drug, although he did introduce one important element into the therapeutic journey. Probably through his conversations with Hofmann and from the results of self-experimentation which had taken place among Hofmann's colleagues, Sandison understood that the LSD experience was not simply determined by the action of the drug on the brain. Whether the experience was benign or malevolent also depended on what the user expected to happen, either based on whether they were anxious or relaxed about taking a new drug, past experience of use, experiences of others they knew or (later on) media reporting, and also the environment in which the drug was being used, for example with trusted friends or a roomful of strangers. This came to be known through the work of American psychiatrist and psychoanalyst Norman Zinberg as the experience triangle – drug, set and setting – although it mainly seemed to apply to hallucinogenic drugs with their complex and percussive impact on the brain rather than drugs with a more predictable effect such as heroin, cocaine or amphetamines.

Fierce Chemistry

In non-western cultures where hallucinogenic plants are used in rituals, the initiate is helped through the experience by a guide (usually the priest or shaman) who may or may not have also taken the drug. Many years ago, I attended a seminar given by two shamans from the Amazon region who were very experienced in the use of a hallucinogenic brew called ayahuasca, made from Banisteriopsis caapi vine and other ingredients, for the rite of passage ceremony taking young boys into manhood. Apart from weeks of preparation in the jungle isolated from family and friends, the boys were helped through a shattering experience by their shaman. But as one of them said, as these boys grew up, leaving the tribe to build a life in the city, some tried ayahuasca and other drugs outside the boundaries of tradition and ritual, where the experiences were not as they expected.

By the same token, Sandison ensured his patients had assistance with the help of a nurse who, as Sandison explained, 'has to understand and yet not comment on the patient's experience; she must not trespass on a delicate situation with bright and diverting remarks; she may answer but not ask questions, she must be prepared to be at the patient's side if needed and to play an intuitive, passive, vigilant part.'

Sandison carried on with LSD psychotherapy for the next twelve years before leaving Powick Hospital in 1964 and ending his association with LSD. In 1968, Dr Nicholas Malleson conducted a survey of psychiatric use of LSD in the UK on behalf of the government's Advisory Committee on Drug Dependence. In all, he found that around 5,000 people were administered some 50,000 doses of LSD. While it proved impossible to untangle all the circumstances, Malleson could only uncover 3 suicides, 20 attempted suicides where LSD might have been implicated and 37 psychotic reactions lasting more than 48 hours. This with other inconclusive results of LSD benefits led the committee to conclude that there was no compelling evidence that in therapeutic terms, LSD was either especially useful or dangerous.

LSD therapy continued in the UK into the 1970s, but the ban on recreational use in both the USA and UK in 1966 and the attendant media reporting made it much harder to use for therapeutic purposes. When the UK Misuse of Drugs Act came into force in 1973, LSD was categorised as a drug with no proven therapeutic application and while a researcher could obtain a Home Office licence for research purposes, clinical use of the drug dried up.

But that wasn't quite the end of the early medical history of LSD. In 1997, 43 ex-Powick Hospital patients sued the local health authority claiming that their lives had been damaged by the LSD they had received between 1950 and 1970. The patients were treated for various forms of depression (for which LSD was not effective) and schizophrenia. The problem for the complainants was the passage of time and, by Sandison's own admission, the standards of due diligence which attended experimental treatments back in the day were very different to those in place by the late 1990s. Eventually the case was settled out of court to the tune of £195,000, way below what was claimed. The patients also had their legal fees amounting to £400,000 covered. That was far less than the estimated £3 million in fees if the case had gone to trial, which is why the NHS settled even though no liability was admitted. There was one intriguing aspect to this case.

In 1995, two years before the patients sued the local health authority, the case was taken by the late Ken Purchase, Labour MP for Wolverhampton East, who had been approached by constituents complaining about their LSD treatment. Purchase raised the issue in the House of Commons, only to be told by Health Minister John Bowis that there was no evidence anybody had received LSD as a treatment. This was quickly shown to be untrue and was followed up by a local BBC reporter, Chris Green, who fronted a feature for the BBC Radio programme *You and Yours*. 'There was one patient interviewed for the programme who said there were Americans present during her therapy session, but she wasn't the only one. They all had the feeling they were guinea pigs.'[3] So who were these Americans? This is where the medical history of LSD in the UK possibly merges into the second LSD track: the military.

Since the start of the Cold War, both the Russians and the Americans had been looking at ways to undermine opposition armed forces using chemicals and brainwashing techniques. The idea was both to find a truth drug for use in interrogations and to establish if there was a drug that could disable troops but leave the ordnance undamaged. Beginning in 1953 with an order of 10 kilos of LSD from Sandoz, the CIA established a number of secret trials under the codename MK-ULTRA in which soldiers and even other CIA operatives had their bar drinks given to them by prostitutes spiked with LSD. The men were then followed home to see what would happen, occasionally with tragic consequences.

What was not so well documented until a *New Statesman* article of October 1994 and subsequent Parliamentary questions, was the involvement of the UK government in similar testing through the Ministry of Defence-run Chemical and Biological Defence Establishment at Porton Down. Could there have been a link with Sandison's work at Powick?

From 1954 to 1956, Sandison was treating his LSD patients in the main hospital building. But for reasons which are unclear, he wasn't happy with this arrangement and applied to Birmingham Regional Hospital Board requesting the building of a special unit. Not only was the funding for an entirely experimental and unevaluated intervention immediately granted, but within two years, at a modern-day equivalent cost of nearly £1.2 million, the unit was up and running. Did a local authority hospital board really have that amount of money to spend on a project like this? Who else had an interest in seeing a special unit built away from public gaze?

Sandison was supported in his bid by Dr Joel Elkes, acknowledged as the father of neuropsychopharmacology, the study of the neural mechanisms acted upon by drugs to influence behaviour. In 1951 he set up the Department of Experimental Psychology at Birmingham University and in 1953 published in the *Journal of Physiology* what might be the first UK article looking at the effects of LSD in healthy volunteers. Elkes had become fascinated with LSD, attended a lecture by Sandison on the subject and the two became friends. Although Sandison knew that Elkes had signed the Official Secrets Act, he said he didn't know why or that Elkes was an adviser to the Ministry of Defence, specifically in matters concerning the potential for the use of LSD as a chemical weapon. In 1955, Elkes wrote to *The Lancet* expressing concern that LSD medical trials were being undertaken with day- and out-patients, whereas he felt such trials should only take place with in-patients so they could be closely watched. Some former patients did tell Chris Green they often went home on the bus after their treatment with no support. But Elkes may have had an ulterior motive for wanting patients closely supervised. Because of his links with both the medical and military use of LSD, it is perfectly feasible that arrangements were made for US military personnel, the 'Americans', to witness LSD psychotherapy sessions at Powick, having perhaps contributed to the building of the unit.

Both the American and the British military gave up on LSD, but like the Powick court case, the repercussions reverberated down the years. In 1976, the family of a US scientist, Frank Olsen, settled with the US government who had maintained for years that Olsen committed suicide by jumping out of a New York hotel window. In fact, Olsen was one of those surreptitiously dosed with LSD by his colleagues and he thought he was going mad. The family continued campaigning in the belief that Olsen may have been murdered by the CIA simply for knowing too much, but had their case dismissed in 2013. The film *Wormwood*, which examined several aspects of the case, was shown on *Netflix* in 2017.

Closer to home, in 2006, MI6 reached an out-of-court settlement with three servicemen who did volunteer for the trial, but were not told what to expect, believing instead they were testing a cure for the common cold. One of the soldiers, who said he'd had flashbacks for 10 years after the tests, remembered a nightmarish experience when he hallucinated for a long time. He saw 'walls melting, cracks appearing in people's faces ... eyes would run down cheeks, Salvador Dali-type faces ... a flower would turn into a slug'. But the main legacy of LSD in the 1960s was neither its medical nor military application but what might be termed the mystical; the role played by this catalytic chemical in creating an unprecedented chapter in British cultural history: the sixties.

* * *

With some 80 British doctors using LSD experimentally in psychotherapy sessions from the 1950s onwards with Sandoz LSD imported into the UK, it was inevitable that LSD would leak onto the streets. A small-time drug courier, Dave Cunliffe, told author Andy Roberts that limited amounts of LSD were circulating the usual Soho haunts between 1956 and '59 and LSD gets a very brief mention in Terry Taylor's novel *Baron's Court: All Change*. Interviewed by *The Spectator* magazine in 2010, author Michael Moorcock recalled obtaining LSD' on prescription from the London pharmacists John Bell & Croyden, although under what circumstances a doctor would prescribe LSD were not explained.

While Timothy Leary, the maverick academic, became the media-savvy poster boy of the psychedelic revolution with his Californian sun-bleached good looks and iconic catchphrase, 'Turn On, Tune In and Drop Out', it was actually a bunch of English ex-pats living in the America who laid the groundwork for Leary's fame and notoriety.

As LSD trials were underway in the Sandoz laboratories, there was interest in other plant-derived hallucinogenic drugs. Experiments followed the same principle that maybe these drugs could mimic psychosis and that to understand a condition such as schizophrenia, it would help to replicate something of the patient's experience which accounts for some psychiatrists trying these drugs out on themselves. Humphrey Osmond, an English émigré working in Canada, was interested in mescaline, the active ingredient of the peyote cactus first synthesised in 1919 for a possible study into schizophrenia. In 1953, his friend Aldous Huxley, who had emigrated to the USA in 1937, piqued Osmond's interest in using mescaline not just for trying to unlock the secrets of a serious mental health condition, but also to perhaps expose an alternative reality to the one which Huxley believed was the product of rampant materialism. In May 1953, Osmond gave Huxley some mescaline to try resulting the following year in the publication of Huxley's ground zero text of the counter-cultural revolution, *The Doors of Perception*, the title inspired by William Blake's observation that, 'if the doors of perception were cleansed, everything will appear to man as it is, infinite'. But as overwhelmed as he was by the experience, Huxley did perceive a problem that he conveyed to Osmond who, stuck for a categorisation of the LSD experience, coined the term 'psychedelic' combining two Ancient Greek words for 'mind' and 'clear'.[4] The problem was that the experience could leave you like a rabbit in the headlights, just endlessly staring into space trying to make sense of it all, to the detriment of getting on with life.

Notwithstanding his misgivings, Huxley and the philosopher Gerard Heard, another US-based British ex-pat, began spreading the word among their friends about mescaline-derived consciousness-raising. Huxley's book produced mixed reactions, especially among theologists who objected to the idea that an artificially induced chemical experience could in any way be compared to religious transcendentalism. One stern critic, the orientalist R. C. Zaehner, took mescaline himself, but while admitting experiencing some sort of mystical visions declared them 'a world of farcical meaninglessness'.[5]

Huxley and Heard first took LSD in 1955 and were ready converts. Heard introduced the drug to Alcoholics Anonymous founder Bill Wilson, whose positive experiences resulted in developments in LSD psychotherapy tailored for those with serious alcohol problems. For his part, Huxley departed life under the influence of LSD in 1963.

Another hallucinogenic drug of psychotherapeutic interest was psilocybin derived from the *Psilocybe mexicana* mushrooms. On 13 May 1957 *Life* magazine published an article by R. Gordon Wasson documenting the use of psilocybin mushrooms in religious rites of the indigenous Mazatec people of Mexico. Wasson was a Vice-President at JP Morgan bank and an unlikely mycologist who had become fascinated with the study of ritual use of mushrooms while on honeymoon in Mexico. He went back to Mexico to conduct further study which (apparently unknown to him) was funded by a CIA front organisation using money from the MK-ULTRA budget. The *Life* magazine article introduced the wider public to the 'secret of the magic mushrooms'.

Timothy Leary had led a highly troubled life as a teenager, soldier, college student and husband. His wife committed suicide in 1955 in the wake of his multiple infidelities and their mutual alcohol abuse. Troubled past aside, in 1957, he was director of psychiatric research at the Kaiser Family Foundation while his book *The Interpersonal Diagnosis of Personality* was hailed as the 'most important work on psychotherapy of the year' by the *Annual Review of Psychology*. In 1959, he was a lecturer in clinical psychology at Harvard University where a colleague, Anthony Russo, told him of his experiments with the mushrooms on a trip to Mexico. In August 1960, Leary travelled to Cuernavaca, Mexico, with Russo and consumed psilocybin mushrooms for the first time, an experience which drastically altered the course of his life. He later claimed he learned more about psychology in the 5 hours after taking these mushrooms than in 15 years of clinical study.

Leary returned from Mexico to Harvard in 1960, and he and his associates (notably Richard Alpert, later known as Ram Dass) began a research programme known as the Harvard Psilocybin Project, analysing the effects of psilocybin initially on prisoners and then on theology students. But as time went on, Leary's Harvard colleagues became increasingly uneasy about these experiments, especially when other students not in the programme started using the mushrooms. Eventually both were fired and instead set up organisations to further their interest and growing evangelism in praise of the power of hallucinogenic drugs. The disaffected, rebellious young and wealthy often become enamoured of counter-cultural activities; heirs to the banking and industrial fortune of Andrew Mellon helped Leary acquire a rambling mansion called Millbrook, which became the headquarters for the International Federation for Internal Freedom and the Castalia Foundation. It was here that another peripatetic Brit proved critical in the propulsion of LSD into public consciousness.

It is a popular misconception that there is a homogenous entity called the 'drug scene' encompassing all those who partake of illegal drugs. This idea was plausible up to the early sixties when the UK scene was largely confined to those who frequented Soho haunts. Soon, though, there were many scenes across London – Notting Hill, Chelsea, Brixton, Hampstead and Camberwell – where the scenes overlapped. People would drift from one to the other, often located in private houses rather than clubs, which were more prone to being busted. Some were overseen by what were known colloquially as 'Faces' – intelligent, devious, usually older men, fixers who had connections to celebrities, to the young, rebellious and wealthy, to gangsters, or to all three. Often they were not the best of people, cloaked as they were in a sort of negligent charisma, gathering to themselves groups of young acolytes who were invariably treated badly but who nonetheless found these men fascinating, charming and captivating, perhaps bathing in a pool of reflected glory and vicarious experience, circling in the orbit of the deliciously dangerous.

One such person was Michael Hollingshead. Born in 1931, Hollingshead's real name was Michael Shinkfield. Although he spent time in a school for bright but troubled boys, he led a fairly conventional life, working for the travel agents Thomas Cook once he had completed his national service. He shared a London flat with the psychologist Dr John Beresford, who, as a paediatric specialist, may have come across Hollingshead in his troubled youth.

Beresford moved to New York and became Assistant Professor in Paediatrics at New York Medical College but became very interested in LSD and resigned his post in 1961 to set up the Agora Scientific Trust to investigate the effects of LSD using supplies imported from Sandoz. Hollingshead went to New York ostensibly as part of a short-lived enterprise called the British-American Institute for Cultural Exchange, which had all the hallmarks of another CIA front organisation but was drearily unexceptional apart from boasting W. H. Auden on its board. Hollingshead again moved in with John Beresford, then sampled LSD for the first time. Hollingshead phoned Aldous Huxley who had first put him onto LSD to tell him of his experience and the author suggested he might like to contact Timothy Leary who had yet to try the drug. Hollingshead appeared at Leary's apartment where the jazz trumpeter Maynard Ferguson and his wife were staying. Hollingshead produced a mayonnaise jar containing a paste mixture of distilled water, sugar and around 5,000 doses of powdered LSD. All three took a trip joined by the initially wary Leary and from then on, despite grave misgivings from his close psychedelic research friends, Leary devoted his life to acid evangelism.

However, while appreciative of the introduction to LSD, Leary was hearing all kinds of bad news about Hollingshead, one contact calling him a 'con artist', another a 'sociopath'. Hollingshead began to make himself a general nuisance around Leary and so Leary's opt out was to send Hollingshead back to the UK to be the advance guard of the acid prophet's arrival, spreading the gospel of LSD. Seeing Hollingshead off as he boarded a ship in New York, Leary commented to Alpert, 'Well, that writes off the psychedelic revolution in England for at least ten years.'[6]

Hollingshead returned to London in October 1965 and set about establishing a miniature version of Leary's Millbrook at 25 Pont Street, in fashionable Chelsea, which he named in typically overblown fashion The World Psychedelic Centre, financially backed by an Old Etonian friend, Desmond O'Brien, who made his money as a Lloyds underwriter.

Hollingshead seemed to start off with all good intentions: he was fully aware of the importance of a calm and supportive environment when taking LSD and set up the Pont Street flat with the necessarily subtle décor, furnishings, music and incense to facilitate the journey. Hollingshead's idea was to attract as many famous people to the centre as possible who might then be influential in any public debate about the law and also offer support for the continued use LSD for medical and research purposes.

The plan worked: members of the young affluent Chelsea set, such as Victoria and Julian Ormsby-Gore, and a bunch of Old Etonians, Playboy Club founder Victor Lowndes, writers William Burroughs and Alex Trocchi, film maker Roman Polansky and actress Sharon Tate, musicians Eric Clapton, Donovan and Paul McCartney all came to sample the wares.

Other LSD scenes popped up around the capital in similarly well-heeled circumstances: the Chelsea flat of antiques dealer Christopher Gibbs and a flat in Cadogan Lane, Belgravia, where Joey Mellen lived. Educated at Eton and Oxford, Mellen confounded family aspirations and instead went on a psychedelic journey which led him to the ultimate head trip: trepanning (boring a hole into the skull). He was the partner of another trepanning enthusiast, Amanda Feilding, whose aristocratic ancestors could be traced back to the Hapsburgs. Both were deeply interested in altered states of consciousness and through her Beckley Foundation, Feilding became a staunch supporter of drug law reform and psychedelic drug research.

Alex Trocchi, another one of those Faces around whom the vulnerable and gullible fluttered like moths, lived at 101 Cromwell Road, South Kensington, a crumbling Regency terrace near the West London Air Terminal linking Heathrow Airport to the centre by coach. The house became a first stop for several people coming into London looking to be part of the swinging city and also a centre for LSD use and dealing. Trocchi found fame with his 1960s novel *Cain's Book* detailing the life of a heroin user in New York, based on his own experiences in the city. He became notorious for encouraging people to try heroin as a statement of personal alienation. Although his main drug interest was heroin, he was up for trying anything, experiencing his first LSD trip in America under the supervision of the psychotherapist Oscar Janiger and had some contact with Leary and Hollingshead.

Terry Taylor, having written *Baron's Court: All Change,* moved to Tangier to write the follow-up, but instead smoked copious amounts of hashish and formed some kind of 'magic' group with local Berbers. In 1964, back in London, he carried on his interest in magic, overseeing an LSD-infused circle to include his girlfriend Detta Whybrow, who earned a living selling sex. The fascination with the drugs–magic dynamic, exploited originally by Aleister Crowley, developed its own cadre of deluded followers.

An altogether more respectable acid advocate, but no less controversial, was R. D. Laing, who become enamoured of LSD and would take doses alongside his patients like Sean Connery, gathered at his Wimpole Street practice. But unlike Sandison and others conducting LSD therapy sessions out of the spotlight, Laing (like Leary) revelled in being an outlier among his professional colleagues, shocking them with both his public statements in support of LSD and his equally well-known antipathy towards conventional psychiatry as expressed in his book *The Divided Self* (1961). Consequently, he drew into his orbit high-profile patients and enjoyed circulating among the new aristocracy of London musicians, fashion designers and photographers. Between October 1965 and into the early months of 1966, LSD was still an elitist secret until, ably assisted by lurid media reporting, the secret was out.

Unfortunately for Hollingshead, rather than a place of quiet LSD contemplation, revelation and therapy, his World Psychedelic Centre rapidly descended into an acid free-for-all with growing numbers of bodies draped everywhere, out of their skulls on LSD-laced punch. One of Hollingshead's less endearing traits was to spike the drinks of women he fancied, revealing one of the dark and contradictory sides of the sixties – the exploitation of women ('chicks') who, while clearly enjoying the freedoms allowed them by the contraceptive pill, were often expected to be willing participants in the hippie notion of 'free love' (a convenient cover for rape in some cases) and denounced as frigid if they weren't. Numbered among those away with the fairies were undercover police officers who had been keeping the place under watch following neighbour complaints about hippies playing loud music.

As Leary predicted, Hollingshead's mission to lay the groundwork for a visit from the Acid Messiah himself quickly disintegrated. In Michael's rambling and generally unreliable ghosted autobiography, *The Man Who Turned On the World*, he was, however, honest about the drug morass he sank into; he was shooting speed several times a day, smoking huge amounts of dope and dropping LSD doses in excess of 500 micrograms. He admitted, 'There was a problem, a self-indulgence of mine which earned me some social suspicion if not social ostracism, and which led me – though against all my instincts – well over that line which divides the normal from the abnormal. I refer of course, only to my taking of Methedrine.'[7]

The inevitable knock on the door came during the week beginning 14 March 1966. Hollingshead had his Methedrine on prescription so was busted on account of the cannabis he actually had in his possession, although there were quantities found all over the flat, so he was also accused of allowing his premises to be used for the smoking of cannabis. This was a recent law change which until 1964 only applied to opium specifically to target opium dens.

While the police had Pont Street under surveillance, and although it seems that some undercover officers were unwittingly 'dosed', it is hard to know how much if any intelligence they had about LSD. But legal or not, once the drug and its effects were publicised, the repercussions were entirely predictable.

The fall was precipitated by the overweening arrogance or stupidity of Hollingshead's main financial backer Desmond O'Brien. In the mid-1960s, *Tatler*, a glossy magazine of high life, fashion, the arts and celebrity interviews aimed at the middle and upper classes, was in some financial trouble and was briefly rebranded as *London Life*, a sort of upmarket *Time Out*. In November 1965, capitalising on celebrity fascination with the underworld, *London Life* ran a very innocuous feature profiling the Krays. As *London Life* staff and World Psychedelic Centre visitors moved in the same circles, eventually the magazine's editor, Mark Boxer, got to hear about LSD and sent two reporters to conduct what turned out to be a 9-hour interview over 2 days at the Hyde Park Hotel with O'Brien. Describing himself very unwisely as 'Mr LSD', he went on to explain how you could take control of the country inside 8 hours using LSD to dose the water supply of Whitehall, Buckingham Palace and a few other key establishments. He stated that 10 grams of LSD would fetch £25,000 (nearly half a million pounds today) and that there was enough of the drug being made in Britain 'to last a lifetime', but refused on both occasions to reveal anything about sources of supply. He also explained the therapeutic value of LSD but admitted that LSD use was out of control: instead of being confined to exclusive use by intellectuals and creatives he said, it was reaching 'the long-haired types and the coffee-bar sets'.

The article was published on 19 March 1966. But instead of what Hollingshead naively hoped would be a sympathetic article, it was headlined, 'LSD, the drug that could become a social menace'. The *London Evening Standard* wrote:

LSD — THE DRUG THAT COULD THREATEN LONDON

Just for kicks, some famous artists, pop stars, and debs are 'taking a trip' on LSD – one of the most powerful and dangerous drugs known to man. It produces hallucinations. It can cause temporary insanity. Kicks like this may be bought at the appalling cost of psychotic illness or even suicide. It is banned in America and elsewhere [*sic*] – but is still available in London, quite legally. Still more appalling – just half an ounce of LSD could knock out London. Socially, the stuff is dynamite. *London Life* magazine has investigated LSD fully and has uncovered a social peril of magnitude which it believes demands immediate legislation ... to stop the spread of a cult which could bring mental lethargy and chaos. *London Life* reporters have also traced the man who calls himself Mr LSD. He has given them an astonishing series of interviews. Read all about him, and about LSD, in this week's *London Life*.

Then came a double whammy. The very next day on 20 March, *The People*, a national Sunday broadsheet, but a tabloid in all but name, trumpeted:

THE MEN BEHIND LSD — THE DRUG THAT IS MENACING YOUNG LIVES....

The drug is LSD-25 – Lysergic Acid Diethylamide. It is by far the most dangerous drug ever to become easily obtainable on the black market. LSD, which is said to give 'visions of heaven and hell' is used legitimately by psychiatrists to produce carefully controlled hallucinations.

In the wrong hands, the hallucinations it produces can lead to utter irresponsibility, disregard for personal safety and suicidal tendencies. IT IS, IN FACT, A KILLER DRUG.

We have obtained evidence of 'LSD parties' being held in London. We have discovered an alarming group of people who are openly and blatantly spreading the irresponsible use of this terrible drug. These men run what they call the Psychedelic Centre.

The fact that *The People* article appeared the very next day after the *London Life* feature suggests the paper had separate strands of intelligence leading them to 'gain entrance' to what they described as a deserted house littered with needle and syringes, ampoules and pills, no doubt the detritus of Hollingshead's drug habit. As the police were already onto the centre before the press, it is likely *The People* was tipped off by the police once they had busted the place.

While Hollingshead (and some of his friends including Joey Mellen) were arrested for cannabis possession, the police were also on the lookout for LSD despite its legality. They couldn't find any and may not have known what they were looking for anyway. If they had, it would have been seized. Yet on what grounds could anybody be charged at that time for being in possession of LSD when it was not controlled under any controlled drug legislation?

Back in 1958, Dr Donald Johnson, of reefer madness fame, was the Conservative MP for Carlisle. On 11 December that year he had an exchange in the House of Commons with Conservative Home Secretary R. A. Butler. Johnson asked Butler if he was 'aware of the dangerous hallucinogenic properties of such new drugs as mescaline and lysergic acid diethylamide; and when he proposes to bring these drugs under the Dangerous Drugs Acts'. Butler replied 'Yes, Sir. I am informed that there is no evidence that these drugs are addiction-producing; it would not, therefore, be appropriate to control them under the Dangerous Drugs Act 1951.' Said Johnson, 'Is my Right Honourable Friend aware that, in spite of what he said, the first of these drugs is what one might call a somewhat fashionable drug today, owing to the unusual visual experiences which it produces, while the second is a very powerful drug which is in frequent use at psychiatric clinics and gives most unusual effects? Will he watch the use of these and related substances very closely?' Butler replied, 'I will gladly receive any information given by my Honourable Friend. These drugs could not appropriately be brought under the scope of the Pharmacy and Poisons Act, 1933, and I am not sure that to list them as poisons would not tend to draw attention to them and stimulate demand. I am doing my best to control distribution, and I shall value any information which my Honourable Friend can give me.'

By 1965, however, LSD, mescaline and psilocybin were included in the Act that Butler mentioned, but because the Act was passed before LSD was invented, when the first actual prosecution for LSD took place the law appeared to be very grey indeed. The poet John Esam had the dubious honour of being the first person in the UK to be arrested on an LSD charge. Esam had been one of the organisers of the International Poetry Incarnation held at the Royal Albert Hall in 1965 where a packed audience heard readings from the illuminati of the radical poetry world including Beat icons Allen Ginsberg, Lawrence Ferlinghetti and Gregory Corso.

Esam was another resident of 101 Cromwell Road. Following surveillance and a tip-off that Esam was dealing LSD from the flat, on 21 February 1966, the police burst in. Esam tried throwing LSD-laced sugar cubes out of the window, only for them to be caught by a waiting policeman. As he wasn't a chemist, Esam was charged with conspiring to sell the 'poison' LSD and another powerful hallucinogen, DMT, in contravention of the poisons legislation.

However, the prosecution came up against a problem of definition because the Dangerous Drugs Act only referred to the alkaloids and homologues and there was a legal dispute over what those terms actually meant, whether lysergide was a homologue of lysergamide and whether lysergamide occurs naturally in ergot. Esam faced two trials with experts disagreeing as to whether LSD came under the technical definition of a poison or not. The prosecution expert at the second trial in January 1967 was none other than Albert Hofmann, who argued that LSD could be regarded as a poison. Eventually it was left to the jury, who found Esam not guilty. But some people did fall foul of what was probably a charge of doubtful legality. In May 1966, freelance photographer Roger Lewis didn't fight the charge and was fined £25 for being in possession of thirteen sugar cubes soaked in LSD.

In terms of cannabis possession, Hollingshead was only caught with very small amounts, but made the huge mistake of taking LSD before he went into court, defended himself and joked all the way through the proceedings. In May 1966, he ended up in Wormwood Scrubs serving a 21-month sentence, which might have been a hardly less draconian 15 months had he not played the joker. His prison visitors included Richard Alpert and the legendary American underground LSD chemist Augustus Owsley Stanley, who provided Hollingshead with a supply of hash and LSD. In his book, Hollingshead claimed he turned fellow inmate George Blake on to LSD, before the spy escaped to Russia having served 5 years of his 42-year sentence. After a few months, Hollingshead was sent to Leyhill Open Prison and on release wandered around the world trying unsuccessfully to establish himself as a writer, ending up in Bolivia where he died of natural causes in July 1984.

The revelations of a doomsday drug which could wreck young lives and paralyse the country saw *The Sun* (10 June 1966) demand in an editorial that 'A loophole in the law affecting the hallucination drug LSD should be closed quickly. The dangerous effects of LSD when it is improperly used have only recently been realised. As a result, it is now an offence in Britain to buy or sell it without a doctor's prescription. But it is not an offence to import it or possess it.' The editorial and the article in *The People* (which also included reporting about the London drug scene generally) were used to highlight the view that the drug situation was symptomatic of a country going to the dogs. On 20 February 1966, *The People* reported that one of its intrepid investigators had perpetrated a buy/bust scam involving a dealer who was selling morphine and heroin and raking in several thousand pounds a week. *The Sun* editorial continued, 'The Ministry of Health and the Government are approaching the whole problem of drug addiction in too lenient a way.'

So, faced with a very public LSD scandal, the government moved quickly. On 4 and 5 August 1966, parliamentarians in the House of Lords and the House of Commons respectively debated the Drugs (Prevention of Misuse) Act 1964 Modification Order 1966, which banned possession without a prescription, banned imports except under licence and required manufacturers (turning imported LSD into medicinal products) to register with the Home Office. By April 1966, thirty-one UK companies, mainly chemists and drug manufacturing companies, had licences to import without specifying reasons. This was changed so that the reason for importation had to be specified such that by January 1967 only Brocades GB had the necessary licence.

In presenting the Bill, reference was made to yet another article, this one in *The Times* which reported on increasing recreational use of LSD with stories of people flying out of windows (in the Lords debate, Lord Stonham suggested that he had known those who thought they could fly after four pints of beer) and an editorial in the *British Medical Journal* (18 June 1966) which recommended some level of control similar to that for amphetamines. The Order was passed and from 9 September 1966, a month before the USA, LSD possession was banned in the UK.

Meanwhile, the London underground scene had completely outgrown the pioneers. The packed gathering at the Albert Hall in 1965 had been the first public outcropping of a nascent counterculture and while it gave free rein to the surrealistic and the avant-garde, it still had links to a more culturally acceptable heritage of poetry and literature. What happened in music was more revolutionary and would have a more lasting impact.

Up until The Beatles released *Revolver* in August 1966, the top British pop bands including The Rolling Stones, The Animals, The Yardbirds and The Beatles themselves took their repertoire and inspiration largely from black American blues and R&B. For The Beatles, *Revolver* marked a huge leap forward in creativity and an aesthetic derived now more from their drug experiences and their growing interest in eastern religion, most obviously on Lennon's 'Tomorrow Never Knows'. John Lennon and George Harrison's first LSD experiences were spiked drinks at the home of a London dentist: the drug had a profound effect on Lennon, who became a regular tripper. The very first line of the song is a straight lift from Timothy Leary's book *The Psychedelic Experience*: 'Turn off your mind, relax and float downstream'.

The impact of LSD on The Beatles played out on different levels. Firstly, they were celebrities, constantly in the public eye, and with more wealth than they could possibly have imagined growing up in the suburbs of Liverpool. They had given up live performances in August 1966 – screaming teenagers and the general chaos that followed them around made playing concerts pointless. In tune with other members of the new aristocracy of the young, rich and famous, they felt a certain shallow emptiness as the glitter wore off the glamour. One effect of LSD (and cannabis) is to promote a stillness, allowing time for reflection as time itself appears to stretch. Into that space new ways of thinking emerged and for George Harrison in particular, a search for a more spiritual existence. Arguably too, the effects of the drugs brought to the surface a surge of nostalgia that was firmly embedded not in Americana, but in a romantic view of a very British past. All of these feelings outcropped in *Sergeant Pepper's Lonely Hearts Club Band*, which rewrote the book on popular songwriting and the sonic possibilities of the studio, as George Martin recreated those psychedelic experiences on vinyl.

As we shall see, the police and the media were all over pop stars as the latest iteration of the Pied Piper, so it was a brave decision by Paul McCartney to confirm in a TV interview filmed in his back garden and broadcast on 19 June 1967 that he had tried LSD 'about four times'. McCartney had first revealed this in *Queen* magazine. The quote was reprinted in *Life* magazine on 16 June in which he said, 'After I took it (LSD), it opened my eyes. We only use one-tenth of our brain. Just think what we could accomplish if we could only tap that hidden part. It would mean a whole new world.' The TV interviewer questioned the wisdom of McCartney's on-air admission, to which McCartney replied that he had been asked a question about LSD and he just answered honestly and if they were going to broadcast the interview on network TV, then the company was far more culpable of spreading this information than he was.

The publicity given to McCartney's revelation – the first pop star to admit taking LSD, and a loveable mop top at that – plus all the speculation about the inspiration for 'Lucy in the Sky with Diamonds' saw LSD reach wider British consciousness. The music business very quickly adopted all the trappings of psychedelia, flower power and the hippy revolution; from the dreamy incomprehension of 'A Whiter Shade of Pale' to the Graham Bond Organisation playing the same R&B – 'psycho-dalek music' as Bond dubbed it – but wearing funny shirts. Probably the band most associated with the meeting point of mainstream pop and the underground was named after two bluesmen whose records Syd Barrett had in his collection: Pink Anderson and Floyd Council.

Music producer Joe Boyd and John 'Hoppy' Hopkins, one of the scene's iconic figures, collaborated in December 1966 to open the UFO in the vast basement of the Blarney Club in Tottenham Court Road. The club was the first of the psychedelic dungeons which sprang up around the West End in the following months – an externalised LSD experience with bands, light shows, films on different walls and an audience that was mostly on Planet Zog. Pink Floyd was the house band, moving very rapidly from R&B cover mode to something very different, driven by Syd's love affair with LSD.

Syd Barrett's acid lyrics looked to outer space with 'Astronomy Domine' and 'Interstellar Overdrive', both on their debut album *The Piper at the Gates of Dawn* but also to inner space – a pastoral world in harmony with nature and populated by childhood fantasies and fables. Their debut album was named after chapter seven of *The Wind in the Willows*, while many of Barrett's songs captured a sense of wistful idyll like 'The Scarecrow', 'See Emily Play' and 'Bike' (complete with a homeless mouse and gingerbread men).

There was much talk of LSD opening people's eyes to the world as it 'really was', as if the true nature of the world had been hitherto hidden from public gaze. But everybody knew how the world really was: baby-boomers' parents had fought and died fighting Nazism; the Cold War brought the threat of nuclear annihilation, which during the 1962 Cuban Missile Crisis seemed far more than just a threat; Kennedy was murdered in 1963; and the case of John Profumo signalled the beginning of the end of the age of deference. So, the visions of LSD did not reveal the present nor were its users in tune with the future – Harold Wilson's aspiration of a nation basking in 'the white heat of technology'. Instead they tuned out into a childlike Arcadian yearning for a past painted in the LSD primary colours of the nursery. The Doors of Perception were the Doors of the Wardrobe to Narnia. Youth fashions revisited a bygone era with boutiques such as I Was Lord Kitchener's Valet and Granny Takes A Trip selling fantasy Edwardian-style dandified clothes to men while the women floated around in pre-Raphaelite finery.

The sights and sounds of LSD drifting through the days of summer in 1967 were a unique if fleeting moment in British culture. For a while, there was a broad church of feeling among thousands of young people in London that change was possible, that there was a route back to a simpler life. For all the later (and often justified) criticisms of the period, the ecology movement grew out of these desires and quickly expressed very real concerns about global warming and the general state of the planet. And like it or not, it was the drug culture that helped focus the mind towards these more weighty and spiritual matters, probably the only period in British drug history before or since where altered states of consciousness delivered more than just idle moments of intoxication. But the hopes and aspirations were very short-lived. Reality quickly kicked in.

One reality was that LSD was not a drug to be trifled with. Thousands of people took thousands of trips emerging unscathed having enjoyed the hallucinogenic experience, and some genuinely felt they had undergone a life-changing experience even if it only extended to swapping a job in the City for a yurt in Wales.

But conversely, and while it is impossible to cite evidence, it is likely that the press played its part in subjecting acid novices to bad trips by creating fear and trepidation through sensational reporting. One of the most widely reported LSD horror stories of the period concerned not one but two sets of American students allegedly going blind by looking at the sun while tripping on acid. The first report appeared in the *Los Angeles Times on* 18 May 1967:

> Four college students have suffered permanent impairment of vision as a result of staring at the sun while under the influence of LSD, according to a spokesman for the Santa Barbara Ophthalmological Society. One of the youths told his doctor he was 'holding a religious conversation with the sun.' Another said he had gazed at the sun 'to produce unusual visual displays.' The students, all males, suffered damage to the retina, the sensory membrane which receives the image formed by the lens. In the same way that a piece of paper will burn when bright light is beamed through a magnifying glass, a pinhead-size hole was burned into the retina of each eye of the students as sunlight passed through the lens. What this has left the students with is not total blindness but a blind spot in the center of their vision. As a result, the victims have lost their reading vision completely and forever, the ophthalmological spokesman said.

As the fact-checking site snopes.com pointed out, nobody was named in this story at all, and apparently readers were asked to believe that four students, none of whom apparently knew each other but were from the same Santa Barbara college, all looked at the sun on the same day while they were all separately on LSD.

Then about eight months later, this story hit the wires. This is an Associated Press dispatch as it appeared in the *Los Angeles Times* on 13 January 1968:

> Six college men suffered total and permanent blindness by staring at the sun while under the influence of the drug LSD, it was learned Friday. The six, all juniors at a western Pennsylvania college that officials decline to name, lost their sight after they took the hallucinatory drug together last spring. Norman M. Yoder, commissioner of the Office of the Blind in the Pennsylvania State Welfare Department, said the retinal areas of the youths' eyes were destroyed.

The story was presented as breaking news: it actually referred to an incident that supposedly happened in April 1966. Except it didn't happen at all.

Five days after the story 'broke', Dr Yoder, blinded himself as a child due to an accident, admitted he had made the whole thing up because of his 'concern over illegal LSD use by children'. Who planted the hoax *LA Times* story remains a mystery – and few, if any, corrections were published.

Another major LSD story claimed that the drug caused chromosome breakage which would result in deformed babies. The government's Advisory Committee on Drug Dependence on amphetamines and LSD report published in 1970 detailed some evidence of chromosomal damage in mice and fruit flies but failed to find any evidence of any damage in humans. But never allowing the facts to get in the way of a good story, the press gleefully reported pregnant LSD users could end up with deformed babies.

Several stories also claimed that people had fallen out of windows believing they could fly. None of these stories could be substantiated, although it was perfectly feasible that under the influence of any drug, including alcohol, an accident of this type could occur. There were occasional murder cases where the perpetrator had supposedly unwittingly killed somebody while under the influence of LSD.

One such UK case received national coverage in 1967. On 17 September Claudie Delbarre, an 18-year-old variously described as an au pair, model, club hostess and prostitute, was discovered by her landlord in her bedsit in Walpole Street, Chelsea, with serious head injuries and a length of sheeting stuffed in her mouth. As the investigation unfolded it became clear that Claudie had a string of boyfriends, sugar daddies and clients. For the press, the link between Chelsea as the hub of 'Swinging London', a murdered good-time girl and rich clients was enticing enough. Then it was revealed that the main suspect, Robert Lipman, the son of a rich American property developer and a heavy drug user and drinker, had been extradited from the States to face a murder charge claiming he was under the influence of LSD. The case eventually came to court in October 1968. Bobby Lipman said he had met Claudie at a flat in Chelsea the previous day, and went back to her flat at 4.15 a.m. They both took a trip. He said in court,

> I felt myself speeding through space and I felt the earth opening and I went right down to it, into the centre of the earth, and found myself in a den of monster snakes which I was fighting off and battling with. They were [a] huge prehistoric type, scaly and with fire shooting from their mouth [*sic*]. I felt I was fighting for my life. I am not sure how I dealt with the fire coming from their mouths.

Lipman claimed that when he came down from the trip, he saw that Claudie was dead and could not understand how or why. He left the flat immediately and was seen running down Walpole Street. He returned to the hotel he was staying at in Knightsbridge, gathered some things together, settled his bill, checked out and flew out of Heathrow back to the States.

Lipman's solicitor, David Napley (who later defended Jeremy Thorpe in the Norman Scott case), both at the time and in his memoir believed not only was his client innocent of murder, but even manslaughter, based simply on his intoxication. Did he really expect Lipman to walk free? If he did, he was disappointed; the jury cleared Lipman of murder, but as Lipman knowingly took a dangerous drug, he was found guilty of manslaughter and sentenced to 6 years in jail.

Writing about the case on 29 June 2008, on the Crime Time website, Anthony Frewin raised some serious doubts about Lipman's account of what happened. If Lipman was randomly thrashing about trying to ward off snakes, this doesn't quite square with Claudie being battered and suffocated with a sheet. Lipman also stated he arrived at Claudie's flat at 4.15 a.m. and left at 7.30 a.m. perfectly able and lucid enough to affect a normal-looking getaway without rousing suspicion. Did he really take LSD at all?[8]

Finally, there were those well-publicised cases like Syd Barrett and Fleetwood Mac's Peter Green – and presumably many undocumented examples of those who took a trip too many and never really came back down to earth. However, more than any other drug, LSD has generated a stock of urban myths. For several years, the organisations I worked for received reports on genuine-looking police force-headed press releases that LSD-laced tattoos were doing the rounds of UK schools – each one a hoax.

***

As the case against Lipman was being played out in court, a deep malaise had infused itself within the counterculture as violence, riots and assassinations took the place of peace and love.

Richard Neville was an Australian who started a satirical magazine called *Oz* with fellow Australian Martin Sharp, a graphic designer whose most famous artwork was the fluorescent-coloured cover of Cream's album *Disraeli Gears*. They brought the magazine to London where its main rival was *International Times*, which shortened the title to *IT* after barely credible legal threats from the publishers of *The Times*. *IT* was launched in October 1966 at a party where guests were handed LSD-laced sugar cubes like canapes at a cocktail party. The newspaper was in general terms a forerunner of *Time Out*, giving the London underground community information about events while at the same time publishing articles about underground politics, music and the other creative arts. *Oz* took its inspiration more from *Private Eye* and from early on took a less reverential view of the counterculture. Neville and Sharp created a character called Mervyn Limp, 'a bank clerk, who visits Indica [bookshop], reads *IT*, tries a joint ("are you *sure* it's trendy?") and is instantly transformed into Frisco Ferlinghetti, the beat poet, "happening" artist, underground film maker and space cadet who gets himself trepanned and hitchhikes to Kathmandu where he finds nirvana and dies of dysentery'.

Despite Neville's emblematic status as the ultimate countercultural rebel, prosecuted in August 1971 under the Obscene Publications Act[9] along with others for publishing the Schoolkids issue of *Oz*,[10] he was never wholly committed to the acid-driven alternative society. By November 1970 in issue 31 of the magazine and in the wake of the Manson Family's murderous spree, the violence at the Altamont music festival, political assassinations, student riots, the gun-toting rhetoric of the Yippies (radicalised hippies) and the deaths of Brian Jones, Jimi Hendrix and Janis Joplin, he gave expression to the disillusionment and disappointment at the demise of the hippy dream,

> The flower child that *Oz* urged readers to plant back in '67 has grown up into Bernadine Dohrn [leader of the American terrorist group The Weather Underground]; for Timothy Leary, happiness is a warm gun. Charles Manson soars to the top of the pops and everyone hip is making war and loving it ... It was tempting if naïve to hope that with the intake of Id-liberating rock, lateralising dope, the emerging group tenderness, communal living style and an intuitive political radicalism that from all this a qualitative change in the conduct of human relationships might develop.

He railed against 'lengthy endorsements of acid's ability to transform shits into (revolutionary) saints' and 'Yippie heavies [like Abbie Hoffman] drooling enthusiastically over Leary's fiftieth birthday present, a gun.' Neville documented that while hippies were supposed to be against the 'bread heads' who thought only of money, there were just as many bread heads in the underground as in the City of London. A good example was the benefit concert at Alexandra Palace held in December 1967 to raise money for *IT* after the offices were raided. Of the £4,000 worth of tickets sold, only a quarter of that found its way to the *IT* bust fund; Neville's view that many of those involved on the scene were 'dope dealers with the morals of the marketplace'. Which takes us on the last stages of the journey from Laboratory to Love-In to Cash-In.

* * *

Until the passing of the Misuse of Drugs Act in 1971, which came into force in 1973, LSD was not controlled under the Dangerous Drugs Act 1965, which was little changed from the Act of 1951. Instead, like amphetamines, it was controlled under the Drugs (Prevention of Misuse) Act 1964 as modified in 1965 to include LSD, mescaline and psilocybin. LSD was also included in the poisons legislation although, as we have seen, there was some dispute as to whether LSD counted as such. The penalties of the 1964 Act were less severe than those in the 1965 Act, meaning LSD and amphetamine were regarded as less dangerous than cannabis. But in neither Act was there any mention of illicit manufacture, the assumption being that either drugs found their way onto the streets through factory, pharmacy thefts or diverted from legitimate prescriptions or, like cannabis, imported from abroad. Under the 1964 Act, there were penalties for anybody involved in importing or distributing drugs or being in unauthorised possession which constituted the 1966 ban. Because the drug was legal and because the British authorities had no intelligence on unauthorised distribution, the first major UK distributor of LSD for non-medical purposes went entirely unnoticed.

Michael Charles Druce worked as a clerk in London merchant offices and became a chemical broker. From this he gained a knowledge of LSD, got to know Leary's financial backer, William Mellon Hitchcock, and began supplying LSD to the USA using LSD purchased from the Czech state-owned company Chamapol via their London trading office Exico. Chamapol were the main suppliers of LSD in Europe once the Sandoz patent had expired. Druce also sold his LSD through London, Oxford and the Home Counties, purchasing some 9 kilos of LSD from Exico in the period 1964–65. Druce pulled out of the UK business in 1966 but kept on exporting LSD to the States and became a very important supplier once the underground chemist Augustus Owsley was busted and out of the picture. Owsley's supply of the basic precursor chemical ergotamine tartrate was running out and his successor chemists Grateful Dead engineer Tim Scully and Nick Sand had great difficulty obtaining new supplies from Europe. The only use for the chemical was to make LSD, so the US Bureau of Narcotics and Dangerous Drugs (forerunner of the Drug Enforcement Administration or DEA) was keeping a close watch on any shipments coming into the country. Druce's LSD was reimported back into the UK in various formulations.[11] The 1970 report on LSD from the Advisory Committee on Drug Dependence stated that 'the evidence suggests that the illegal market in LSD in this country is supplied by illegal manufacture. Clandestine laboratories manufacturing the substance have been discovered here, but probable the bulk of it is smuggled from the USA. We were told that users preferred the American LSD and regarded the English product as inferior.' Little did they or the users know that much of that LSD came from the UK in the first place.

In November 1967 and acting on intelligence, police uncovered the UK's first LSD laboratory. One of Detta Whybrow's clients, Victor James Kapur, was a chemist. She persuaded (or possibly blackmailed) Kapur into cooking up LSD for use in Terry Taylor's magic circle, but the chemist quickly realised he could seriously cash in.

In August 1967, Alexander Davidson was arrested at Heathrow trying to smuggle LSD to the USA. Police learned that the drug had been made in a lab based in north London and quickly identified the key suspect as Victor Kapur. They set up a surveillance operation and finally arrested Kapur and another associate, Harry Nathan, in a West End pub after Kapur had handed over about 19 grams of powdered LSD in a condom, enough for nearly 100,000 strong doses. Ten others were arrested and two laboratories discovered, one in the back of Kapur's pharmacy shop and another in a rented garage. Detta Whybrow was among those arrested and as the investigation unfolded, she emerged as a key player in the operation, selling Kapur's product on to street-level dealers, although the police had no direct evidence of her involvement. Following a paper trail, the police found that Kapur had been sourcing his base chemicals from Germany and had been active from around the time that Druce dropped out of the market, making some 15 million doses from September 1966 to the time of his arrest.

The case came to trial in May 1968. At that point, there was still no law specifically outlawing the illegal manufacture of LSD, so Kapur was charged with multiple offences under the Drug (Prevention of Misuse) Act 1964, which added up to a 9-year sentence. The man he was arrested with, antiques dealer Harry Nathan, named by the police as a main distributor, also received a hefty 7-year sentence. Detta Whybrow however got off with

2 years' probation and there was some suspicion that she had done a deal with the police. There was an interesting sidebar to this story.

In his book about the Krays, John Pearson writes about Nathan's son-in-law Alan Bruce Cooper who it was claimed was strong-armed by the US Bureau of Narcotic Drugs to try to persuade the twins to get into drug trafficking, which they declined to do. Cooper was known to be manufacturing and distributing LSD and this was used as leverage by the Bureau. In July 1968, Cooper gave evidence in court against the Krays while at the same time denying he had given the police any information about Harry Nathan's involvement with Kapur. But in his autobiography, Detective Chief Superintendent Leonard 'Nipper' Read, whose Metropolitan Police murder squad officers arrested the Krays, painted a picture of Cooper strongly suggesting that he, and not Nathan, was the major LSD distributor of Kapur's products, making Nathan a very minor player who did not deserve a 7-year stretch.[12]

Earlier that year, a Hungarian student chemist named Kalniczky and his associate, Davies, were caught running an LSD factory in the East End. They told the police they obtained their chemical from industrial chemist Malcolm Sinclair, who was also exporting chemicals for ultimate LSD manufacture to the States with the help of Ken Lee, who had contacts there. Another key figure was a club owner John Conway, whose phone calls with Sinclair were intercepted. On the strength of what they heard, the police arrested both men, but the case collapsed because being in possession of the base chemicals was not an offence, unlike LSD itself of which the police found no trace. LSD investigations were especially tricky for the police – even finding a lab with all the equipment and precursor chemicals was not enough to secure a conviction. The drug itself was very easy to hide and officers could just as easily touch minute quantities left behind – enough for an exciting trip to never-never land, as the drug was equally active absorbed through the skin.

Irrespective of how much LSD might have been in circulation in the UK up to 1970, it paled into insignificance compared with the activities of two chemists working in Wales and London whose product came closest to turning on the world. The story of Operation Julie has been covered from all possible angles in an array of books, book chapters, articles and a TV mini-series. It became the most famous UK drug operation of all time. The headline numbers of the story are that between 1970 and the final bust in 1977, Richard Kemp and Henry Todd produced around 30 million doses of LSD which, according to police estimates, accounted for about 90 per cent of all the LSD in circulation in the UK during that period; even more astonishingly, it represented between 40 and 60 per cent of all the global demand for the drug. On the morning of 26 March 1977, 800 detectives raided nearly 90 addresses and arrested 120 people. The 15 key defendants appeared in the dock and between them landed a total 120 years in prison. Despite exhaustive searching across continents, only about 10 per cent of the estimated £10 million proceeds were ever recovered as the money trail revealed a tangled global web of bank accounts and financial portfolios into which cash could easily disappear.

From the police point of view, it was a landmark operation involving officers from 11 forces working together in a hand-picked squad of the type never before seen in British policing, engaged in long-term undercover work, phone tapping and 24-hour surveillance operations.

Of all the tales told and retold about Operation Julie, three key points emerge. Firstly, this was probably the last throw of the dice for LSD as a counter-cultural force. While most of those involved were just in it for the money, Kemp and his girlfriend, Dr Christine Bott, genuinely believed in the power of LSD to bring about a change in societal attitudes, to recalibrate the world away from rampant materialism and the careless attitude to the state of the planet. Secondly, there was no hint during the whole of the investigation that there was any violence associated with this highly lucrative venture in stark contrast to what was to follow in the decades ahead on UK streets. Thirdly was the disappointment that followed for Operation Julie leader Detective Inspector Dick Lee and his closest colleagues. Lee had seriously hoped that the success of Julie would pave the way for national drugs squads along the lines of the US DEA. But his pleas fell on deaf ears; the squad was broken up and returned to mundane policing duties, while DI Lee and others quit the force in disgust.

In a way, Lee should not have been that surprised at the complete indifference to his viewpoint. Back in 1974 as head of the Thames Valley Drug Squad and so responsible for policing the early rock festivals, he knew there was far more demand for LSD than the meagre official police seizure records showed. Lee took his concerns to the Central Drugs Intelligence Unit (CDIU). The CDIU was based at Scotland Yard and was supposed to be collating and circulating relevant drug intelligence, not just to the Metropolitan Police but to all the forces around the country. The CDIU said there was no intelligence about widespread LSD distribution. It transpired they were being less than honest: while they were supposed to be a nationwide support unit, they owed all their allegiance to the Metropolitan Police who in turn were highly uncooperative from the start, regarding drugs as their patch and any officers from outside London as 'swedes'. The CDIU even went out of its way to discourage police in Wales from cooperating with Dick Lee. Eventually it took the intervention of Britain's most powerful policemen, both high up in the Association of Chief Police Officers and backed by Bing Spear at the Home Office, to finally clear the way for Operation Julie to get underway. In the end, rather than back the idea of a national police force, the attitude of those managing the individual Julie officers was in effect, 'Play time is over. You've had your fun. Now get back to ordinary policing.' The drug remained a favourite of those attending the Free Festivals of the early 1980s and among members of the Peace Convoy travelling between the festivals.

In the end, maybe because it was a drug of individual introspection reaching for an unobtainable nirvana and known to carry very real dangers, that for all the talk of LSD providing the road map to an alternative society, it was never the focus for drug reform campaigning or wider political and social protest. The story of cannabis in the UK was very different.

6

Pot, Politics and Pilchards

At the outbreak of the Second World War, the League of Nations collapsed, to be replaced in 1946 by the United Nations. America emerged from the war as a world superpower and was therefore the dominant force in the new configuration of nations, no more so than when it came to international drug control. During the interwar years, having walked out of the 1925 Geneva Convention talks and refused to sign the 1936 Convention because they failed to secure criminalisation of all non-medical production and distribution, the Americans had been largely side-lined. Now they were back in their full prohibitionist glory led by none other than Harry Anslinger. Still the head of the US Federal Bureau of Narcotics, he was also the USA's prime mover in its attempt to construct one overarching prohibitionist-inspired convention that would bring together all existing international legislation covering opium-based drugs, the more recently developed synthetic opioids, cocaine and cannabis.

Although the bureaucratic structures of international drug control had changed, much of the politics remained the same insofar as the USA and UK were still the key players in the new landscape, backed by nations sympathetic either to the British or American approach. From the earliest post-war days when work on what became the Single Convention on Narcotic Drugs began, Anslinger and an inner core of equally messianic officials had their sights set on nothing less than the total eradication of all the main plant-based controlled drugs. The Americans harboured a fundamentalist self-interested belief that the only way to deal with the homeland drug problem was not just harsh domestic law enforcement, but to stop any of these drugs being produced anywhere in the world for any purpose. The main stumbling block between the British and the Americans in the early years of the century had been British economic colonial interests regarding opium and cannabis production, mainly in India. Those colonial interests no longer applied but now, in the interests of domestic pharmaceutical and medical interests, the British were not going to be pressured into accepting invasive international regulations. On the other hand, the British again did not want to appear uncooperative in the yet-to-be-named 'war against drugs'. In the end, and after a decade of bureaucratic and diplomatic wrangling, the Single Convention on Narcotic Drugs 1961 actually represented a victory for British-inspired regulation and control over the worst excesses of American anti-drug zeal. However, compromises needed to be negotiated and the easiest ground to cede for Britain and other like-minded nations was over Anslinger's desire to bring cannabis into the Single Convention, thereby sending the message that the international community viewed cannabis to be just as dangerous as heroin or cocaine, with the intention that every signatory should introduce harsh penalties for supply and possession.

As Bureau chief, Anslinger had pretty much written the playbook on the evils of cannabis, or 'Indian Hemp' as it was called in most official UK documents. However, his efforts to translate that into international law were not without much initial disagreement over the real dangers of the drug, its medical value and the problem of trying to enforce laws against a drug embedded in the rituals and customs of countries like India. Moreover, cannabis grew like weeds everywhere; it was not an agricultural crop like opium whose yield could be easily monitored and cultivation bans enforced. Anslinger was even having to face down unpalatable medical evidence in his own backyard.

In a largely forgotten small study, back in June 1931, at the request of the Commanding General of the US-owned Panama Canal Zone, a committee was designated to investigate the effect of marijuana on military personnel, with a view to securing additional evidence that might possibly be used as a basis for regulations forbidding the cultivation, possession, or sale of marijuana in the Canal Zone. The Governor designated members to serve on the committee from Health and the Army and Navy Medical Corps. The committee agreed that the best method of securing reliable information would be to hospitalise soldiers (thirty-four in the end) who were known marijuana smokers, allow them to use it, withdraw the drug and then have a psychiatrist observe what happens. They used cannabis grown in the Zone which was a described as 'a mild stimulant and intoxicant' and not addictive. The psychiatrist reported back that he failed to observe any mental or physical deterioration from smoking marijuana. This was the first, albeit small-scale, US study to challenge what became later in the 1930s Anslinger's reefer madness narrative.

Far more threatening to his world view were the results of a 5-year study of cannabis use in New York prepared by the New York Academy of Medicine on behalf of a commission appointed by Mayor Fiorello LaGuardia, a feisty, charismatic character whose achievements in his three-term reign as a left-leaning Republican marked him out as one of America's greatest local officials. Among the report's conclusions were that smoking cannabis does not lead to addiction of itself nor is it a gateway to morphine, heroin or cocaine; is not a major factor in determining crime; is not associated with juvenile delinquency; nor is used widely used by schoolchildren. The killer punchline was that all the publicity (much of it generated by Anslinger's office) about the catastrophic effects of cannabis was unfounded.

Anslinger was not impressed. He slated this first extensive and objective study of cannabis in America undertaken by no less a body than the

New York Academy of Medicine as 'unscientific' and at the very first meeting of the newly formed Commission on Narcotic Drugs (CND) called their views 'extremely dangerous'.[1] The continuing calls from CND delegates for new evidence about cannabis prior to coming to a decision had little to do with honouring the evidence base and everything to do with finding as much incriminating evidence as possible. The baton was passed to the World Health Organisation (WHO) to come up with a definitive statement on the mental and physical effects of cannabis. The WHO obliged with a report written by Pablo Osvaldo Wolff, a former secretary of the WHO's drug addiction committee, entitled *Marijuana in Latin America: The Threat It Constitutes* and presented to the CND in 1955, which relied heavily on newspaper articles about the dire effects of the drug where the scientific evidence failed to deliver the necessary goods.

In his 1971 book *The Marijuana Smokers*, American sociologist Eric Goode offered this analysis of Wolff's book: 'Rather than a study, it is another enumeration of crimes supposedly caused by marijuana, along with extravagant declarations as to marijuana's baleful effect.' Goode quoted Wolff: 'With every reason, marihuana ... has been closely associated since the most remote time with insanity, with crime, with violence, and with brutality', and further noted,

> Again one searches in vain for a systematic analysis of the criminogenic effect of this supposedly deadly drug. Instead, we are greeted with a barrage of rumor, distortions, blatant falsehoods, and dogmatic assertions. Although we have been assured by Anslinger in the foreword that the author is 'impartial', and the monograph, 'painstaking ... erudite, well-documented ... comprehensive ... accurate ... extensive ... well-rounded ... convincing' we are perplexed by the bombastic and otiose language which casts considerable doubt on its author as a reliable, impartial observer. We are assured that 'this weed ... changes thousands of persons into nothing more than human scum,' and that 'this vice ... should be suppressed at any cost.' Marijuana is labelled 'weed of the brutal crime and of the burning hell', an 'exterminating demon which is now attacking our country'; users are referred to as 'addicts' (passim) whose 'motive belongs to a strain which is pure viciousness.'[2]

As Anslinger wrote the foreword to the book, in turn endorsed by the French CND Chair Charles Vaille, that pretty much sealed the fate of cannabis as a drug with no therapeutic value, and as there were no commercial interests involved there was no substantive argument about cannabis after 1955. If anybody was left in any doubt that scientific and clinical evidence played little part in international control decisions over cannabis, Charles Vaille told a 1973 CND meeting, 'The question of the relative harmfulness of different varieties of cannabis, of taking the drug in large or small doses etc., was doubtless of theoretical and clinical interest and WHO should certainly continue its investigations along those lines, *but such investigations should not be allowed to influence international control measures in any way whatsoever* [author's italics].'[3]

There has been an over-interpretation of the Convention: there was no obligation on Parties to imprison people for possession of any of the drugs listed. Article 36 required Parties to adopt measures against 'cultivation, production, manufacture, extraction, preparation, possession, offering, offering for sale, distribution, purchase, sale, delivery on any terms whatsoever, brokerage, dispatch, dispatch in transit, transport, importation and exportation of drugs contrary to the provisions of this Convention', as well as '[i]ntentional participation in, conspiracy to commit and attempts to commit, any of such offences, and preparatory acts and financial operations in connexion with the offences referred to in this article'. Article 36 did not directly require criminalisation of all the above; it stated only in the cases of (unspecified) serious offences that they 'shall be liable to adequate punishment particularly by imprisonment or other penalties of deprivation of liberty'.

A 1971 amendment to the Article granted nations the discretion to substitute 'treatment, education, after-care, rehabilitation and social reintegration' for criminal penalties if the offender is a drug 'abuser'. A loophole in the Single Convention is that it requires Parties to place anti-drug laws on the books, but does not clearly mandate their enforcement, except in the case of drug cultivation.

***

Throughout the 1950s, cannabis use in the UK was confined to immigrant groups living in major cities, especially port cities like Liverpool and London where there was also a community of itinerant sailors. In London, of course the drug found favour with the usual coterie of Soho outliers. Apart from the flurry of interest generated by Donald Johnson's book, the media did not seem to think cannabis was a serious medical problem in itself, rather a moral issue as it apparently encouraged that always vicariously thrilling notion of white girls mixing with black men, a view typically expressed by *The Times* of 15 July 1957. The headline was 'Haunts of the Reefer: Hemp is Britain's biggest drug problem', but the article by the paper's unnamed 'special correspondent' informed readers that while there were plenty of seizures to report around the country and that cannabis trafficking was obviously a crime, 'the problem ... is not one of addiction' and suggested that depriving a hemp smoker of his drug was at best no worse that depriving a smoker of his tobacco. The writer's main concern was that use would spread more widely to the white community coupled with the 'moral danger' that young white girls might find themselves in, 'which is the greatest concern to the authorities'.

Regarding the medical authorities, a government committee was convened in June 1958 and chaired by the neurologist Sir Russell Brain, recently retired president of the Royal College of Physicians, to review the workings of addiction treatment since Rolleston. However, not until October 1959 did this first Brain Committee consider cannabis in the wider discussion of how 'addicts' in general were identified. In their deliberations and final report, they concluded that while there was cannabis use among immigrant groups, this was simply part of their 'normal way of life' and while use might pose a social problem (and was incidentally decided to be without any therapeutic value) they found no evidence of medical problems and in particular no evidence that cannabis was addictive in the sense they understood addiction to heroin or morphine. As far as the committee was concerned, this was simply a matter for the Home Office and the police and there was nothing in their terms of reference that demanded they make any recommendations about cannabis.

Nor did the police think it worth allocating extra resources to deal with cannabis in addition to everyday duties. The attitude of the police to the cannabis issue infuriated the one agency that did seem bothered, the Home Office, and one official in particular, Bing Spear. In 1960, he wrote a detailed internal memo on the cannabis situation in the UK since 1950. In the early part of the decade, cannabis was mainly arriving into UK ports either direct from the growing regions of south-east Asia, particularly Burma, Ceylon or from transit countries such as Cyprus. It was assumed that most of the importation would be used by the growing numbers of immigrants from the West Indies, India and Pakistan. But as the decade wore on, signs emerged that the rise in the number and quantity of seizures and the discovery of cannabis in both leaf and resin form coming through the post and inside flight passenger luggage suggested use of the drug was spreading beyond those immigrant groups as shown by the testimonies of Raymond Thorp, Terry Taylor and numerous first-hand accounts of the Soho jazz scene of the period. The data suggested, again as Thorp indicated, that the trade was quite well organised albeit in absolute numbers still serving a relatively limited clientele. Bing was even able to confirm the existence of Thorp's 'Mr Smith', the white cannabis trafficker who imported his cannabis from Ceylon.

The main thrust of Bing's memo was to establish that the cannabis trade was increasingly significant in terms of the numbers of seizures and the quantity of each one. He cited a number of individual cases of seizures and prosecutions, one on the largest being the seizure of around 80 kilos of cannabis from the merchant ship *Worcestershire* at Tilbury Docks in April 1957. The Metropolitan Police Drug Squad had passed information to the Port of London Authority police who found 200 blocks of compressed cannabis hidden in the engine room ventilator shaft. Police in Liverpool had been tipped off that four men from the city had gone to London to take delivery of the consignment. When they were eventually picked up with some of the ship's crew, all denied any knowledge of the cannabis, but the police were able to charge two of the men with cannabis possession, which earned them both a prison sentence. This and other similar cases demonstrated to Bing that there was an organised distribution network for cannabis across the UK taking in not only London and Liverpool, but Glasgow, Swansea, Birmingham, Manchester, Nottingham and other cities. What irked Bing in all of this was that the number of convictions was not rising to correspond with the growing evidence of (relatively) large-scale dealing. Using his own information sources, he had no confidence in any of the official police statistics and, for example, was incredulous that given the presence of a significant immigrant population in Bradford and Leeds, the police there did not record a single cannabis conviction.

Eventually in 1957, a note was sent to the Chief Constables' Conference making the very point that while recent months had seen some large cannabis seizures, it was surprising that convictions had been falling steadily since 1954. The note suggested that rather than waiting for tip-offs, 'there may be some justification for taking more direct measures to gain information about the movement and use of the drug'.

Following their meeting, the Chief Constables replied,

> ...members ... did not accept that the recent increase in the quantity of cannabis seized indicated a growth in use of the drug. It might reflect a keener vigilance of the ports. Nor did a decline in the number of prosecutions necessarily mean that police measures were less effective. The police had not relaxed their efforts ... If these large amounts had been seized on ships, it could not be agreed that the circulation of the drug within the United Kingdom had increased.

Musing on this response, Bing concluded that 'the Chief Constables disposed of this item with the minimum of thought and preparation. For this reason alone their views are worthless.' He also remarked that the Chief Constable of Liverpool asked where all these seizures had been made, apparently with no knowledge that in 1957 there has been 18 seizures in his own city totalling nearly 100 kilos.

Bing worked in the Home Office Drugs Branch where the subject was front and centre of every working day, so it was not surprising that he was critical of those he saw as not being concerned as he was about drug problems. There were very few specialist drugs police officers; the Metropolitan Police Drug Squad, the first in the country, had only come into existence in 1954. Bing did buy into the gateway theory, but he reserved some of his deeper concerns at what he saw as the growing use of the drug among young white people. He wrote, 'In recent years, persons have been found in possession of the drug at such unlikely places – unlikely in view of the absence of any appreciable coloured population – as ... Oxford, Cambridge.' What these places had in abundance, though, were students.

* * *

While music, drugs and fashion gave 'the sixties' its most public expression, arguably it was post-war government education policies which ultimately helped create the environment for alterative and counter-cultural blossoms to bloom, a shifting in society's tectonic plates opening up an even wider fissure between the generations which in turn the Establishment would find so threatening. The 1944 Education Act introduced by R. A. Butler, Minister for Education under Winston Churchill, aimed to reconcile the huge disparity between the choices open to working-class children as opposed to those higher up the social scale. In the pre-war period working-class children often left school at 13 as they were needed to boost family income. The day-to-day financial struggles of poorer people were somewhat ameliorated by the creation of the Welfare State and the NHS, which helped relieve some of the pressures forcing children prematurely out of school. Those who devised the Education Act were looking not only to keep children in school longer – to 15 – but also introduce them to subjects such as music, art and literature. The school-leaving age was raised and, importantly, fees for state secondary education were abolished (but many grammar schools charged for entry). Local authorities were now obliged to provide free school meals and milk, which again helped the children from poorer families for whom school dinners might be the main meal of the day. The main beneficiaries of the Act in terms of access to higher education though were middle-class children; surveys showed the more literate the parents, the better the child performed in school.

The Conservative government then turned its attention to higher education. The Robbins Report recommended the immediate expansion of universities. York and East Anglia Universities were established in 1963 while the incoming Labour government in 1964 continued the expansion and development of the so-called 'plate glass universities' with Essex, Kent, Lancaster, Sussex and Warwick opening their doors. Following on from the Robbins Report, the government also introduced a means-tested grant system enabling not just the public school elite to go to university, although certainly the Oxbridge colleges continued to draw heavily on the privately educated.

Then there were the Art Schools. Interviewed by Jonathan Green for his book on the English cultural underground movement in the 1960s *Days in the Life*, graphic designer Pearce Marchbank believed that these institutions were crucibles for the counterculture:

> If you want to try and find somewhere from which you could say the whole sixties culture comes from, it was the art schools. Art schools in the sixties really were the laboratories that were making rock musicians and designers and painters, they were the real universities of the sixties. Hundreds of rock stars started off as art students; Lennon, Townsend, Clapton … The thing was that you were bombarded with a lot more than just the set syllabus. You had this thing called Liberal Studies and the people who taught were often very interesting. A. S. Byatt used to teach me literature.

Others interviewed by Green concurred: 'The art-school scene was the key to young bohemia,' said one. 'Art school – that's where it all came from' said another.[4] The point about art schools was that they were locally based and served as entry points into higher education for working- and lower-middle-class kids; the ones who didn't want a 9–5 job, but might not have been right for, or had no interest in, the university academic life.

Taken together, these developments in education policy paved the way for more young people to go to university and college to be exposed to radical philosophies, politics, literature, music and drugs they might never have come across going from school to work. The expansion of universities in the 1960s also gave young people, both boys and girls, the chance to escape from home – and the prying eyes and ears of parents – something previously only national service or marriage would have permitted.

Like the white Jewish jazz musicians who felt an affinity with the new immigrants, the middle-class rebellious teenager felt a similar affinity with those who society treated with disdain because they were different, which for some also read across to left-wing politics and its cries on behalf of the struggling and oppressed working classes. Hugely attractive too was the music, the snappy dressing and the general 'coolness' of West Indian men to young people still smothered in Beige Britain. The cannabis leaf became the cultural logo representing rebellion, affinity with the black community, a political statement for the 1960s, the lightning rod of sixties protest in default of our own US-style civil rights and anti-war movements as the Campaign for Nuclear Disarmament (CND) had lost momentum by the mid-sixties and British youth were not being sent to fight a needless war in a far-distant land.

A portent of the generational clash over cannabis came on 12 March 1962 with the raid on the Peace Café in the Fulham Road, south-west London. The café was owned by Dr Rachel Pinney, a pioneer in therapy for autism, an ardent peace activist and CND supporter. The Peace Café was an unofficial local headquarters for CND supporters. The police raided the café and arrested the café manager and some employees on charges of possession of cannabis and opium, and allowing the premises to be used for the smoking of opium. There were a couple of young people living upstairs from the café who did experiment with opium smoking, but there was no evidence presented in court as reported by *The Times* (26 March and 4 April 1962) that the place was a regular haunt of cannabis smokers who, as CND supporters, would have been mostly white and middle class. Despite lack of any hard evidence, the prosecution claimed that 'drugs [were] being administered to young people who supported that [CND] campaign and congregated there', as if the café clientele were somehow passive recipients of drugs like hospital patients. Sentencing the café manager, the magistrate described the café as 'a den of absolute iniquity and debauchery'. The extravagant language suggests that the magistrate and prosecuting counsel were as much outraged by the very existence of an anti-establishment, anti-nuclear movement of young people acting to undermine the defence of the realm as they were about drug use. The case came to trial barely six months before the world was brought the brink of annihilation by the Cuban Missile Crisis of October 1962.

A Metropolitan Police report dated 1961 gave the police view of the emerging young white cannabis consumer who, in fact, had been present in Soho since the end of the war: 'Of the white users of the drug they are mainly in their late teens or early twenties and are of the type frequenting the jazz clubs and coffee bars of the West End where this activity is mainly confined. There are signs however, of it spreading to whites of similar tendencies in Brixton, Kensington, Chelsea, Paddington and Notting Hill area.' In his Home Office memo of the previous year, Bing Spear cited a number of cannabis possession cases which played to the public image of the young white drug user – the drug itself being immaterial – usually either unemployed or in very low-skilled jobs and not very bright, making Godfrey Glubb appear out of the ordinary. The 20-year-old son of Major General Glubb was convicted of cannabis possession in April 1960. Glubb had run away from Wellington public school to become a student in the 1960s at the School of Oriental and African Studies, part of London University.[5]

The year 1964 was significant for UK cannabis history – the year the Single Convention came into force and in December, a new amendment to the UK drug laws making it an offence to allow premises to be used for the smoking of cannabis to align cannabis with the existing law relating to opium. This had nothing to do with the Single Convention, rather a response to the rise in the number of police raids in both clubs and some student accommodation where packets of cannabis would be thrown on the floor so that individuals could not be charged with possession. The premises' owners had an 'absolute' liability, meaning they were guilty of the offence which carried a prison term, whether they knew about the drug use or not. As originally conceived, it was unlikely that somebody would set up an opium den and then not know what was going on, but this did not necessarily apply to cannabis. The more significant development which would eventually get the attention of politicians, was that for the first time, there were more white cannabis offenders, 284, than non-white, 260. By 1967, those figures were 1,737 and 656 respectively: the public image of the typical drug user as some low-life immigrant criminal was seriously challenged by a scandal emerging from inside our most prestigious hall of learning.

Born and raised in Chicago, Steve Abrams was an Advanced Student in Parapsychology at St Catherine's College, Oxford, from 1960 to 1967, heading the parapsychology laboratory of the university's Biometry department. He had a written a sensible and balanced overview of cannabis intended as a chapter in a book called *The Book of Grass* edited by cannabis activists George Andrews and Simon Vinkenoog. The article found its way to the *Sunday People*, which published it without permission on 29 January 1967 under the headline 'Drug Sensation at Oxford'. Alongside his general information on the drug, Steve had also conducted a piece of informal qualitative research to find out about cannabis use among the students. He wrote:

I live in Oxford where there are several hundred undergraduates and an increasing number of Dons on the 'pot scene'. The observations I have been able to make are probably biased in various ways, and I accept that their validity may be called into question. But I am obliged to report what I have seen and the conclusions I have drawn in the hope that they may, in a modest way, assist in the determination of public policy and the planning of properly controlled experimental research...

It is very difficult to estimate the number of members of the University who make use of cannabis. At one time I kept a list which grew to 257 names before I decided that it would be prudent to destroy the list in fairness to my informants. I am continuously surprised by meeting someone for the first time at a party, a university society or a coffee house and learning that he smokes cannabis and does so with a group whose existence had previously been unknown to me. *Without any claim to accuracy I should think that there are at least 500 junior members of the University who smoke cannabis when it is available. In addition, the drug is now being used by a few dozen of the younger Dons, though it has not yet been smoked in the Senior Common Rooms* [emphasis added]. Some of these Dons were undergraduates when cannabis was introduced to Oxford, but others have been 'turned on' by their students. Some of the older and more eminent Dons have also experimented with cannabis. Most of these Dons are people who have taken LSD, mescaline or other hallucinogens and regard cannabis as a comparatively innocuous drug to be taken out of curiosity or to find out whether it is safe for one's students.

The University vehemently denied any such goings-on, with rebuttals published in *The Times* and *The Daily Telegraph*. Even so, the University Commission on Student Health quickly convened to discuss Steve's findings and accepted that cannabis smoking took place, but in its report published on 3 April pointed out that there were cannabis smokers in several universities. Prior to publication on 28 February, the Vice-Chancellor of Oxford wrote to Home Secretary Roy Jenkins urging that the government undertake a review of the drug situation in the UK, but one that was based on science and not prejudice. However, the exposé of student drug use at Oxford was immediately overtaken by an even more explosive drug scandal.

In his article, Steve Abrams wrote,

Undergraduates introduced the large-scale use of cannabis to Oxford in the autumn of 1963, about the time that pop music, pop art and pop culture became a country-wide intellectual fad. The standards set by the leading pop groups are not merely sartorial. This is an open secret, as should be obvious from the names of some of the groups, and the titles and words of many of their songs.

***

These days, revelations of drug use by rock and pop musicians hardly raise an eyebrow, although perceptions have changed insofar as more recent deaths such as Michael Jackson, Prince and George Michael have been associated with prescription medication often supplied by doctors rather than illegal drug dealers and so to that extent addiction has gained a more respectable and excusable veneer. Back in the 1960s the idea that the nation's favourite pop stars, surrounded by screaming teenage girls, used drugs was generally not known. And it was not known to the fans nor, equally importantly, to their parents who were stumping up the pocket money for the records, because the industry PR machine kept it that way. By 1966, though, the atmosphere was beginning to change, and media focus began to shift. As Decca PR boss Tony Calder observed,

As the sixties developed, the national newspapers which had taken rock and roll to the front pages became more and more interested in rock stars ... they'd spent years being utilised by people like [the Stones PR man] Andrew Oldham to build up their artists, now they were interested in trying to bring them down ... It was an open secret among music and entertainment journalists that musicians were using drugs, but now there was a more concerted attempt to try and find some printable evidence.[6]

The main rivals here were the experts in Sunday breakfast sleaze, the *News of the World* and the *Sunday People*. The latter had a scoop exposing a football match-fixing operation. The *News of the World* set up an investigative team including a journalist pinched from the *People* who had not only scored with the football story, but also obtained scoops concerning both the Profumo Affair and the Great Train Robbery. So long as you looked the part, gaining access to pop parties was not difficult as people drifted in and out of these events unnoticed. The *News of the World* had form on drugs, having previously gone into overdrive about Mods and amphetamine and the antics of London's various self-appointed kings of acid. The team might have been on the ball exposing soccer players taking backhanders and clerics with their trousers down, but they knew little about drugs, an ignorance cruelly exposed when having wandered lonely as a cloud around UFO, one breathless reporter from *News of the World* claimed he saw 'couples injecting reefers'.[7]

On 29 January 1967, not coincidentally one suspects, the same day that their rival published the story about drug use at Oxford, the *News of the World* started a series headlined 'Pop Stars: Facts That Will Shock You'. The first instalment zeroed in on Donovan, who in July 1966 became the first pop star to be prosecuted for drugs and fined £250 for possession of cannabis. Donovan did himself no favours by openly smoking dope for a documentary (*A Boy Called Donovan*) screened the previous January. The raid was conducted by the officer who became notorious for deciding that, in true Anslinger-style, busting musicians for drugs would be top of his hit list, although given the level of corruption in the Metropolitan Police at the time, this was more to do with publicity seeking and downright envy than moral outrage.

Norbert Clement 'Nobby' Pilcher brought with him into the Metropolitan Police Drug Squad the off-radar and often unorthodox practices of his previous posting in the Flying Squad. The squad was set up in 1918 as an elite mobile force who would go out and about on the lookout for criminal activity. A major success was the capture of 17 of the Great Train Robbers in 1963. In order to achieve some of its spectacular results, it often sailed very close to the line and crossed it more than once. The Flying Squad relied heavily on paid informants; transferring that to the Drug Squad meant working with drug dealers, some of whom became in effect 'licensed', allowed to operate in exchange for information. According to the authors of *The Fall of Scotland Yard* corruption exposé, dealers not in the loop might be set up to be arrested. Pilcher's mentor in the Flying Squad was Vic Kelaher who would later take over the Drug Squad. In the spirit of the times, both would eventually do time for falsifying evidence in a drug case.

There was a knock of Donovan's rented flat and a troop of policemen barged in. The singer was arrested for possession of cannabis, although Donovan later claimed the hash he and his girlfriend were smoking was all gone by the time the police burst in. Donovan's manager and his wife were raided the same night and similarly charged. They were all taken to Marylebone Police Station and as they were let out at 4 a.m., Pilcher asked Donovan for an autograph for his daughter. Pilcher would go on to nab Brian Jones, John Lennon, Yoko Ono and George Harrison in a blaze of media glory, first tipping-off the press that the raids were going down. He missed Eric Clapton, warned in advance apparently by a police contact of Cream drummer Ginger Baker, as Pilcher and company raided Clapton's Chelsea flat. Lennon immortalised Pilcher in 'I Am the Walrus', referring to him as a 'semolina pilchard'. It must have irked the fishy copper to miss out on the most highly publicised pop star drug bust ever.

In preparation for the second instalment of their pop star scoop published on 5 February, the *News of the World* reporters cornered Brian Jones at Blaise's, a celebrity hangout in the basement of the Imperial Hotel in London. Jones babbled on about drug-related stuff which the journalists duly reported. However, these clueless media hounds thought they were talking to Mick Jagger, who was away in Italy at the time. Incensed to read all about his drug use, Jagger hit the paper with a suit for libel. The bosses knew they didn't have a leg to stand on and faced paying out thousands in damages, so they resolved to find a way of crippling Jagger's chances of winning. Eventually, through an informer who was never formally identified, the paper discovered the Stones were having a gathering at Keith Richards' country home Redlands, West Wittering, Sussex, with a very good chance that a smorgasbord of drugs would be there for the seizing. The paper's editor-in-chief approached the Drug Squad headed by John Lynch, who said he wanted nothing to do with it on the grounds that if he arrested Mick Jagger for smoking cannabis, every kid in the country would want to experiment and his job was to try and keep a lid on the drug problem not fan the flames.[8] There may also have been a territorial issue as the West Sussex police would not take kindly to the Met turning up on their patch for a high-profile drug bust.

What happened next went down in rock history; suffice to say, and leaving aside fake news about Mars Bars, Keith Richards was arrested for allowing his premises to be used for smoking cannabis, Mick Jagger for possession of four amphetamine tablets and art dealer Robert Fraser for possession of heroin tablets. Richards fell foul of the cannabis premises law whose absolute liability element was eventually overturned consequent on the outcome of a far less famous case involving Stephanie Sweet. A student teacher at the time, she rented out a farmhouse and was charged under the premises law when police conducted a drugs raid and found cannabis, about which Ms Sweet knew nothing. The case was taken up by parliamentarians and the press as grossly unfair and the conviction was finally quashed by the House of Lords in 1969.

Keith Richards of course had no such defence and despite Jagger saying his drugs had been prescribed by a doctor, on 29 June, the jury found them both guilty having considered the case thoroughly for all of 5 minutes. Responding to the sentences of 12 months in jail for Richards and 3 months for Jagger, *Times* editor William Rees-Mogg penned his famous editorial, 'Who Breaks a Butterfly on a Wheel?' (1 July), the title taken from a satirical poem by Alexander Pope which translated into modern parlance means using a hammer to crack a nut. Rees-Mogg's key point was the judgement on Jagger focused not on the offence which at worst only warranted a fine, but on the accused; a celebrity much admired by young people who was supposedly setting a bad example and posing an existential threat to the nation's youth. However, Rees-Mogg had nothing to say about Keith Richards' ridiculous first-offence sentence of a year in prison.

The initial articles by the *News of the World* resulted in demonstrations outside their offices where an ex-public schoolgirl teamed up with a lawyer to start an organisation to help the increasing number of (mainly white) young people in trouble with the law for the first time in their lives having been caught with cannabis but with no idea of their rights. Caroline Coon was first made aware of the injustice of what was unfolding when she attended the trial of her Jamaican boyfriend who was jailed for 3½ half years for possessing 3 grams of cannabis (but incidentally only 9 months for the gun).[9] Together, with financial assistance from George Harrison, and lawyer Rufus Harris, Caroline Coon set up Release, a 24-hour emergency legal helpline which through many iterations and ups and downs is nevertheless still going and is now the UK's longest-running drugs charity.

The drama around the Rolling Stones, the protest outside the *News of the World* offices, the release on 1 June of the drug-drenched Beatles album *Sergeant Pepper's* and the 'Legalise Pot' rally held in Hyde Park on 16 July all contributed to raising the issue of drug use by young people and whether the drug laws were proportionate. A government committee addressed the issue led by its chair, criminologist and sociologist Baroness Barbara Wootton, which laid the groundwork for the primary legislation under which drugs are still governed in the UK today.

As political concerns about drug use were growing, the government established the Advisory Committee on Drug Dependence in 1966 chaired by Sir Edward Wayne from Glasgow University, who in turn formed sub-committees to consider specific issues. The Sub-Committee on Hallucinogens to investigate both cannabis and LSD started work on 7 April 1967.

According to an unpublished paper by Steve Abrams, the committee began by restricting its discussion to the psychopharmacology of both drugs.[10] Back in February, Abrams had founded the Soma Research Association (SOMA) whose mission was to campaign for the funding to be made available to undertake all the necessary research into the effects of cannabis, research which was being inhibited because of the law. With the convening of the Wootton committee, Abrams saw a chance to influence its deliberations by persuading it firstly to consider cannabis alone, not alongside LSD, and then to widen its brief to go beyond simply the science of cannabis to consider the social aspects of cannabis use and to make specific recommendations for law reform.

Abrams had seen an article in *The Marijuana Papers* in which Allen Ginsberg had suggested an advert in the *New York Times* to be signed by 500 people. In 1966, *The Times* had devoted four pages to an advert appealing for peace in Vietnam: 'I thought if *The Times* will print that, they'll print anything.'[11] A plan was hatched to place a full-page advert in *The Times* which Paul McCartney agreed to pay for, probably because it would deflect attention away from the Beatles and their declared use of LSD and also align the Beatles with more respectable if radical views about drugs. Steve approached those Wootton committee members he judged most sympathetic to the cause of reform, Dr Nicholas Malleson from London University and psychologist Michael Schofield. After some rewrites, both agreed to sign the advert.

Published on 24 July, the advert drew its force from the list of signatories including Graham Greene, Nobel Prize Winner Dr Francis Crick and a host of celebrities including David Dimbleby, R. D. Laing, Jonathan Miller, all four Beatles with their MBEs, and two MPs. The (incorrect) assumption that SOMA's aim was complete legalisation came from the large bold heading which announced, 'The law against marijuana is immoral in principle and unworkable in practice.' The signatories wanted the government to allow all research into cannabis, legalise possession or reduce down to a fine of no more than £10 for a first offence, allow smoking on private premises and commute sentences for all those convicted of possession or allowing smoking on private premises.

Four days later, on 28 July, the advert was the subject of a House of Commons Adjournment Debate proposed by Paul Channon. He delivered a very balanced speech, but most significantly called into question the appropriateness of the law on cannabis as it currently stood under the 1965 Dangerous Drugs Act and how it was impacting on otherwise 'normal' respectable young people (for which read essentially the white middle class):

The argument [about cannabis laws] has come to a head in recent months because there is no doubt that the number of young people smoking cannabis has increased. It was also brought to a head by an advertisement in *The Times* this week in which it was alleged by many distinguished people, including medical people, that the law against cannabis at the moment is 'immoral in principle and unworkable in practice'.

With the latter half of that statement I am beginning to agree. I think that the law is becoming increasingly unworkable in practice. I do not know whether the House realises how many respectable young people indulge in the practice. I am not talking about the lower strata, the people who are so distressed that they have no other form of relief than marijuana. I fear that there are large numbers of respectable people with good jobs, or students, who are taking the drugs, and they represent an intelligent section of our society. For them, repression is not enough. They must be convinced as well as repressed, if repression is the right step.

I want to make it clear that I do not come here today to ask for cannabis to be legalised. What I want is that the evidence should be obtained on which a balanced judgment can be formed, and then we shall know where the truth lies, because people must be convinced at the end of the day one way or the other. I hope that this is a meaningful research project – I think it is – and that at the end of the day people will be able to decide one way or the other.

May I put a point for consideration by the Government: do they consider it essential for marijuana to be on the same list under the Dangerous Drugs

Act 1965 as the more dangerous drugs, such as heroin and the hard drugs? At the moment it is possible to receive a sentence of ten years' imprisonment for being in possession of cannabis. It is precisely the same sentence as that for heroin, and yet I cannot believe that any Honourable Member does not draw a big distinction between those two categories … I have also been informed … that there have been several cases – I can think of two – in which, for the first offence of being in possession of the drug, people have been sentenced to imprisonment of up to a year. Does the House think that wise?'

In response, Minister of State Alice Bacon had little of value to say other than pulling a figure out of the air that 97 per cent of those known to the Home Office as heroin users had started on cannabis; to compare Paul McCartney unfavourably with Lulu who had gone public with her anti-drug views, but also that the sub-committee would take on board the wide variety of views about cannabis.

On 31 July, the sentences on Keith Richards and Mick Jagger were quashed and reduced to conditional discharges respectively, which in Richards' case was remarkable as he had no means to argue against the charge as cannabis had been found on premises he owned, so the move must be regarded as political rather than judicial.

As signatories to the advert, Malleson and Schofield were the most vociferous in trying to persuade their committee colleagues to consider cannabis issues more broadly. Barbara Wootton did take some persuading, but despite some hard-line protests, she agreed.

Although the UK cannabis law was 40 years old, this was the first time there had been an evidence-based consideration of the health effects of the drug since the Indian Hemp Commission Report. Paragraph 29 of Baroness Wootton's final report cited that very study and LaGuardia from 1944 in concluding that 'the long-term consumption of cannabis in moderate doses has no harmful effects'. Paragraph 67 dismissed the 'reefer madness' narrative: 'There is no evidence that this activity is causing violent crime or aggressive anti-social behavior or is producing in otherwise normal people condition of dependence or psychosis, requiring medical treatment.' Paragraph 51 dispensed with the evidence for the 'gateway effect' to heroin concluding, 'It can be clearly argued that on the world picture, cannabis use does not lead to heroin.' Nor could they find any specific evidence relating to the gateway effect in the UK that would justify retaining undue 'control over this drug'.

Having brushed aside the myths about the worst effect of cannabis, they arrived at the nub of the matter – what to do about the law. They began their discussion with a consideration of the prospect for outright legalisation. They concluded it was not practicable 'in the near future' (SOMA came to a similar view), but did concede 'we do not entirely discount the possibility that properly organized research may one day produce information which could justify further consideration of the practical problems of legalization'. (Para 72.)

Given all the scientific and clinical evidence they had reviewed and the evidence of all the witnesses who presented, the committee concluded it was not tenable for cannabis to be treated as if it were as dangerous as heroin and that the penalties for possession and supply were 'altogether too high'. The report recommended there should be a distinction made between different drugs on the basis of evidence-based harm; that nobody should go to prison for possessing small amounts of cannabis and that overall penalties for cannabis offences should be significantly reduced. This hardly seems groundbreaking now but given existing laws made no differentiation between drugs, and the subject was so highly charged, the notion was radical even though the recommendations for penalty change relating to cannabis were quite modest. Under the 1965 Dangerous Drugs Act, the maximum penalties in a magistrate's court for possession, sale or supply were a £250 fine and/ or a year in prison. If the case went before a judge and jury, this escalated on conviction to £1,000 fine and/or 10 years in prison. The Wootton Report recommended that the maximum fine and prison should be reduced to £100 and/or 4 months and an unlimited fine and/or 2 years respectively. In practice, if heard before a magistrate's court nobody would go to prison for a minor possession offence because under the Criminal Justice Act 1968, sentences of less than 6 months would automatically be suspended.

Finalised in June 1968, the report was submitted to Home Secretary James Callaghan in November. He was not legally obligated to publish it and might have squashed it but for threats of resignation from the committee, revealed in the *London Evening News* shortly after the report was handed in. There were several newspaper articles trying to second guess the contents of the report while at the Conservative Party conference in October 1968, Shadow Home Secretary Quintin Hogg commented rather confusingly on the summer's pro-cannabis activities saying he was 'profoundly shocked' by those who wanted to change the law: 'I must frankly describe the arguments in favour of an alteration to the law in this respect as casuistic, confused, sophisticated and immature. Of course, we must make no mistake about this; it is all or nothing. There is no halfway house in this matter. There can be no encouraging the drug up to a point. You either sell it over the counter or you prohibit it altogether.'[12] Even before the report was officially published, Callaghan was saying that he would take much convincing about changing the law. When the report was finally published on 8 January 1969, the tabloid headlines reflected both the views of some senior politicians and the predictable editorial line of the papers:

'Row looms over plea for pot' *Daily Mirror*
'Storm over pot smokers charter' *Daily Express*
'Clash over soft line on drug taking' *Daily Mail*

Press reports were overwhelmingly hostile with the exception of the *Daily Telegraph*, while the *British Medical Journal* (supporting a law change) and *The Lancet* (against) took polar opposite views.

Before the Commons debated the report on 27 January, Callaghan had already made his view publicly known in answering a request put to him by Arthur Blenkinsop MP on 23 January to make a statement about the report and give the House an assurance that 'he does not accept the recommendation of the … Committee that the present maximum penalties for possession and supply of the drug [cannabis] are altogether too high'.

In reply Callaghan said he thought MPs should read the report and that it did contain lots of useful information, but,

> On the other hand, I cannot reconcile the view expressed by the main Committee that the wider use of cannabis should not be encouraged with the proposal that legislation should be brought in to reduce the existing penalties for use. Nor has the Advisory Committee made any forecast of the consequences of such legislation. But, in our opinion, to reduce the penalties for possession, sale or supply of cannabis would be bound to lead people to think that the Government take a less than serious view of the effects of drug-taking.
>
> That is not so. It would be entirely contrary to Government policy to allow this impression to spread, nor would such a view accord with the resolution of the United Nations Commission on Narcotic Drugs, which the Government accepted last year, recommending that all countries concerned increase their efforts to eradicate the abuse and illicit traffic in cannabis. Accordingly, it is not the Government's intention to legislate to reduce existing penalties.

When the report was debated in the Commons four days later in the full knowledge that both the press and politicians were clearly against reform Callaghan launched a scathing attack saying,

> I think that it came as a surprise, if not a shock, to most people, when that notorious advertisement appeared in *The Times* in 1967, to find that there is a lobby in favour of legalising cannabis. The House should recognise that this lobby exists, and my reading of the Report is that the Wootton Sub-Committee was over-influenced by this lobby. I had the … impression … that it was compromise at the end; that those who were in favour of legalising 'pot' were all the time pushing the other members of the Committee back, so that eventually these remarkable conclusions emerged that it would be wrong to legalise it but that the penalties should be reduced. The existence of this lobby is something that the House and public opinion should take into account and be ready to combat, as I am. It is another aspect of the so-called permissive society, and I am glad if my decision has enabled the House to call a halt in the advancing tide of so-called permissiveness.

The reference to 'permissiveness' revealed the real issue here was not cannabis *per se* rather drug use as symbolic of what was going 'wrong' in society. Callaghan was drawing a red line on taking a more liberal stance on the issue of reform not least because the next General Election was looming. There was a sense among many politicians, media commentators and religious and moral campaigners that social reform had gone too far and that while young people might need protecting (for example, Mary Whitehouse and the Clean Up TV pressure group), they were also becoming more of a threat to the social order. Taking a moral stand on drugs was an easy win for any politician guaranteed to gain the support of parliamentarians, press and the public at large.

There was a raft of social reforming legislation beginning in 1959 with the Obscene Publications Act, which although much later would be used to try and prosecute (largely unsuccessfully) pro-drug literature of the 'how to grow cannabis' type, meant that publishers could escape conviction if a work was deemed in court to be of sufficient literary merit. This new law saved the publishers of *Lady Chatterley's Lover* at the end of the famous trial of 1960. That same year saw the passing of the Betting and Gaming Act, which legalised high street betting shops; previously gambling on horses and dogs was only allowed at the track. In 1961, oral contraceptives were available on prescription on the NHS, which was a major step forward in allowing women more control over their own sexual lives. The first laws against racial discrimination in 1965 made it illegal to refuse housing, employment, or public services to a person on the grounds of colour, race, ethnic or national origins. Hanging was abolished in Great Britain (but not in Northern Ireland until 1973). In 1967, the laws on abortion and homosexuality were relaxed and theatre censorship abolished in 1968. Reform of the divorce laws and the introduction of an Equal Pay Act would come in 1969 and 1970 respectively.

In the face of this plethora of social reforming legislation from both Conservative and Labour governments, the only exception was drugs; amphetamines were controlled in 1964 along with the cannabis premises legislation; LSD in 1966 and new regulations on GP prescribing of controlled drugs in 1968 (*see* next chapter). Moreover, concerns about 'permissiveness' were certainly dialled up over Mod/Rocker violence, the rise of hippies and the counterculture, student sit-ins and the confrontation outside the American Embassy over Vietnam in 1968.

In his book *The Drugtakers*, published in 1971, sociologist Jock Young shone a light on the lives and attitudes of cannabis smokers living in Notting Hill and the way the media deliberately amplified deviance to the level of creating moral panic. Writing about the media in *Drugs and Society*, he said,

the mass media portrayal of the drug taker is not a function of random ignorance but a coherent part of a consensual mythology ... The myth of the drug taker is rooted in moral indignation; it supports the hypothetical world of the normal citizen; it blinkers the audience to deviant realities outside the consensus; it spells out justice for the righteous and punishment for the wicked. Although much of its world view is fantasy, its effects are real enough. By creating moral panics over drug use, it contributes enormously to public hostility to the drug taker and precludes any rational approach or solution to the problem. It also provides a bevy of convenient scapegoats onto whom ... moral discontent can be directed.[13]

The following year, Stan Cohen published his book about the creation of Mods and Rockers as 'folk devils'. Cohen defined a moral panic as those moments in history when, a condition, an episode, a person or group of persons emerges to become defined as a threat to societal values and interests; its nature is presented in a stylised and stereotypical fashion by the mass media; the moral barricades are manned by editors, politicians, bishops and other right-thinking people; socially accredited experts pronounce their diagnoses and solutions; ways of coping are evolved (or more often) resorted to; the condition then disappears, submerges or deteriorates. Sometimes the object of the panic is quite novel and other times it is something which has been in existence long enough, but suddenly appears in the limelight.[14]

So, did these societal constructs push politicians to ditch the Wootton Report? Quite the contrary: the report laid the foundation for the Misuse of Drugs Act 1971.

On 1 February 1970, *The Sunday Mirror* published the unlikely news that Callaghan had done a U-turn: 'Drug Law Shock. Jim changes his mind. Penalties for pot; smokers to be cut'. Did he really change his mind? No. Secretary of State Richard Crossman kept a set of diaries during his time in office and about cannabis law he wrote that Callaghan came to the cabinet with the proposal 'not to have any reduction at all in any penalties on cannabis'. A row ensued and it was put to a vote. Significantly, 'every member of the Cabinet who had been to university voted one way and everyone else voted the other way'. Callaghan lost the vote.

Callaghan published his Misuse of Drugs Bill, which set out the now familiar A-B-C classification of drugs on the basis of relative harms; differentiated between possession and possession with intent to supply; and did reduce the penalties for cannabis possession, not to the level recommended by Wootton, but lower than then existed under the Dangerous Drugs Act. Additionally, the idea of having an expert panel to advise the government on drug laws was enshrined in the legislation with the creation of the Advisory Council on the Misuse of Drugs (ACMD) to replace the Advisory Committee. However, Callaghan never got the chance to push the Bill through Parliament because Labour lost the 1970 General Election to Edward Heath's Conservatives and it was the new government who hurried the Bill through unchanged to become the Misuse of Drugs Act.

Once the Act came into force in 1973, Quintin Hogg, now Lord Hailsham, and Lord Chancellor, made a telling intervention about cannabis possession. Having been vehemently opposed to showing any leniency to cannabis smokers back in 1968, he was now urging magistrates 'not to "dive off the deep end" when confronted with cases of cannabis possession'. Users of 'soft drugs' (by implication not just cannabis) should be treated with 'becoming moderation ... Look at the background of the offence ... [and do not] deal unduly harshly with the offender'. (*The Times*, 13 October 1973)

The comment was telling because it reflected the dramatically changed cohort of cannabis smokers now revealed to be the university- and college-educated sons and daughters of the professional middle classes, including the offspring of parliamentarians. Ministers-to-be in Margaret Thatcher's government had by no means been anti-cannabis hardliners. Briefed by Steve Abrams, Paul Channon had been opposed to harsh cannabis laws;

Michael Havers had defended Mick Jagger; Norman St John-Stevas had spoken in favour of legalisation; while Timothy Raison sat on the Wootton Committee.

The sixties are often referred to as the period when recreational drug use exploded across Britain. In truth, it wasn't until the 1970s that drug use, especially cannabis, became ubiquitous in towns and cities and rural areas across the country. Accurate estimates of the number of the cannabis smokers were impossible to come by. Given the intense interest in the drug, many surveys were undertaken to try to establish the cannabis landscape. The Wootton Committee heard conflicting evidence estimating the extent of regular use at anything between 30,000 and 300,000. A survey commissioned by the BBC suggested that 50 per cent of those aged 17–34 living in inner London had tried the drug; other surveys indicated 15 per cent of London University students had smoked cannabis, while another put the national consumption figure at 3.8 million. Whichever way you looked at it, the cannabis numbers were large: convictions went from 544 in 1964 to nearly 10,000 by 1974 while the amount of cannabis seized soared through the seventies. The drug was big business and once cannabis became embedded in the counterculture, while some of the literati were pushing cannabis politics, others were simply pushing cannabis.

* * *

Wootton devoted just a couple of paragraphs to cannabis supply. The report spoke of 'individual cases of highly organised smuggling', but that most of the smuggling was in 'small amounts carried by persons returning from holidays abroad or sent – mainly to immigrants – by post from their home countries'. The report mentioned that 'amateur smuggling' was becoming 'more organised with a standardised drug in the illicit market'. Lebanon, Pakistan and Cyprus were mentioned as major sources. It was suggested that hashish formed some '80 per cent of the market'. 'Within the United Kingdom, we were told the competition of the amateur smuggler has made the illicit traffic a very loosely organised and often casual activity not exploited to any significant extent by professional criminals.'[15]

That's certainly how it started out. Although there was some cannabis resin around in the 1950s, the cannabis market was dominated by herbal cannabis shipped in from various source countries including the West Indies and Africa. This began to change in the early 1960s for two reasons: many of the newer white smokers were wary of going into black cafés like The Rio in west London whose atmosphere could be quite intimidating and so they began to look for their own source. Much of this came from that group who went off on the hippy trail to Nepal, Afghanistan and North Africa, returning with a pound or two of hash in their rucksacks. Until 1973, Nepal was the only country in the world where cannabis was legal and where the government controlled both cannabis production and sale. More enterprising students would conceal some hash inside their camper van. VW vans became synonymous with drug smuggling and on arrival back in the UK were regularly stripped down to the rivets by bored customs officials.

As the market grew, there was clearly some serious money to be made, even if for some it was still a 'righteous' anti-establishment type of law breaking and was still largely 'amateur' in its execution. In the early 1960s, well before it became the melting pot for the rave scene, Ibiza was a bohemian hideaway populated by the dissolute and the damaged, the arty, the creatives, those on the run and those needing a break from the hotbed of London life. One such resident was Damien Enright, who wrote a classic memoir of the times, *Dope in the Age of Innocence* (2010). In 1964, Enright took a massive risk in smuggling just 5 kilos of hash out of Turkey, concealed in his VW van. He got as far as the Spanish border on his way back to Ibiza when the haul was discovered. Enright's travelling companion was busted, but Enright managed to get away on foot. That this bust made headline news as Spain's largest-ever cannabis haul was a sign of just how small the European market for hash was back in 1964. As Enright and his island friends spent much of their time smoking dope, it suggested that the resin would have been mainly for personal consumption although some low-level sales might have eased Enright's hand-to-mouth existence. His name cropped again in the story of another amateur smuggler, although one who was more ambitious if no less disorganised.

Francis Morland was born in 1934 into a well-off Quaker family and was sent to Leighton Park, the Quaker Eton. During National Service, Morland was singled out as an excellent skier and represented Great Britain. A promising sculptor, he rose up in the London art world and was spoken of in the same breath as New Generation artists such as Peter Blake and David Hockney. His work was well regarded but not well paid, and as part of Princess Margaret's 'fast set' he had an extravagant lifestyle to fund. Morland realised that among his clique, cash for drugs was never in short supply and that a childhood sailing hobby could also come in handy. Slowly, he built a small outfit running resin up from Morocco and across from Lebanon. In his autobiography *The Art of Smuggling* (2015), he recalled, 'the wholesale importation of cannabis was still in the hands of relative amateurs who had stumbled into the business during the sixties more because of opportunity than criminal breeding'[16] without sharing the 'hippy complacency that cannabis smuggling was an evangelising adventure which only a few "pigs" cared about'.[17]

By 1966, Morland was travelling abroad, sometimes in the company of Enright, to bring cannabis resin to the UK, although he says he found Enright a '24-carat paranoia king who nevertheless has dabbled in a nervy way with drugs'.

Before hash really lit up London in the mid-1960s, Morland counted as a major player, reckoning he controlled about 10 per cent of the still relatively small 1-ton UK resin market, mainly distributed around the capital.

The first of five busts over 20 years which put Morland behind bars for three quarters of that time came in 1969 when Mr Pilcher knocked on his door. Morland was charged with his wife Susan, American pilot Robert Palacios and Fulton Dunbar, the Third Secretary at the Liberian Embassy in Rome, of smuggling £150,000's worth of hash into the UK with a plan to ship a further ton to the States via the Bahamas. On that occasion Morland skipped bail; in court he was described by the Crown prosecutor as running 'a highly professional and organised smuggling ring' (*The Times*, 23 March 1971) whereas the way Morland organised his business was more like the gang who couldn't shoot straight. Without naming Morland, Enright said in his book, 'Recently I met an English friend of mine, an upper-class old lag who'd served time for botched cannabis deals in many countries and had just come out of an open prison in the UK at the age of 72. I asked him why the hell he hadn't given up the business long ago. "Because when it's happening, it's so exciting – it's like being in a movie," he said.'[18]

In reviewing Morland's book for *The Guardian* (28 January 2016) and talking about the 'gentleman smuggler', Ed Cummings wrote, 'Our hero must be intelligent and cheeky. There can be little hard violence, few hard drugs, few deaths. Run-ins with the law must have a light quality. Nothing too heavy in other words. There must be no risk of readers coming away with the impression that they are dealing with anything other than a loveable scamp.' Step forward Oxford University graduate Howard Marks.

Marks had been dealing a few pounds of hash a year when his Oxford friend Graham Plinston was busted at the Swiss/German border with 45 kilos hidden in his car. This was Howard's opportunity to enter the wholesale smuggling market and he took cannabis smuggling to a whole new level. His book *Mr Nice* reads like a spy thriller – and indeed he was for a short time recruited by MI6 – criss-crossing the world armed with a plethora of fake passports, multiple identities, offshore bank accounts and setting up front companies, living the rock star life with the millions of pounds that passed through his hands. Yet he always needed one eye over his shoulder, facing the imminent threat of arrest as the DEA in particular became mightily pissed off that they couldn't catch him. Until they did.

Marks quickly realised that to build up a global network needed more than just a few college chums and a camper van. Over time, he was dealing directly or indirectly with corrupt foreign diplomats, police, border guards, customs officials, airline and ground staff. He needed to do deals with professional criminals who had those connections and in one case an IRA operative who could secure Shannon airport to receive multi-ton consignments of hash. For example, in 1980 Howard was on remand in Brixton prison having just lost 15 tons of hash, one of the biggest consignments ever to be seized in Europe. The prison housed some serious criminals including Great Train Robber Thomas Wisbey and members of the Arif family, one of the leading UK drug-trafficking crime families during the 1980s. Marks connected with a fellow prisoner, a non-drug serial offender who said he had contacts working in airports and docks. Marks wrote,

This was typical of the many conversations I and other dope dealers had with more traditional British criminals in British prisons at the end of the 1970s and the beginning of the 1980s. The money we had made in our profession tended to dwarf that made by robbers, fraudsters and thieves. Accordingly, many heavy criminals had begun to deal dope, all kinds ... Some of the results were predictable. A lot more ruthlessness and violence was injected into dope-trading activities. Rip-offs and guns became more common. Inevitably a customs officer was shot and killed while busting a container of Moroccan cannabis ... Instead of seeing this tragedy as an obvious consequence of drug prohibition (high profits attracting criminal organisations) the authorities seized upon it as proof of an association between drugs and violence.[19]

Marks said that some of his dope-smoking friends wanted cannabis to remain illegal to underline their anti-establishment stance – not a view he shared.

The implications of a growing and highly profitable trade in cannabis reached all the way back to the producer countries. Lebanon was a major supplier of the world's hashish market. In 1975, the country was plunged into civil war causing a complete breakdown of law and order and allowing drug production to soar, the income from which was used by all the warring factions to fund the armed struggle. In 1990, the DEA estimated that the war had upped drug production to annual totals of more than 2,000 tons of hash and around 10 tons of heroin.

During this period, the Americans put increasing pressure on producer countries to do more to tackle the drug trade, which made the business even more risky as British teenager Timothy Davey found out when in 1972 he was sentenced to 6 years in a Turkish jail for trying to sell 37 kilos of hash. This highly publicised arrest served to mask the reality of international cannabis smuggling; widespread bribery and corruption allowed multiple tons of cannabis to reach the UK, of which customs and police took out only a fraction.

There had been warnings in the UK that a growing market would attract more serious criminal organisations. Wootton Committee member Peter Brodie, the Metropolitan Police Assistant Commissioner, had written a minority report arguing against reducing supply penalties. Concerns about infiltration by criminals with no previous connection with drugs continued to be raised during the 1970s by the Home Office. By the early 1980s, while multi-ton weights of cannabis coming into the UK were more likely in the hands of what we would now regard as organised crime as opposed to Raffles-type chancers, there was a far more serious drug problem heading our way, the full extent of which reverberates to this day.

7

Too Much Monkey Business

In 1926, the Rolleston Committee decided that as a measure of last resort, it was legitimate medical practice for a doctor to prescribe controlled drugs such as morphine and heroin to two 'classes' of patient. One set comprised patients for whom complete withdrawal would cause severe distress and 'even risk to life'. But there was another set where 'experience showed that a certain minimum dose of the drug was necessary to enable patients to lead useful and relatively normal lives and that if deprived of this non-progressive dose they became incapable of work'. These rather vague definitions left some key questions unanswered.

It was more than 30 years later in 1958 that the government decided to review this decision by establishing the previously mentioned Interdepartmental Committee on Drug Addiction chaired by Sir Russell Brain, which became known as the First Brain Report or Brain 1. How had the opiate scene changed in that time to warrant a review?

Despite the passage of time and the outbreak of war, there was a significant degree of continuity in the illicit scene, although the main focus of Rolleston's deliberations was not to consider 'pleasure-seeking' groups but the most appropriate intervention for those single individuals largely from the professional and middle classes who had unfortunately become addicted to drugs originally prescribed, for example for chronic pain – so-called therapeutic addicts. These patients continued to be seen quietly and privately by GPs around the country until the law change in 1968, without either the patient or the doctor coming to the attention of the authorities. One patient and one doctor worth mentioning in this context, although the patient led anything but a normal life, was the writer Anna Kavan and her doctor of 20 years, Karl Theodore Bluth.

Anna Kavan was born Helen Woods in 1901, the child of a wealthy family. At just 4 years old, she was abandoned into the care of relatives while her parents went to live in America. To compound her sense of betrayal, she was sent to boarding school aged 6 where she stayed feeling lonely and isolated until her early teens, often forced to remain alone at school during the holidays. Once her parents returned to the UK, she was only allowed to visit her mother for 10 minutes before dinner. Her father committed suicide by jumping off a ship bound for South America and she was left in the clutches of a hostile and manipulative mother who persuaded Anna not to take up an Oxford place, but instead to do what her mother had done, and marry for money to which she duly submitted.

In her early adult life, she endured two unhappy marriages, dominated by abusive alcoholic husbands which produced a son she couldn't look after who eventually died in the First World War, a daughter who died in infancy and a third child lost to an abortion. Given such a ruptured, loveless life she grew up to be an obsessively private, untrusting woman destroying most of her personal papers and diaries. She also suffered acute mental illness and made more than one suicide attempt, which saw her frequently admitted to psychiatric hospitals.

As Helen Ferguson (her first married name), she sublimated all her misery in a number of semi-autobiographical novels which in their detail about her abusive relationships and her contempt for men later became regarded as pioneering examples of feminist fiction. She retreated still further into her imagination in 1940 by adopting as a pseudonym the name of one of her characters, Anna Kavan, as both her writing and legal name until her death in 1968. With her new identity, her writing moved from social realism to entirely experimental. J. G. Ballard wrote, 'the brilliance of Anna Kavan lay somewhere between poetry and madness', while journalist and author Virginia Ironside noted that 'Anna Kavan, with her frightening glimpses of the dark sides of life, is one of the world's best kept secrets'. Anna's biggest secret, never revealed in her lifetime to the general public, was her lifelong addiction to heroin.

As she destroyed most of her personal documents and was engaged in an activity which while medically legitimised was nonetheless still regarded as morally suspect, her biographers found it hard to track the trajectory of her heroin addiction. There are those who would argue that you should distinguish between the life of the artist and their work, but in this case, heroin was the source of much of Kavan's creativity (and a curse that could thwart it) and while she rarely mentioned it in print by name, she used the glacial and dystopic inner geography she traversed in her fiction as a metaphor for her numbing heroin experience. This was best expressed in her most famous novel, *Ice*, published in 1967 in which the brutalisation of women by men is framed in a frozen post-apocalyptic ice sheet threatening to smother the world.

She did suffer a congenital spinal condition, although there is no record of this actually causing chronic pain: instead a French tennis coach may have introduced her to drugs in the late 1920s by giving some cocaine following an ankle injury which did plague her in subsequent years. One biographer, Jeremy Reed, made the mistaken assertion that Kavan did not register with the Home Office so must have found a dealer to supply her both with heroin and a supply of clean needles. Patients did not personally register with the Home Office. Doctors informed the Home Office on a voluntary basis although most of the information held by the Home Office on the numbers of those in receipt of controlled drugs came from the police inspection of pharmacy records. Despite being the right age, Anna Kavan was never a member of London's Bright Young Things. However, some of the very few friends she had (mainly gay therefore 'safe' men) may well have had helpful West End connections and it is perfectly possible that she was in receipt of private prescriptions from a doctor who also dispensed the drug, meaning her name would not appear on pharmacy records.

Anna's supply line became more stable in 1943 when she met Dr Karl Theodore Bluth, a radical anti-psychiatry psychiatrist presaging R. D. Laing. Dr Bluth worked at St Stephen's Hospital in London where Kavan was sent following yet another suicide attempt. They formed an intense, platonic, almost telepathic connection that went way beyond the conventional doctor/patient relationship and Bluth regularly prescribed her heroin until his death in 1964. They were both existentially isolated individuals who deeply understood each other. Bluth took an entirely sympathetic view of Anna's heroin addiction, seeing it as a source of creativity and her way both of dealing with chronic suicidal depression and of insulating herself from the world.

Before he became a doctor, Bluth studied literature and philosophy and wrote in support of the use of drugs such as opium by German Romantics as an aid to unlocking the creative spirit. He wrote about opium and its role in the romantic imagination, 'the drug described by physiologist and painter Carl Gustav Carus as the crystallised substance of the unconscious, able to carry a soul home to its dark origin. It was the spirit of night that the poet and author Novalis found in the "magic oil" of its brown juice. To these people opium was not a dangerous drug nor a symbol of delusion, but a draught of reality.'[1]

In his study of Britain's opiate culture from 1916 to 1960, Christopher Hallam categorised the prescribing doctors into three categories: compassionate, eccentric and transgressive. The evidence suggests that given his liberal views on drug use by artists, Dr Bluth could be all three, but certainly veered towards the eccentric. For Anna Kavan's migraine, he recommended the full palette of amphetamines: Dexedrine, Methedrine, Benzedrine and Ephedrine. The poet David Gascoyne wrote that during the war he was 'under the control of a refugee I will refer to K. T. B.' who was prescribing for him high doses of amphetamine, causing the poet one Christmas Eve to find himself outside Buckingham Palace declaring he had an important spiritual message to deliver. Included in the amphetamine injection Gascoyne received that day was added ox blood and Vitamin B. Gascoyne reported when he turned up once at Bluth's surgery in Notting Hill, he was greeted by Bluth hammering away at a piano before injecting him with a mixture of ox blood and methadone, a bizarre concoction also visited upon Anna Kavan and the German actor Conrad Veidt, best known for his 1920 role in *The Cabinet of Dr Caligari*. On being consulted by the poet George Barker who complained of hearing peacocks screaming in his head, Bluth told him he was a religious maniac and prescribed Methedrine.

Anna Kavan spent much of her life on a chemical carousel trying LSD and cocaine and attempting suicide with a whole plethora of sleeping pills which she took regularly. Sleeping pills were also administered to her during numerous attempts at detoxification because while the writer knew how much she depended on heroin just to work, she had times when she really felt desperate to be rid of the habit. The technique of narcosis (later revived under the label [ultra]rapid opioid detoxification) involved either putting the patient to sleep or at least severely sedating them for days so they could get through the withdrawal phase with as little discomfort as possible. But as Charlie Parker famously said, 'They can get the drug out of your body, but not out of your mind,' and while Anna might have been physically detoxified, the cumulative mental distress she had suffered all her life, primarily a fear of going mad, was left unaddressed.

There is no evidence that Dr Bluth ever came to the attention of the Home Office. His generous amphetamine prescribing would not have warranted a visit because it was not a controlled drug, nor does it seem that his long-standing prescribing of heroin attracted any visits either. Much to Anna's deep distress, Bluth, who had a chronic heart problem, died in 1964. Where she then sourced her heroin was a mystery because when she was found dead on her bed in December 1968, apparently from a heart attack – a loaded syringe was found by her side. The attending police reported that she had stockpiled enough heroin 'to kill the street'. Anna Kavan died as quietly dependent on heroin as she had lived in life, bothering nobody while producing a body of crystalline, dark and unsettling work which now enjoys cult status.

What about then those groups of users who according to Rolleston's typography were using drugs simply to 'satisfy an addiction'.

There was a Chelsea set of whom Brenda Dean Paul was the leading light, a group that continued well into the 1950s and 1960s. The group mainly comprised women (including a subset of lesbians) like Brenda of the 'better class' who were determined they were not going to conform to what society expected of women of their status and upbringing, to the point of publicly injecting morphine in smart restaurants and nightclubs. The supply came from doctors, although there was evidence of the group receiving small illicit consignments from Paris. Like Brenda, as well as making political statements, it is likely that some of the women were also self-medicating unhappy and unfulfilled lives while their husbands used alcohol to battle their own demons.

There was a second 'continuity set', a more disparate and less connected group working in Soho's night-time economy: musicians, restaurant and bar staff, nightclub hostesses, dancers, actors and prostitutes. They largely relied on stolen or smuggled supplies of drugs: there existed a supply connection through the street grapevine allowing for information exchange and dealer contacts. Bing Spear reckoned the Chelsea set never numbered more than about 30, while the numbers of users living and working in the West End and their customers was unknown but given the decline in pre-war prosecutions, probably not significant. However, because the numbers were so small, it only took one or two key individuals to keep the drugs flowing. For the Chelsea users it was Brenda; for the pre-war West End fraternity, it was Gerald O'Brien, nephew of Irish nationalist fighter Desmond Fitzgerald, father of Garrett Fitzgerald, Irish Taoiseach in the 1980s.

Although he trained as an accountant, O'Brien became bored and looking for a more exciting life began a venture running bottle parties (similar to blues and rent parties) in Mayfair flats as a way of circumventing the licensing laws and was also acquitted of trying to swindle a jeweller out of cash, ostensibly to be used to buy a club. Becoming ever more immersed in the Soho nightlife, he became addicted to drugs in the company of Bella Gold, a hostess O'Brien met at a nightclub. They chose not to try to source drugs from doctors, but instead from Paris where they established some underground connections. On 30 June 1937, O'Brien was arrested by customs at Newhaven in possession of 6 grams of heroin and he was sentenced to 6 months' imprisonment. Bella's flat was raided in October that year where police found packets of heroin, cocaine and cannabis from the same French connection. When she appeared in court, the police were at pains to state that not only was she one of a 'network of addicts', but was regarded by police as a 'trafficker', not just on account of the drugs found but because a stash of letters discovered made oblique references to drugs such as 'getting high'.[2] The police also made the connection between Gold and O'Brien whose 6 grams of heroin marked him out as a major trafficker. But Gold's defence played the therapeutic addict card and won, saying Bella had a chest problem, tried heroin in Paris as a cure and was then in the clutches of dealers. The same judge who sent Brenda Dean Paul to prison instead gave Bella 2 years' probation.

The casualties suffered by the civilian population during the Blitz demanded increasing supplies of morphine to be readily available, raising concerns at the Home Office about large-scale pilfering by both recreational users and addicted medical staff. But while some drug users found an enthusiasm for volunteering as Air Raid Precaution wardens – including Brenda Dean Paul's brother – and there were cases of drug thefts, Home Office fears of a morphine epidemic did not materialise.

Soho's nightlife did not entirely shut down during the war and the arrival of US servicemen boosted the numbers of those who would be active in London's post-war drug scene where numbers started to rise as a new type of using culture began to develop and the 'scenes' themselves began to merge and overlap.

There were two sources of illicit heroin; one was thefts from pharmacies, wholesalers and manufacturers. The most significant case to come to court involved Kevin Patrick Saunders, also known as Mark. He had been a porter at All Saints Hospital in Chatham and after leaving the job went back to steal 144 grams of morphine, 30 grams of heroin and 56 grams of cocaine, which were sold on to West End customers. Saunders helpfully kept a notebook listing all his customers' names by initials, some of whom told the Home Office they had switched to heroin because of a shortage of cannabis.[3] This chimes with a conversation I had with poet and lyricist Pete Brown who was very much part of the London 'Beat' scene. He told me that a number of musicians he knew were using heroin at the time in preference to cannabis simply because they could get it legally from a doctor. When the Home Office checked through all the names in Saunders book, they found only 2 users out of 63 who were known to officials. One was Barry Ellis, who like Brenda Dean Paul became something of a media celebrity through his highly unreliable autobiography, *I Came Back from Hell: the Barry Ellis Story*, written by journalist Alistair Revie and published in 1964. The book blurb gives a flavour of the content:

I Came Back From Hell is the story of Barry Ellis, a one-time drug addict who managed to cure himself of the worst illness known to man. Known internationally as the daddy of all junkies, Ellis had taken more drugs than anyone else alive. It is on record at two London chemists that in 18 years he used 46,000 grains of heroin and a not much smaller quantity of cocaine. Enough to kill a normal man 250,000 times!!!

Born in 1925, Ellis said his violent father married his mother for money, but her family went bankrupt before the inheritance came through. Shunted around to numerous schools, he later found employment at The Whitehall Theatre. Despite being just 16, he was soon promoted to stage manager, but decided to volunteer for the army in March 1942. After being injured and shell-shocked, Ellis said he got hooked on the morphine found in the medical kits used to treat injured soldiers. Ellis was eventually invalided out of the army, although he might have been court-marshalled and possibly also jailed for stealing morphine ampoules. Back on the Soho scene, he got some minor acting roles. He hooked up with Maureen Wyndham-Wilson, one of Brenda Dean Paul's associates, sharing both her bed and her heroin. He drifted through the fifties' and sixties' Soho drug scene, hanging out with Alex Trocchi, was virtually a down and out by the 1980s and still on a script, eventually dying in 1995 following a fire at his flat when he fell asleep holding a lit cigarette.

The Mark case heralded a sign that the user population was larger than any official data at the time was showing. But alongside thefts of this kind was the trade in forged prescriptions, and oversupply from the post-war generation of what become known in the Home Office as 'script' or later in sixties tabloid-speak as 'junkie' doctors.

The pre-war cases of Drs Connor, Grant and Boddy were the reasons why Delevingne needed some medical adjudication on legitimate medical practice. But there were no guidelines, let alone enforceable laws, as to what constituted the types of prescribing identified by Chris Hallam – the compassionate, the eccentric and the transgressive. What was a legitimate dose and for how long? Nor was there any clear-cut idea of the difference between a 'therapeutic addict' and somebody 'gratifying an addiction'. The headline assumption was that the first was just dealing with an organic condition while the second was just pleasure-seeking. But the waters were well muddied when Rolleston distinguished that second group who simply need a controlled dose of a controlled drug to lead a relatively normal and useful life. On that basis, anybody leading a stressful and anxious life, such as those on the West End drug scene or even a life that could put you in immediate danger such as prostitution, could be deemed in need.

As it turned out, in the 1950s there emerged a small group of doctors whose prescribing practices were, as far as the Home Office was concerned, clearly in the 'transgressive' category and where the difference between different types of patient was entirely moot. Taken as a group, these doctors were not making any attempt to negotiate a cure with the patients, not reducing but in many cases increasing dosages, not seeing patients regularly, but instead being willing to send prescriptions in the post, in some cases actually phoning the patient to say a next prescription was due, signing blank prescriptions for the patient to fill in – essentially seeing addiction treatment as a financial transaction. However, the Home Office could do little about it while the medical establishment was reluctant to act.

The Home Office did have the power to revoke a licence to prescribe controlled drugs, but only if the doctor had been convicted under the Dangerous Drugs legislation. Such prescribing, however out of control it might seem, was not *per se* against the law because it could be justified on the grounds of the doctor's professional judgement. The only leverage the Home Office had was to prosecute a doctor for not keeping proper controlled drug records. That only applied to those doctors who dispensed drugs from their surgery (as many did then), not those who simply prescribed. And even if a doctor was convicted of failing to keep records, it usually only warranted a fine. A conviction could in theory trigger some action by the General Medical Council which had disciplinary powers, but it didn't want to take up any cases on the grounds the members felt it was a police matter. One avenue as recommended by Rolleston was to establish a Medical Tribunal under the auspices of the Home Office comprising two doctors and a legal adviser to investigate prescribing practices that were causing concern. Much to Bing Spear's disgust, this option was never taken up until the Misuse of Drugs Act came into force in 1973 because the view among senior Home Office officials was that witnesses could not be compelled to attend; that no evidence from a drug user was reliable and, in any case, why would a user give evidence against the doctor who was prescribing exactly what was wanted?

The first post-war case involved Dr Mark Ripka who had been noticed by the Home Office as a generous prescriber since 1935. He was actually extremely cooperative with the Home Office, telling them who his patients were, and admitting that he often increased dosages because he was 'soft-hearted'.[4] Even though he was a classic candidate for a tribunal hearing, for reasons cited above, that never happened. Instead, Ripka made the mistake of sending heroin prescriptions abroad to another user in Saunders' little book, Angela Wyndham-Wilson, for her to pass on to a former Ripka patient living in Malta. He pleaded guilty, was fined and undertook not to see any more user patients.

The older pre-war patients were seeking out doctors primarily to support their own use, but a new breed of user came along looking to secure large amounts for sale onto the illegal market. Probably the most compliant doctors in that respect was the practice partnership of Drs Maguire and Rourke. It wasn't so much that they were seeing many patients, but the amounts they were prepared to prescribe meant quantities of heroin and cocaine were leaking onto the illicit market. Their patients were able to 'double script' between them because both would state they had no idea that the patient was obtaining drugs from the other. Rourke for example, was prescribing more than 1,000 mg of heroin a day with additional prescriptions on top to one of his patients. One patient carried around a few blank signed NHS prescriptions but was still paying the doctor up to £10 a week. All this came to light at the overdose death inquest of Nigerian jazz musician Broderick Walker who had two prescriptions obtained separately from the two doctors on the same day. Attempts to prosecute the two doctors failed again on the grounds that this was all a matter of professional judgement Rourke carried on prescribing until he died in 1960.

One significant group on the London post-war heroin scene were the jazz musicians. They were inspired by the advent of the bebop jazz revolution creating a whole new subcultural aesthetic around heroin among the musicians and their camp followers who hankered after the 'jazz life' – an over-romanticised image of the urban cowboy, the anti-establishment existential hero. The heroin-using jazz musicians on the scene included some of Britain's finest jazz drummers – Dick Devere, Phil Seaman, Red Reece and Ginger Baker – and other stellar musicians such as Tubby Hayes and Graham Bond. Collectively they formed an inner circle of coveted shared secrets.

By common consent, Dicky Devere sat at the top of the pile of drumming talent; even the legendary Phil Seaman sometimes stomped off in disgust at failing to replicate one of Devere's drum patterns. Dicky was tricky and had a few stunts up his sleeve when it came to acquiring drugs. For a start Dicky Devere was not his real name; it was simply an onomatopoeic handle replicating a fast drum pattern. His real name was Derek Paul Rainbird and he obtained drugs from various doctors using both names. He also had links into the Chelsea users through Brenda Dean Paul, one indication that the various drug scenes should not be regarded as totally discrete and unconnected.

During a police surveillance operation in 1956, Dicky was seen entering Brenda Dean Paul's Chelsea flat; an informer had told Drugs Branch chief Len Dyke that Paul supplied drugs from there. At various times, she was in receipt of prescriptions from four different doctors including Dr Rourke, but at the time of the surveillance, was seeing Dr Hugh Freeman who was described by police as 'comparatively young and inexperienced' from whom she had received just under a ½ ounce of cocaine and 1 gram of morphine daily with an unsubstantiated allegation that what was going between doctor and patient was more than just prescribing. Freeman's relative youthfulness contrasted with many of the script doctors; those that weren't deliberately venal were often elderly doctors working alone who could come under enormous pressure to prescribe.

Freeman was prescribing around 14 grams of pharmaceutical-grade cocaine every day, so it was hardly a shock that Brenda would be selling some on as her finances were often precarious. Paul also introduced Devere to Dr Rourke. His position as Britain's top jazz drummer notwithstanding, he was a heroin evangelist who possibly introduced Phil Seamen to the drug. Devere's friend, musician and roadie Pete Bailey described Devere to me as an 'evil little bastard'. What he lacked in inches he made up for in causing as much mayhem as possible. He would often barge into a club, go right down the front where the band was playing and shout out that he was a much better drummer and they should hire him. But when he was under police scrutiny, he was unemployed, having dropped out of the scene in 1953, re-emerging briefly in 1959. Unfortunately, heavy drug use made Devere unreliable and unemployable. Ill for much of the 1960s, he died in 1970 aged 42 from an overdose in a hospital toilet, not of heroin, but an anaesthetic, which led the coroner to conclude that Dickie Devere committed suicide. Death from drug overdose or complications arising from drug use was a fate which befell most of those musicians on the 1950s heroin scene including Phil Seamen and Tubby Hayes, but with the notable exception of Ginger Baker.

Heroin use played a complicated role in the life of jazz musicians, elements of which would be entirely alien to the totally medicalised view of addiction. Aside from the cultural positioning of the wandering minstrel, there was an understanding that the 'ego release' of heroin would dampen down inhibitions as an aid to the central role of improvisation in modern jazz. No musician could play blind drunk; plenty played well while stoned on heroin. However, the belief you had to have a habit big enough to fell an ox in order to play like Charlie Parker was the classic mistake made by many of his acolytes – what bassist Jack Bruce called 'the Charlie Parker death wish'. What they failed to see or chose not to comprehend was that Bird played brilliantly on heroin because he was dependent on it. That was the only time he felt well enough to play normally; in other words, better than anybody else.

This was borne out by American psychologist Charles Winick in 1954 in the only study ever carried out on the use of drugs by jazz musicians. He interviewed 409 New York musicians, 32 per cent of whom thought a heroin-using musician would often play under the influence of the drug. Just over half thought heroin a dangerous drug, but many also viewed it as a 'working drug'.[5]

Heroin had other functions in the erratic and poorly paid life of the jazz musician where even those working regularly could not afford to miss a gig through illness. Musicians were especially prone to colds and flu, moving as they often did from a freezing cold tour bus or train into a sweltering club environment and then back outside into the night air, for weeks on end. This was a particular problem for singers; if their voice went, the whole gig could be in jeopardy. But nobody on heroin gets flu, colds or coughs because heroin dries out the membranes and suppresses the cough reflex. Phil Seamen started out as an occasional heroin and cocaine user but told saxophonist Dick Heckstall-Smith that he took a conscious decision to carry on using for purely pragmatic reasons even though he knew it would shorten his life.

Popular accounts of heroin addiction like Thorp's and Sunday tabloid exposés such as the story of Mandy Taylor in *Empire News and Sunday Chronicle* (29 March 1959) who had been in and out of trouble with the law as a teenager, came to the bright lights of London, worked as a waitress, but ended up as a high-class prostitute to pay for her heroin habit, followed a familiar trope of the Barrie Ellis-style 'my drug hell' cautionary tale to ensure payment for the type of story that the paper wanted to print.

Alongside these accounts and the evidence provided by the occasional script doctor or forged prescription court case was the memorandum written by Bing Spear in 1955. He raised concerns there was a growing illicit market in heroin involving younger 'non-therapeutic' users fuelled by overprescribing and reminded his bosses about the Rolleston recommendation of using a Medical Tribunal to discipline those doctors viewed as overprescribers. His bosses were not convinced, but there was a view taken that a review of Rolleston might be in order because of some American medical views that opiate withdrawal was not life threatening, which might undermine the argument for maintenance prescribing and because there were some new synthetic opiates on the market which could add to the problem.

There was also a political imperative suggesting a review of treatment might be expedient. Negotiations were still underway concerning the Single Convention on Narcotic Drugs. Britain had already seen off an attempt by the Americans to ban heroin in 1955 and it would be in British interests to demonstrate that legal heroin prescribing was helping to prevent the mess the Americans were in. But at the same time, it was important not to suggest that heroin use was slipping out of control. Other senior officials disagreed, suggesting the Americans would never believe such a government-led review would be independent. Eventually, in June 1958, two-and-a-half years after the idea was first raised, the government appointed Sir Russell Brain to investigate the matter with a very restrictive brief. It took until April 1961 to produce a slim report, which essentially said the situation since Rolleston remained stable with no evidence of a growing illicit heroin scene fuelled by overprescribing doctors, just a small group of isolated therapeutic users dotted around the country. They took no evidence about the illicit scene and were also misled by the apparent falling numbers of 'notified addicts'.

Since 1933, in order to provide data to the League of Nations, the Home Office had kept a card index of all those known to be in receipt of prescriptions for morphine, heroin and cocaine and their respective doctors. The idea was to try to prevent users 'double scripting' from doctors and to monitor numbers. Notification by doctors to the 'Addicts Index' was voluntary, to which was added information from the pharmacy records collected by specialist police known as Chemists Sergeants. On paper the numbers had fallen from 616 in 1936 to 359 in 1957, adding to the committee's view that the system was working so no change was necessary. What the Home Office failed to point out was that the way of calculating the figures had changed, which affected the statistics and because the committee heard no evidence about the illicit scene, would not have taken into account there were users unknown to the Home Office.

However, Sir Russell Brain was soon to be embarrassed by the shortcomings of his own report and the revelation the Home Office had withheld evidence that there was a growing illicit heroin scene. Brain previewed his report findings at a meeting of the Society for the Study of Addiction shortly before publication. Irving Benjamin, a pharmacist at John Bell & Croyden, one of London's two all-night pharmacies, stood up and said that,

Sir Russell's optimism amazes me. A short while ago I came across an addict who was completely unknown to the Home Office. He presented his prescription for something like 30 grains of cocaine (about 1,900 mg) and 40–50 grains of heroin (about 3,000 mg). This was repeated on several different occasions, in several quantities. This was prescribed by a doctor who I know for a fact was making every effort to treat these people ... That patient was obviously obtaining supplies illicitly on such a scale as to get used to those quantities ... As to the suggestion that there seems to be no large centre of addiction, I can personally record forty or fifty cocaine, heroin and morphine addicts in the London area alone.[6]

By the time the Brain Committee was reconvened again in July 1964, there was no ducking the issue of fast-evolving changes on the London heroin and cocaine scene. The Home Office figures of users known to the civil servants were indicative of what was happening. As evidence of the changing situation, the Home Office started to separate 'non-therapeutic addicts' from the rest. In 1959, there were 47 in this category with 9 new users added that year. By 1961, the figures read 112 and 54 respectively and by 1964, the numbers had jumped to 329 and 160, including the first notifications of users under 20.

Within these figures were other younger emerging groups. Raymond Thorp was one example of the early post-war generation of heroin users – an ordinary bloke who came from an ordinary, unremarkable, untroubled suburban background, but somehow feeling he just didn't fit with the 'straight' world and eventually drifted into heroin use because it was there. He would not be alone on this journey.

Bob was a teenager on the early sixties music scene, hung out at the World Psychedelic Centre and knew all the Soho celebrities from Alex Trocchi to Christine Keeler. Amphetamine was his initial drug of choice, 'but dope, speed, heroin, it was just what you did. There was a lot of casual heroin use. Many more people used heroin than bothered to go to a doctor to be registered. It was a bit of a burden; you were then known by the authorities – and that was uncool even though it meant you were largely free from prosecution.' Bob's heroin habit took many years to conquer; it was eventually achieved at the Phoenix House therapeutic community.

Peter left home at 15 and agrees with Thorp that much of the appeal of the drug scene and the characters that went with it was a reaction against boredom and of not fitting in with the world his parents expected him to inhabit. Like Bob, Peter was a speed freak and found heroin useful to come down from all the amphetamine and Methedrine he was consuming. Methedrine was the trade name for methamphetamine produced by Burroughs Wellcome as white 5 mg tablets and 30 mg liquid capsules. Although methamphetamine metabolises into amphetamine once ingested, the difference in chemistry between the two drugs meant that Methedrine was far stronger and more long-lasting than amphetamine. Peter's introduction to heroin was the sort of casual affair referred to by Bob. A famous artist and designer on the music scene 'dared me to try heroin'. Peter's subsequent drug career took him down the murky lanes of serious dealing but, like Bob, he ended up in the seventies at Phoenix House and both went on to work in the voluntary sector drug treatment field.

Back in the sixties, Peter and Bob knew an eccentric character called Billy whose access to family money and seemingly endless supplies of doctor-prescribed Methedrine helped create a new younger drug-using Chelsea clique to succeed that which swirled around Brenda Dean Paul. This crowd included both the 'new aristocracy', such as the Rolling Stones, Marianne Faithful and Robert Fraser. Like Billy, there were the wayward trust fund kids including Guinness heir Tara Guinness to whom John Lennon dedicated *A Day in the Life* after Guinness died in a road accident in December 1966 aged just 21 and Lord Harlech's daughter Alice Ormsby-Gore, who become Eric Clapton's girlfriend. She scored heroin for him from doctors and died of a heroin overdose in 1995. In his autobiography, *Survival of the Coolest*, William Pryor, Charles Darwin's great-great-grandson, wrote of his years of heroin addiction as he too drifted into the Soho drug milieu on the run from a high-achieving, well-off but emotionally cold family environment and a desperately unhappy time at Eton that left him feeling invisible and unloved.

Between 1962 and '63, the Home Office submitted two reports which together justified reconvening the Brain Committee; one setting out the rising numbers of heroin users and their changing demographic and the other about the specific prescribing habits of one doctor who almost single-handedly seemed to be underwriting London's heroin scene.

As a qualified psychiatrist, Dr Isabella Robertson was one of the first researchers at the Maudsley Hospital in south London to examine the physical aetiology of psychosis. During the Second World War she worked at the Cambridge University's Psychology Laboratory researching the use of dietary supplements to improve the physical performance of servicemen. After the death of her first husband Gordon Cunningham, she married the eminent surgeon Claude Frankau and when he was knighted in 1945, she took the title of Lady Frankau and began mixing in the highest levels of British society. She was in the congregation in May 1960 when Princess Margaret married Lord Snowdon. In the early 1950s, she was engaged in research into the use of electroshock therapy as a treatment for alcoholism. Within her private practice, Lady Frankau was seeing politicians and members of the aristocracy who had a drink problem, when she was consulted by a GP, Patricia Stanwell, based in South Kensington about one of her own alcoholic patients. Dr Stanwell suggested Lady Frankau might want to see one of her drug-using patients as well, as the GP already had a growing number of users coming to see her.

One of Lady Frankau's first patients was Mandy Taylor. Interviewed by Brian Freemantle back in 1986 for his book *The Fix*, Mandy described Lady Frankau as a stern character who wore a monocle and severe black suits and could be equally severe with her patients: 'We couldn't protest or anything,' said Mandy. 'She was a sergeant major ... the worst you ever knew. If we upset her, she'd make us suffer. "Wait until last." Things like that.'[7]

I interviewed Dr Stanwell back in the 1980s and she told me that once she saw her first drug-using patient seeking a prescription in the mid-1950s, she quickly acquired several others: 'The public didn't know what was going on and the medical profession didn't want to know ... at one time I had more than the Home Office knew about. That's when I started writing to the Home Office and getting an acknowledgement so I could show they knew about them.' She gave a strong impression that the Home Office didn't actually want to know that the heroin addiction figures were going up and says that Bing Spear told her that he would acknowledge her letter, 'even if he had to destroy mine'. This resonates with Bing's view that in the run-up to Brain 1, there was a 'cover-up' so as not to give the impression to the Americans and their hard-line supporters at the UN that the Rolleston approach was failing to control addiction, even if that was never its purpose.

Dr Stanwell was trying to cope on her own:

Nobody could offer me an alternative [to prescribing] so what was I supposed to do? The number of vials that fell down lift shafts and went under trains or down the drain, I can't tell you. I didn't believe much of it but when they come in vomiting and shaking, doubled up with stomach cramps, you've got to do something. One Christmas Day I had the station master from South Kensington station banging on the door saying he had a boy who wouldn't leave the station until he got a prescription.

The two doctors began working together; Dr Stanwell from her surgery and Lady Frankau from her palatial rooms at 32 Wimpole Street W1. Initially, Lady Frankau was just seeing Dr Stanwell's NHS patients and signing the prescriptions on behalf of her partner. Together they co-wrote a paper on drug addiction treatment published in *The Lancet* in December 1960.

Working with a cohort of 51 patients, they described a two-phase programme. The first phase involved prescribing 'adequate supplies' of heroin and cocaine to keep patients away from the illicit market. In phase two, dosages would be reduced but combined with prescriptions for tranquillisers to cope with anxiety and insomnia, and vitamins to improve physical health, leading to complete in-patient drug withdrawal.

They claimed a high success rate, but in reality, Lady Frankau rarely reduced dosages or attempted withdrawal and justified prescribing cocaine to those heroin users who had never used it on the grounds that as there was no physical withdrawal symptoms from cocaine, it eased the worst of heroin withdrawal. Other prescribing doctors began to follow her example, all of which increased the amount of cocaine available illegally on the streets.

Bing Spear described her prescribing habits as 'increasingly bizarre': pharmacy data collected by the Home Office revealed just how bizarre; of the 1 million heroin tablets prescribed to users in 1962, 600,000 or 6 kilos came from her pen. This level of prescribing eventually led to a falling out with Dr Stanwell who was far less generous with the prescription pad. 'We disagreed over prescribing. I just felt the whole thing was getting out of control.' The break came in April 1961: 'She thought I'd killed one of her patients while she was on holiday by not prescribing enough drugs for him. I'm not sure what happened, but there was a fire in his flat and she certainly blamed me. She was very self-opinionated and if she thought she was right nothing would stop her.' Dr Stanwell thought it was Lady Frankau's increasing frailty that warped her judgement: 'It's the only thing I could think of. She certainly changed over the period we started working together in 1957 through to 1961.' Once Lady Frankau started seeing her own patients, the records revealed that all strands of London's heroin scene were beating a path to her door, including Brenda Dean Paul and her brother Brian, Raymond Thorp, Ginger Baker, Phil Seamen, Dicky Devere, William Pryor, Michael Hollingshead and Billy. Peter was on her list recalling 'all these guys gouching out in these grand rooms'. And for all her attempts to control her patients like naughty children, Mandy said that Lady Frankau never decided for herself the amounts to prescribe, 'she just asked what we wanted and gave it ... You'd just go there, ask for what you wanted and get it! Marvellous! One girl was referred to her because she was hooked on purple hearts ... She sat in front of Lady Frankau who wrote her a script for heroin and cocaine and gave it to her. The girl came out to us in the waiting room and said, "What's this for?' I don't know what it is." You can imagine the rush to help her!'

From 1959, her caseload took on an international flavour, bringing the number of users on her books to over 100. In December that year, the first of 91 Canadian heroin users came to the UK on the run from American-style prohibitionist drug policies. On arrival at Heathrow Airport, they often went straight to the Home Office to inquire about obtaining prescriptions, but soon learnt through the grapevine about Lady Frankau. Some observers blamed these older, more experienced users for fuelling the London heroin scene or even encouraging people to turn on. They certainly had tales to tell and earned a cachet among young London users, but they tended to keep themselves to themselves and were not heroin evangelists.

Once here, their experiences of the heroin scene were by no means homogenous. Some went home saying they missed the excitement of the illegal heroin scene, claiming strangely that the adulterated street heroin back in Canada was stronger than the pure drug they were getting from the chemist here.[8] But for others it was a revelation. One Canadian user wrote his story for the *Toronto Daily Star* (2 October 1963). Leonard Jordan, 38, arrived in London and went to see Lady Frankau (although he didn't name her directly). She asked him if he could foresee ever coming off drugs and he said he would give supervised withdrawal a go. She wrote him out a prescription for just one day and he described his elation at walking into Boots like any other customer and picking up his prescription in stark contrast to his last unreliable and illegal street purchase in Canada. The article didn't indicate that he did go for withdrawal, but he did get and hold down a job and carried on obtaining his prescription without anybody knowing about his heroin habit. He observed that heroin just became part of his life rather than dominating his daily existence in the endless round of finding the money to buy drugs and waiting for, or hunting down, the dealer.

In 1969, American sociologist Jim Zacune, working at the Addiction Research Unit run by Professor Griffith Edwards, set out to track down the Canadians to find out what happened to them all. He found out that 10 had died in England, 10 more had been deported, 35 voluntarily went home and some had just vanished. He did manage to secure a study group of 25; they were quite a bit older than the English users, had been on heroin for many years longer and were using at least 600 mg a day. While back home, they were generally either unemployed or could barely hold down a job, because they were often in and out of prison. In England the majority had regular jobs, one for seven years washing taxis while using large daily amounts of heroin yet hardly missing a day of work. In 1963 Lady Frankau was in Canada to speak about her treatment which did encourage a few more to come to the UK, but by then the peak of arrivals had passed.

Along with Canadians, some illustrious names from the American jazz scene also obtained their supplies from Lady Frankau, including Dexter Gordon, Bill Evans and Chet Baker, who wrote about her in his diary. He went to see her in 1962 while filming *Stolen Moments* with Susan Hayward: '[She] was about 75 years old ... and very business-like. She simply asked me my name, address and how much heroin and cocaine I wanted each day.' He said he walked away with heroin and cocaine that would have cost him several hundred dollars in the USA.[9]

Despite the evidence of a developing illicit drug scene, especially the growth in recreational amphetamine use among young people, the reconvened Brain Committee, usually referred to as Brain 2, had yet another very narrow term of reference, focusing entirely on overprescribing. In an interview with me, Bing Spear went so far as to say, 'The whole of Brain 2 was set up because of Lady Frankau.' Having interviewed her for 25 minutes, the committee were confirmed in their view that while there might be a few other overprescribers out there, the key to solving the current problem was simply to stop Lady Frankau.

The deficiencies of their tunnel vision were laid bare by the 100-page dossier on Lady Frankau compiled by the Home Office in which, for example, the activities of Raymond Thorp told a contrasting story. He began obtaining legal prescriptions in May 1957 from various doctors, finally arriving at Dr Stanwell's door in October 1958. She began reducing his prescription of 600 mg of heroin and 195 mg of cocaine per day. He soon began seeing other doctors, including Lady Frankau, who were prepared to prescribe more. He eventually hit the jackpot with an unnamed doctor who was prescribing 650 mg of heroin and 380 mg of cocaine daily, which gave him the surplus he was looking for. It earnt him a 12-month sentence in June 1961 for selling heroin outside Boots in Piccadilly Circus. Anybody active on the scene at the time, whether Home Officials like Bing Spear, users or doctors, knew that Lady Frankau was not single-handedly responsible for a heroin epidemic, but it was nevertheless true that relatively few doctors in London were prepared to write prescriptions for patients with a heroin addiction.

The first Brain Committee had disregarded or had not known about the script doctors of the 1950s; now this fact was inescapable. Moreover, the final recommendations of the Second Brain Report reflected some new thinking about heroin addiction – Britain was now dealing with a socially infectious disease, posing a threat to wider society especially young people, not just an issue of individual pathology to be dealt with at the discretion of the doctor. Their set of recommendations signalled the beginning of more State intervention in the treatment and control of drug addiction. Their key recommendations, published in November 1965, were that there should be mandatory notification of users to the Home Office in the same way that doctors were obliged to notify it of patients suffering from infectious diseases, and there should be new specialist NHS treatment centres. The most significant recommendation was that only those doctors working in the new treatment centres should be allowed to prescribe heroin or cocaine to users in support of an addiction.

These recommendations have been interpreted as signalling the end of what might be called the British Approach to drug addiction, rather than any sort of system, although there was nothing in the report calling for an end to maintenance prescribing. In fact, the report recognised that 'some patients may have to remain indefinitely under the care of the treatment centres'. While determined to limit the damage of the overprescribing by 'six doctors', the committee recognised the risk that 'if ... restrictions are so severe as to prevent or seriously discourage the addict obtaining any supplies from legitimate sources it may lead to the development of an organised illicit traffic. The absence hitherto of such an organised illicit traffic has been attributed largely to the fact that the addict has been able to obtain supplies of drugs legally.' The GP was largely written out of the drug treatment script, but the clinical judgement of the consultant psychiatrists who took over the running of the clinics was not challenged by government. As we shall see, what ultimately undermined the ethos of Rolleston was the attitude of those doctors resistant to the idea of maintenance prescribing.

The report received a cautious welcome from the medical profession. Many GPs breathed a sigh of relief that they were now barred from prescribing drugs in support of an addiction. But others thought it was a mistake to change the existing arrangements for the sake of a few supposedly irresponsible doctors and in the process removing the right to prescribe from some doctors who were not only prescribing more responsibly but who had a lot of experience dealing with a difficult and challenging patient group. One such doctor was John Hewetson, not only a GP (who managed to get Kevin 'Mark' Saunders off heroin) but a committed anarchist, a champion of contraception for working-class women and abortion on demand, and author of *Ill Health, Poverty and the State* (1946), a damning indictment of capitalist and authoritarian society and the health gap between rich and poor. He was scathing about the Brain report (he gave evidence to the committee), attacking the committee for their failure to recognise how hard it was for a user to find either a GP who would be prepared to take them as patients or for the GP to secure any kind of assistance from psychiatrists. Moreover, as he wrote for the magazine *Anarchy* in 1966,

> ... it could be ... argued that as these few doctors are the only ones in contact with drug addicts, they are the only people who know anything worthwhile about the problem. These doctors would be enormously helped if they could send their patients at the right moment into adequately

equipped psychiatric units. But these units will have to be staffed by psychiatrists who have learned something about addiction – at the moment there are an even smaller handful of such than of the maligned general practitioners. For the question has to be asked: who *are* the experts? The Brain Committee, in two reports, has sufficiently demonstrated its own ignorance and ineptitude. General practitioners who for years have shouldered the main burden of the work may well be more than a little tired of being sneered at and told what to do by people who have no idea of the problems involved.[10]

Another GP and psychiatrist, Dr Robert Ollendorff, wrote in the *Liverpool Journal of Psychiatry* that the report was 'a total failure … They have neither understood the problem nor obviously been able to provide an answer … to take drugs out of experienced medical hands seems retrogressive and senseless.'[11] Dr Ollendorff was another practitioner who bitterly resented the callous attitude of hospital staff. 'I remember Robert Ollendorf saying to me,' said Bing Spear, 'it would easier to get a camel through the eye of a needle than an addict into hospital.' And even if a GP managed to get a patient admitted, 'within a fortnight they'd be back on the doctor's doorstep'.

Dr Stanwell was equally critical of the decision; the committee, she said, 'was full of all these people who had done nothing to help me when I needed it so what did they know about it?' Lady Frankau was not named in the report but knew only too well at whom the barbs were aimed. As she told the *Sunday Times* (20 February 1966), 'If the Brain Committee thinks it's going to get effective treatment in centres, jolly good luck to them. But if you know anything about these people, you know how scared … they are about society in any form.'

Writing several years later, Bing Spear was surprisingly magnanimous about Lady Frankau. Unlike other 'script doctors', it was obvious that she was not in it for the money and often waived her consultation fee. She apparently gave Barrie Ellis a car and was known to stop her Bentley at a prearranged spot in order to hand over a prescription to a desperate user.

Spear acknowledged that she genuinely believed in her methods, even if she was prepared to take on trust anything she was told about lost prescriptions, did prescribe to some individuals without making any checks to see if they genuinely had a heroin problem and overall refused to acknowledge her role in creating the illicit market she claimed her prescribing helped prevent. Furthermore, and to her credit, like Dr Stanwell and others, she was prepared to see increasing numbers of patients in default of the mental health hospitals and most GPs who wanted nothing to do with a group of patients they regarded as a disruptive, undeserving nuisance. According to Mandy Taylor, for all her eccentricities and the somewhat 'bent' relationship that she had with her patients, she was using the money she charged rich clients to underwrite the costs of seeing those patients who could ill-afford consultation fees, however modest. As something of an outsider himself at the Home Office, Spear had a sneaking admiration for her general disdain of officialdom, bureaucracy and the medical establishment. Lady Frankau dispensed drugs directly to her patients from the US Embassy so that their names would not appear on pharmacy records and when Spear wanted to see her Dangerous Drugs Register, he was told it had been stolen in a burglary.

The idea of the prescribing doctor as an 'outsider' was perceptively noted in the *Sunday Times* article which quoted Lady Frankau and other doctors anonymously, none of whom were seeing drug-using patients privately and thus earning fees. The question was posed, if treating drug users was such a challenge, why on earth would you do it? 'All these doctors had an unusual quality about them – some element of the outsider in their make-up; strong political opinions; the status of the exile or perhaps an unusual degree of professional compassion. And it is possible as a result of this that they succeed in acting as a link between the outcast addicts and normal society.'

* * *

In their report the committee recognised that if addiction treatment was limited to the new treatment centres they had recommended, these had to be up and running by the time the necessary legislation was enacted. Moreover, they noted there would be a significant chance of relapse if people were discharged from community treatment centres without some kind of 'long-term rehabilitation' facilities being available. All of which added up to the need for urgent action. As Sir Russell Brain wrote to Health Minister Kenneth Robinson in July 1965 in submitting the report, 'You will appreciate when you read the report why we regard the matter as one of urgency and the Committee has asked me to express the hope that you will arrange for the publication of the report with the least possible delay.'[12]

So how urgently did the government act on the report? Ken Leech wrote a letter to *The Times* published on 9 November 1966 which neatly summed up the lack of progress:

What has happened in the 12 months since the Brain Report? … the answer is nothing at all. There is much talk and proliferation of writing about drug taking but virtually no action. Treatment facilities remain appallingly inadequate … The Minister of Health's notorious statement of 2 August about treatment centres was received by doctors, social workers and addicts with cynical laughter or with despair. Those who daily face the problems of the young drug taker are finding the obstacles almost insurmountable; hours and days spent ringing round hospitals for admissions; refusals, evasions, and interminable delays; addicts whose condition deteriorates and parents whose hearts are broken; doctors who refuse to prescribe and doctors who prescribe with almost criminal irresponsibility; and an overwhelming sense of hopelessness and despair among those who know the drug scene closest.

The widespread reluctance and refusal of GPs throughout London to prescribe heroin and cocaine even under carefully controlled conditions coupled with the opting out of several well-known doctors has led to a worsening state of affairs.

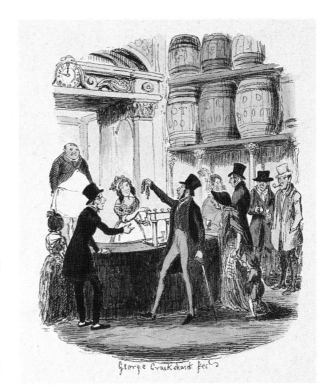

Right: A busy gin palace bar with customers buying drinks. (Courtesy of the Wellcome Collection)

Below: A fleet of opium clippers with other boats and rafts on the Ganges. (Courtesy of the Wellcome Collection)

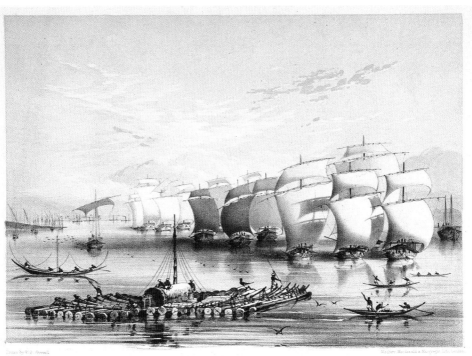

THE OPIUM FLEET,
DESCENDING THE GANGES EN ROUTE TO CALCUTTA

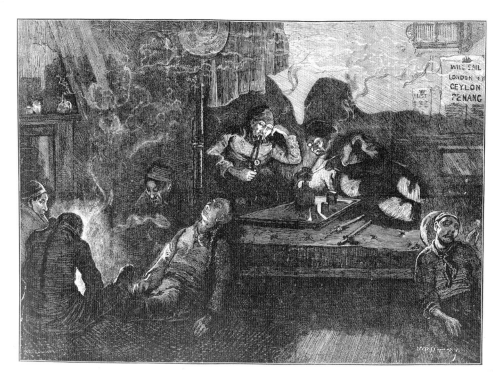

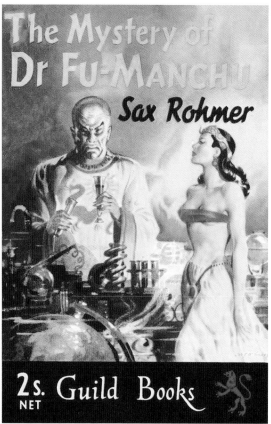

Above: An Opium den in the East End of London, 1874. (Courtesy of the Wellcome Collection)

Left: The Mystery of Dr Fu-Manchu by Sax Rohmer, published 1913. The author's popular novels used themes of opium use and the white slave traffic.

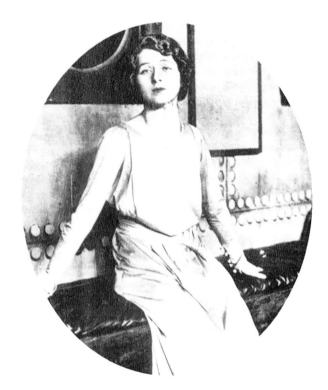

Billie Carleton, whose death in 1918 from a drug overdose was a major scandal.

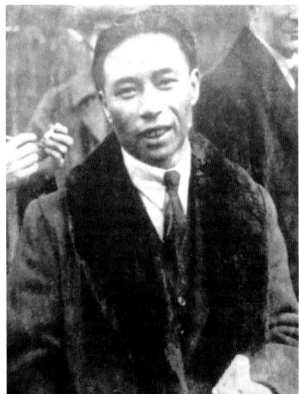

Brilliant Chang, dealer to the stars. He was characterised in the press as London's 'Dope King', perhaps playing on the stereotypes evident in Sax Rohmer's novels.

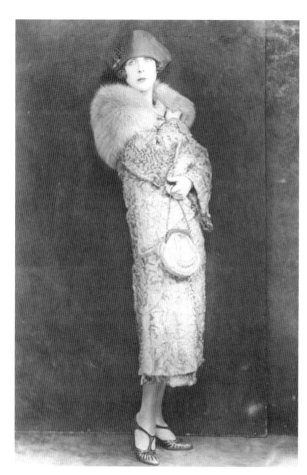

Left: Lady Diana Manners indulged in what she described as morphine 'orgies' with her friend Katherine, the wife of PM Asquith's son. (Courtesy of the Library of Congress)

Below: A flapper affixes a pin to a Cannon Row police officer in the late 1920s. The poster on the railings signals, for some women, a break from the Victorian straitjacket. (Courtesy of Leonard Bentley)

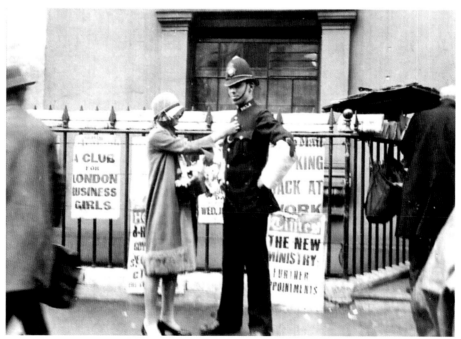

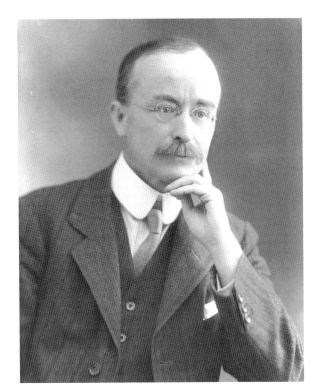

Sir Malcolm Delevingne was the lead official on UK drug control from the mid-1910s to the early 1930s and has gone down in history as the architect of UK drug prohibition. (© National Portrait Gallery)

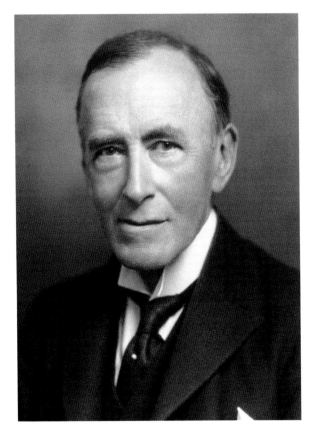

Sir Humphrey Rolleston's eponymous report on drug control, published in 1926, would prove almost a blueprint for much later guidance on addiction treatment. (Courtesy of the Wellcome Collection)

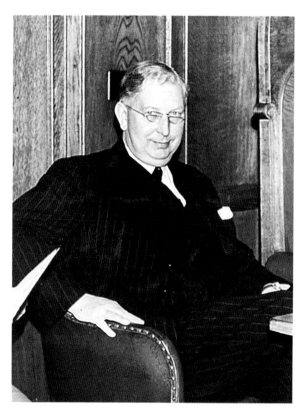

In 1958, neurologist Russell Brain chaired the first major government committee investigating addiction treatment since Rolleston. (Courtesy of the Wellcome Collection)

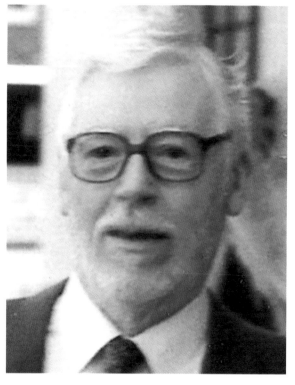

The psychiatrist Ronald Sandison pioneered the use of LSD as a treatment in psychotherapy in the UK.

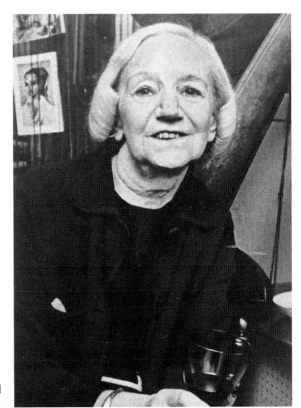

Celebrated author Anna Kavan spent her troubled life on a chemical carousel. Her struggle with mental health and addiction informed her writing.

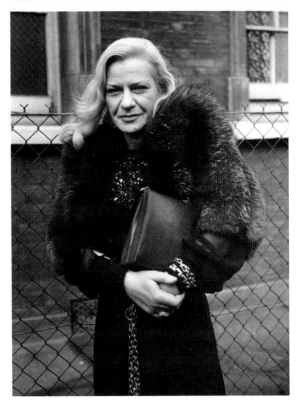

Actress, socialite and Bright Young Thing Brenda Dean Paul became a staple of the tabloid press for her drug addiction. She served terms in Holloway Prison and was committed to various care homes as a result. (© Alamy)

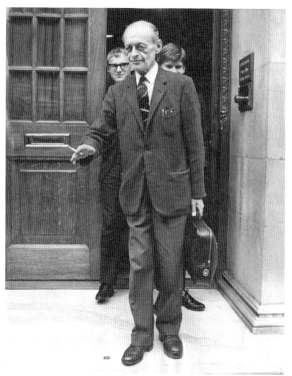

John Petro outside court after denying accusations of 'infamous professional conduct'. Among the charges were that he continued prescribing or supplying Methedrine to a former secretary until she agreed to allow him to photograph her in underclothes or a nightdress.

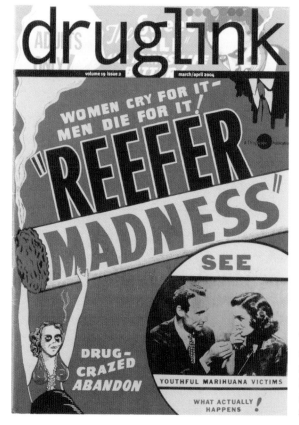

The cover of Druglink magazine, March/April 2004, reproduces the type of 'Shock! Horror!' treatment the US media once gave to marijuana smoking.

THE DOPE CHRONICLES

Fascinating, sometimes funny, *The Dope Chronicles* reproduces actual newspaper pages containing drug stories from 1850-1950. It recreates how we felt about and dealt with the use of opium, cocaine, marijuana, and exotic drugs in our midst. Fifteen major metropolitan newspapers veer in these pages between hysteria over the disintegration of our moral fabric and lurid fascination with the dark underside of the drug world. *The Dope Chronicles* evokes a time when there were no social drugs, just social menaces.

Gary Silver is head of Yellow Press, the antiquarian clipping bureau which has collected several thousand bound newspaper volumes. *Michael Aldrich* is custodian of San Francisco's prestigious Fitz Hugh Ludlow Memorial Library, containing the most comprehensive archives of drug-related literature in the world.

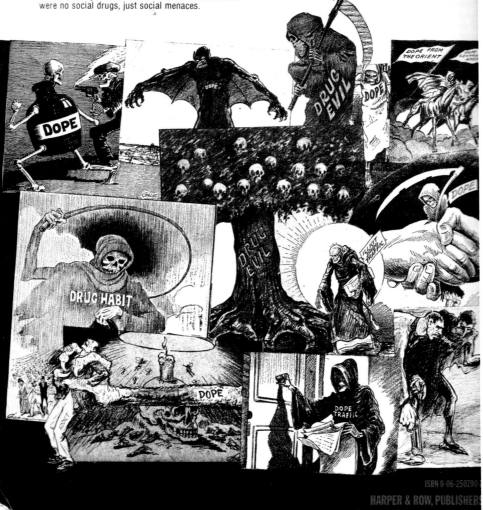

ISBN 0-06-250290-
HARPER & ROW, PUBLISHERS

The Dope Chronicles examined the initial moral panic surrounding drugs and how illustrations gave birth to the myth of the drug fiend.

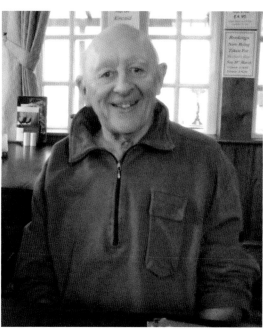

Above: A 1967 photograph showing some icons of the 1960s drug scene. Standing, from left to right: Michael Cooper, Mick Jagger, a pregnant Marianne Faithfull, Shepard Sherbell, Brian Jones. Sitting: Maharishi Mahesh Yogi. (Courtesy of the Nationaal Archief)

Left: Anglican priest Ken Leech served in deprived parishes of London in the sixties and seventies, and was confronted daily by drug addiction and other social issues. After setting up the Soho Drug Group in 1967 to help young drug users, he established the leading charity Centrepoint in 1969.

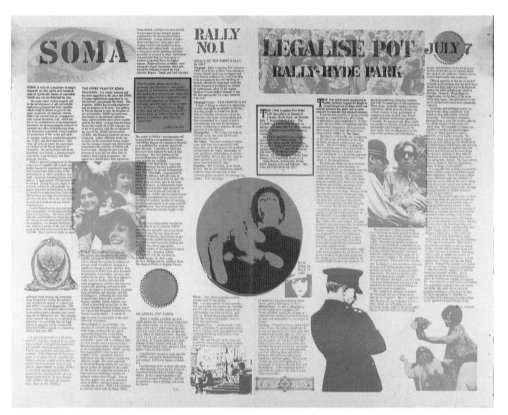

Above: A 1968 feature from the underground newspaper *International Times* reporting on Steve Abrams' drug research project SOMA and its campaign to have the cannabis laws reformed.

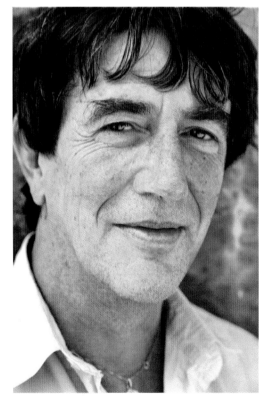

Left: Hugely successful cannabis smuggler Howard Marks, who became famous as Mr Nice and campaigned for changes to drug legislation after completing seven years of twenty-five-year prison sentence. (© Alamy)

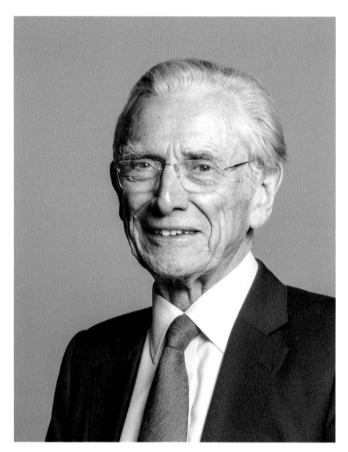

As Health and Social Services Secretary, Norman Fowler was responsible for public safety campaigns concerning AIDS and persuaded Cabinet colleagues to support needle exchanges.

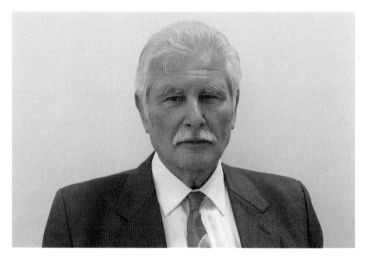

Erstwhile Chief Constable of Yorkshire Keith Hellawell was Tony Blair's choice for 'drugs czar'. Frustrated by his experiences at Whitehall, he would resign four years later, the experiment having proved a failure.

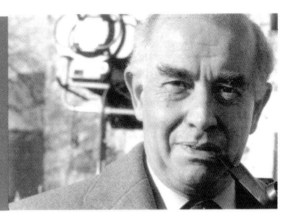

Two major LSD factories were operating in the UK supplying a worldwide market under the noses of the police, until a DI from Thames Valley drug squad became curious. What happened next helped revolutionise the policing of drugs. By **Harry Shapiro**

Druglink magazine's November/December 2004 edition ran a major feature on Operation Julie headed up by DI Dick Lee of the Thames Valley Drug Squad (above). Richard Kemp (below), a chemist who had graduated from Liverpool University, and his student girlfriend Dr Christine Bott represented the last vestiges of a counter-cultural approach to LSD that believed the drug could benefit all.

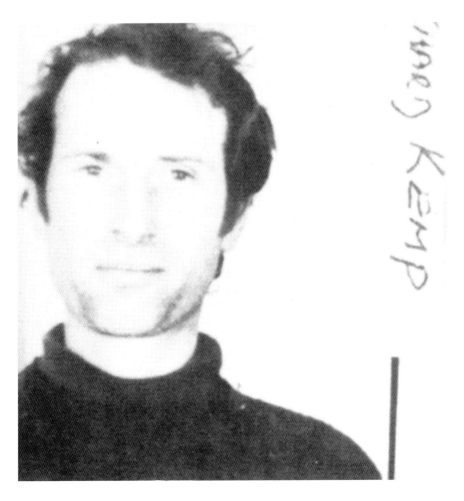

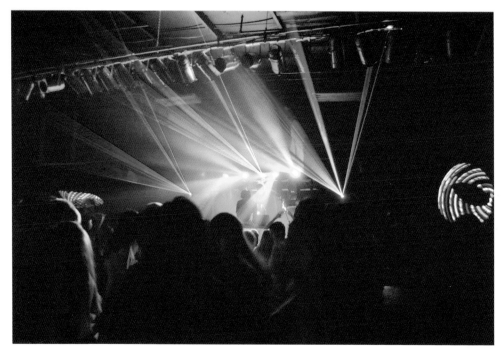

Lights, music, action. A typical rave scene from the 1990s. (Courtesy of Paulina Spencer)

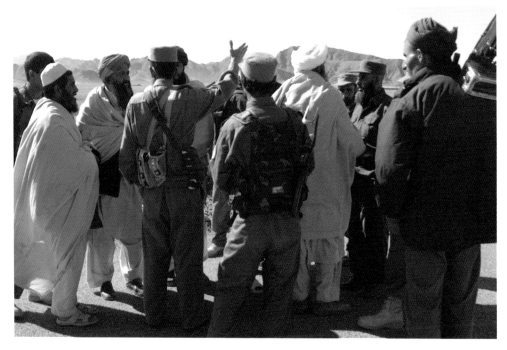

Angry poppy farmers argue with Afghan National Police District Chief Haji Khodadad about the ANP's plans to eradicate their poppy fields in Bala Baluk district on 15 April 2009. (Courtesy of the ISAF)

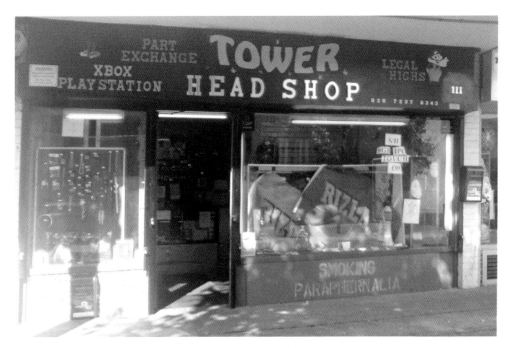

Head shops such as this one in Bermondsey sold legal highs and paraphernalia associated with recreational drug use, bridging the gap between legal recreational pursuits and illegal drug use. (Courtesy of Secret London)

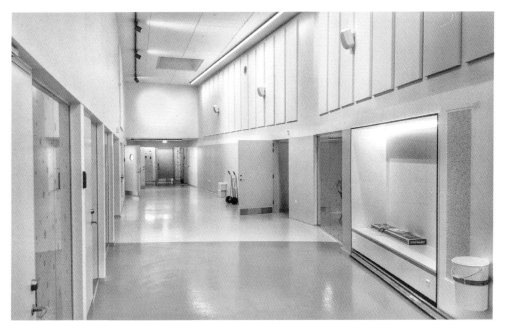

A supervised drug consumption facility in Denmark. UK drug charities have been campaigning for similar facilities to help reduce opioid overdoses. (Courtesy of Steve Rolles)

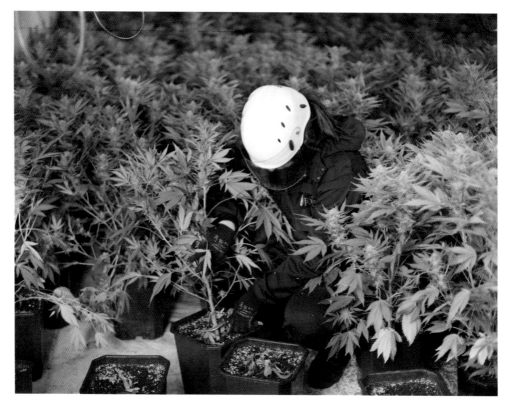

Police dismantle a large cannabis factory in Coventry. (Courtesy of the West Midlands Police)

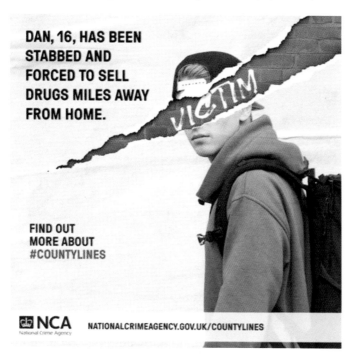

DAN, 16, HAS BEEN STABBED AND FORCED TO SELL DRUGS MILES AWAY FROM HOME.

VICTIM

FIND OUT MORE ABOUT #COUNTYLINES

NCA
National Crime Agency

NATIONALCRIMEAGENCY.GOV.UK/COUNTYLINES

Over the last decade, tackling the County Lines phenomenon has become a key plank UK drug policy.

The small group of 'junkie doctors' whose names and addresses are well known to everyone working in the field have inherited a situation which is now beyond control. It was inevitable that given the post-Brain situation, the black market would develop. The latest Home Office report to the UN comments on the 'significant increase in the number of addicts who have obtained the drug from entirely unknown sources'. The same report insists that 'the illicit traffic in narcotics is not extensive in the United Kingdom...' but how long will that last?

The 'notorious statement' the Reverend Leech referred to came in a reply by Kenneth Robinson to a parliamentary question about progress in setting up treatment centres. He said, 'There were already centres for the treatment of addicts and more beds could be made available if the demand increased.' He went on to say that a conference of doctors 'experienced in the treatment of drug addiction' was being convened in order to pool the medical knowledge on the subject. Except, of course, in 1966, there were almost no such doctors other than those prescribing in the community.

So little progress had been made by the following spring that on 8 May 1967, almost two years after the reconvened Brain Committee Report was signed off and 18 months after it was published, William Deedes MP, who had already raised the matter in the Commons on a number of occasions, complained,

> I get the strong impression that in some official quarters this is all regarded as a very tiresome, troublesome business which must not be allowed to delay other important matters. It is very tiresome and it is also very dangerous. I suggest that after two years we ought to move a little faster than we are moving. We are dealing with a small virulent plague which is being tackled in many places at walking pace.

Interviewed in 1982, Kenneth Robinson admitted, 'I don't think that I ever saw it as the sort of problem that could seriously embarrass the Government as long as we could say we were doing something about it and that initiatives were being taken.'[13]

And for Bing and his officials, the time between the publication of Brain 2 until the first new clinics actually opened on 16 April 1968 'was a period which gave totally new meanings to words like "immediate", "urgent" and "pressing" and saw the overworking of phrases such as "we are still consulting", "we are close in touch with" or "we are keeping the situation under review" – all euphemisms for, "we don't intend to do anything more or faster unless forced to do so by public, press or Parliamentary pressure".'[14] So why was there so little progress? Almost by definition, government bureaucracies are like slow-moving oil tankers. Beyond that, though, this was an entirely new social problem the officials really had no idea how to address. The medical establishment was largely unhelpful in trying to resolve the question of exactly how to get to grips with drug addiction by young 'non-therapeutic' users. The primary goal of the Second

Brain Report was to take prescribing out of the hands of GPs, whom they saw as the main reason for the rise in heroin use, and to restrict prescribing to a cohort of doctors working in new treatment centres, both to stop the spread of addiction and head off the development of an illicit market. That said, it did not specifically rule out other doctors prescribing so long as they had a Home Office licence.

Then the question arose, what do you do about those doctors who continue to prescribe irresponsibly? This was the focus of one delay as the British Medical Association (BMA) were initially unhappy about having to take on a disciplinary role and so it was back to the arguments about a Medical Tribunal. Then in meetings with the Home Office, the Ministry of Health raised the idea that maybe the new clinic doctors should only prescribe methadone, to which the Home Office officials, who had far more experience of the drug scene, responded along the lines of, 'Well, you won't get many people coming forward for treatment then.'

The idea of using methadone to treat heroin addiction was the brainchild of two American doctors, Vincent Dole and Marie Nyswander, who worked at New York's Rockefeller Institute for Medical Research and whose findings were published in the *Journal of the American Medical Association* in 1965. Working with a group of 22 patients for whom all other treatment had failed, they found a once-a-day prescription of methadone hydrochloride, an opiate drug but without the percussive effects of heroin, kept cravings and withdrawals at bay and which (in high enough doses) neutralised normal doses of heroin, enabling patients to get on with their lives. Furthermore, they took a Rolleston view that if this is what it took for heroin users to lead any sort of normal life, then methadone maintenance was clinically ethical. If there was any idea of trying to suggest to the psychiatrists who were due to take over the new clinics what they should or should not prescribe, it was quickly dropped in deference to the monolithic belief in the sanctity of professional medical judgement. But while the government seemed to be standing still in bringing on stream the new treatment centres, the heroin scene was moving on.

As Ken Leech alluded to, in November 1966 one of the major prescribing doctors, Geoffrey Dymond, suddenly pulled out of prescribing, leaving about 80 users scurrying around for a new legal supply. Then in May 1967, the same month that William Deedes was complaining about lack of action to implement Brain 2, Lady Frankau died. Her dozens of patients were also without a legal supply of drugs. Dr Hawes, who was already seeing approximately 400 users, then wrote to all the hospitals which the Ministry of Health claimed were providing addiction treatment, only to be rebuffed by all of them. Into the breach stepped a doctor who in his 18 months of prescribing probably did not dish out as much as Lady Frankau, but who rapidly earned himself the reputation as a solid gold media hate figure.

John Petro came from Poland at the age of 11 in 1916 as John Piotrkowski. An outstanding scholar, he studied at Cambridge and St George's Hospital Medical School and qualified in 1929 having won the coveted Brackenbury Prize for surgery. During the war, he was a naval Surgeon Lieutenant

Commander, had a speciality in dermatology, was seconded to work with Alexander Fleming on penicillin and became an early prescriber of the new wonder drug. Until 1950, he had a GP practice with his brother Alexander.

John Petro desperately wanted to be accepted by the British establishment and he was making steps in that direction. He was on the guest list of a black-tie fundraiser for the treatment of delinquency held at the Savoy Hotel and hosted by the Lord Chancellor. In 1960, he was called as a witness in a libel case involving the Duchess of Argyll where he said he was the Duke's doctor. But his private life was a mess; he went through two marriages and his weakness for gambling left him bankrupt and virtually destitute by the mid-1960s. I recall Petro being pointed out to me as he came into my father's betting shop.

The story goes that in early 1967, he met up with one of the Canadian users in the Golden Nugget Casino in Shaftesbury Avenue who suggested the doctor take on some of his compatriots and others as patients, as Lady Frankau was by then in hospital. Petro went to see Lady Frankau's companion Mrs Clarke, offering to take on the doctor's patients while she was indisposed. He later said that he did this as a favour to Sir Claude Frankau under whom Petro had learned his surgical skills, but the impression he was trying to give that he was a close friend of the family was not borne out when Mrs Clarke checked with Sir Claude himself. And so, according to Bing Spear's detailed internal memo of Petro's initial intervention in the addiction world, while Mrs Clarke was grateful for the offer, she still had grave misgivings about Dr Petro taking over Lady Frankau's caseload.

Initially, though, all seemed above board. When the Home Office first became aware of Dr Petro, he had a consulting room in Wimpole Street and a flat in Marylebone and declared his intentions to cooperate fully with officials, regularly phoning to check the backgrounds of his new patients and providing an initial list of 20 patients, all but one already known to the department.

However, owing to his extremely precarious financial situation, Dr Petro's daily life was as peripatetic and unpredictable as his patients. Almost as soon as he took on his new caseload, he lost both the surgery and the flat and began to prescribe from increasingly unconventional settings, which quickly brought him to the attention of the media. On 7 July 1967 both the *Daily Mail* and *The Sun* ran front-page stories that Dr Petro was seeing patients at the café in Baker Street underground station. The café manager quickly put a stop to this, forcing Dr Petro to cover his tracks from prying media eyes, moving from one seedy hotel to another, making arrangements with patients by phone or telegram to meet in particular cafés and pharmacies. Patients were phoning the Home Office to find out where he was, or which other doctors would be willing to prescribe.

On 10 August, Dr Petro turned up at the Home Office where the conversation centred not on his patients, but on Petro's contention that both the press and the police were conducting a witch hunt against him, after a constable stopped him coming out of a pub and asked him for some identity. He even suggested his phone was being tapped, all of which played to a general impression that having spectacularly failed to achieve the position in British society he craved, John Petro, now 62, combined the arrogance and sense of entitlement not uncommon in his profession with the patina of the fantasist.[15]

He actually asked Bing Spear and his colleague Detective Sergeant Patrick if they thought he was overprescribing, to which the answer was a resounding yes. Petro's patient load was increasing specifically because he was seen as a soft touch and there was evidence that his patients were selling surplus drugs.

From August to December 1967, Dr Petro found the owner of the Winton Hotel in Paddington willing to accommodate him and even provided a separate entrance for the use of patients. However, an article in the *Daily Express* on 17 December revealed that he had been evicted from the hotel resulting in more frantic calls to the Home Office from users seeking his whereabouts. He disappeared to Scotland over Christmas but resumed prescribing in public both from Bayswater and Paddington Station, even asking the Home Office to pass this information on to those who phoned up. His request for the Home Office to be in effect his personal post office was politely declined.

As unorthodox and eccentric as Dr Petro's conduct might have been, he hadn't broken any law, but the storm clouds were gathering. Because he had no permanent address, the Home Office informed chemists that his prescriptions were invalid, and he was buying supplies of controlled drugs without logging the purchases in his Dangerous Drugs Register. By now he had seen some 200 users, for whom in Bing's words 'he has been willing to prescribe in quantities which seem to bear a greater relationship to the addicts' ability to pay than to their actually physical needs'.

Dr Petro continued to complain to the Home Office about unwarranted media attention, but this didn't stop him agreeing to appear on the *Frost Programme* in January 1968 where he faced an unsurprisingly hostile audience. Confronted by patients who told the programme how easy it was to obtain drugs from Dr Petro, he openly admitted not checking patient stories with the Home Office, claiming that a doctor as experienced in the addiction problem as he was, could easily determine the accuracy of what he was being told – a claim also made by Lady Frankau. The interview with Dr Petro and another by David Frost with the corrupt businessman Emil Savundra saw MP Alex Lyon urge that there should be a ban on trial by television as neither man at that point had faced criminal charges. Coincidentally, Savundra died aged only 53, dependent on pethidine for chronic back pain.

Dr Petro was arrested immediately following his television appearance on charges related to his failure to keep proper records of drug purchases and was fined a total of £1,700 on 17 different counts. The fact that he had been convicted of an offence, meant that he was now in the crosshairs of the General Medical Council (GMC). Peter, the user referred to earlier, had crashed his car while high on Methedrine supplied by Dr Petro and was sent to Borstal, an early form of youth custody centre, on an indeterminate sentence. 'GMC lawyers came to see me and suggested they could do something about that. They put a lot of pressure on me, but I wouldn't say a bad word against him.'

The Second Brain report did not name the 'six doctors' who were being blamed for London's heroin epidemic; Lady Frankau was one and it likely that another three were those named by the *News of the World* in its exposé published just two days after John Petro's arrest. The paper named Drs Wood, Mellor and Cohen, who stood accused of the standing operating procedure of the 'script doctor' – overprescribing, not trying to reduce dosages and taking users' accounts of their needs at face value in pursuit of the consultation fee. The doctors were getting the blame for all the concerns about the drug problem.

By the time John Petro faced his peers at the GMC in May 1968, the Dangerous Drugs Act 1967 with the attendant 1968 Regulations had come into force. It banned GPs from prescribing heroin or cocaine in support of an addiction without a Home Office licence. And some of the hitherto mythical NHS London drug clinics had finally opened their doors. Meanwhile, behind the closed doors of the GMC hearings, Dr John Petro was found guilty of infamous professional conduct and ordered to be struck off the medical register but given leave to appeal, not due to be heard until October, during which time he was allowed to continue prescribing. He could no longer prescribe heroin or cocaine, but there was nothing to stop him or any other like-minded doctor from prescribing Methedrine, which he and others prescribed in unwarranted quantities causing chaos on the London drug scene.

Ken Leech wrote in 1973,

Towards the end of 1967 and particularly during 1968 we were caught up in the most significant drug epidemic in the recent history of London's drug culture. [Methedrine] began to circulate on a large scale ... a very powerful cerebral stimulant ... Introduced originally in the late 1930s, its use had been restricted to post-operative conditions, spinal anaesthesia and to some extent abreaction in psychiatry and the treatment of obesity. The use of oral Methedrine became obsolete with that of the other amphetamines (though they continue to be prescribed) and by the time of the epidemic of illicit use, the clinical use of the injectable preparation had become very limited. Injectable Methedrine began to spread among two sections of the drug-taking population. The first was that of heroin addicts who now began to use Methedrine instead of cocaine. The second was the amphetamine users who had progressed from oral to intravenous use of the drug. It was the spread of Methedrine ampoules which above all else brought together the heroin addicts and the wider community of adolescents who were involved with amphetamine use. It was Methedrine which played the 'escalation role' which is often wrongly attributed to cannabis. It was Methedrine which made the process of fixing an integral part of West End drug culture. The West End was not the same after Methedrine: it was more destructive, more hopeless, more needle centred.[16]

The Haight-Ashbury district of San Francisco was hit by a similar epidemic of injectable methamphetamine (and heroin) use, where the slogan 'speed kills' originated. *International Times* issued a warning about the drug in August

1968 calling it 'one of the most dangerous drugs around at the moment' and listing a battery of bad effects, most notably a paranoid psychosis often indistinguishable from paranoid schizophrenia, as well as a general warning about injecting with unsterile needles to a community of mainly LSD and cannabis users unused to injecting drugs. As it happened, your regular hippy wanted nothing to do with Methedrine, but Ken Leech and his co-workers were seeing numbers of very damaged, unstable young people, regularly in trouble with the police and often sleeping rough, who gravitated from Methedrine to heroin.

Based on an internal memo from Bing Spear, it is possible that Dr Petro was the most prolific of the overprescribing Methedrine doctors. By checking through pharmacy records, the Home Office established that in May 1968 alone, Dr Petro prescribed 24,905 ampoules of Methedrine to 110 patients.

Petro was hardly out of court during 1968, turning up to one appearance in a Rolls-Royce and wearing a yellow carnation. He was named in the trial of Sarah Nash, wife of Soho club boss Raymond Nash, on charges of amphetamine possession; his 'secretary', Denise Oran, was jailed for possession; Petro himself was in court charged with stealing a cigarette lighter and two cigarettes. He was eventually struck off in October 1968, but his legal troubles didn't end there. In March 1969, he was fined for fraudulently obtaining credit as an undischarged bankrupt, then arrested as he left the court for failing to pay the £1,700 fine; he ended up in prison for 3 months.

In November 1969, he was caught with a tiny amount of cannabis at Glasgow Airport, after which he dropped out of view, going to work as a volunteer for the Simon Community for homeless people. There was one last court appearance in Brighton in 1975 for obtaining some slimming tablets 'by deception'. In 1980 I tracked him down to a nursing home in Northwood, just outside London, in the hope of an interview, but by then dementia had entirely isolated him from the world and he died a year later. However, I did get a glimpse of some fragments of an autobiography which he said had been commissioned by a Sunday newspaper back in 1968. It was never finished, and he never got as far as his days as a 'script doctor'. He said he was in the States during prohibition and remembered seeing people literally blind drunk from bathtub alcohol and being refused admission to hospital because they were breaking the law, although it was never illegal to drink during prohibition. He cited the failure of prohibition as the natural outcome of interfering with human liberty, which perhaps framed his attitude to prescribing and drug addiction, and his disdain for the medical establishment – its attempt to control doctors, its rigid conservatism and general autocratic demeanour. He believed with some justification that he was being made the scapegoat for the failure to control addiction, although he did court the limelight. Perhaps the ultimate tragedy was that for somebody who obviously craved an association with society headliners, when he himself hit the headlines, it was the beginning of the process by which his career was destroyed.

It is hard to imagine any doctor these days being able to operate even remotely as did Dr Petro. His patients called him the barefoot doctor; he slept on their floors, at Ken Leech's Centrepoint and at the Simon Community and for a while when he couldn't even prescribe from a railway station, he was driven around by a patient offering a drugs-on-wheels prescribing service. While no doubt most of the staff at the new clinics would have had no time for Dr Petro, at least one doctor took a more empathetic view.

In 1973, Dr Margaret Tripp, who ran the drug dependency unit at St Clement's Hospital in the East End, wrote a sympathetic account of the doctor entitled *Who Speaks for Petro* in *Drugs and Society*. One rainy evening she went with Dr Petro down to Piccadilly Circus where a small group of his ex-patients regularly congregated.

> He introduced me to each one and told me the long and complex story of their life ... Standing next to him, I perceived the closeness of their relationship. There was no doubting the genuineness of the affection the addicts had for him. Calling him by his first name, congratulating him on the successful outcome of his last lawsuit, there was no reserve in their replies to his questions. The barrier always present between themselves and clinic staff was gone. He was both their doctor and one of them. Listening to him I realised for the first time how total was his addiction. His committal to the lifestyle was as great as any user in the clinic. He had reached the position where nothing else is as interesting and everything seems less real in comparison. I perceived that although I stood next to him, he was in a different place where, for many reasons, I could not join him.[17]

Soon after this meeting, the powers that be found a way of stopping Petro, even offering some basic primary care, tending injecting wound abscesses down the 'Dilly.

The prescribing doctors of the 1960s were a complex combination of the caring, the compassionate, the naïve and the arrogant. For some, there was a modest financial aspect to this. Then there was Dr Christopher Swan, the lead character in one of more disturbing prescribing stories of this period.

Calling him only Dr X, Dr Jim Willis mentioned Dr Swan in a chapter he wrote on the early days of the drug clinics for a book edited by Professor Sir John Strang and Dr Michael Gossop. 'I attended a court hearing in Southend in which his prescribing had led to disaster and recognised him as a doctor I had met briefly in 1964 when he was a registrar ... He turned out to be a smooth-talking young man who looked and dressed like a car salesman.' Dr Willis went on to describe Dr Swan as thinking he could pass all the necessary exams to be a consultant within a few months.[18]

The recent crisis in US opioid painkiller addiction and overdose was fuelled by doctors setting up what are known as 'pill mills'. These doctors, several of whom had been struck off, simply set up shop handing out large amounts of painkillers for cash and devoid of any medical justification. This is pretty much what Dr Swan was doing from his East London surgery, using local gangsters to dispense the drugs.

Before he was appointed as the consultant psychiatrist at University College Hospital addiction clinic, Dr Martin Mitcheson was a researcher at the Institute of Psychiatry and was the lead researcher of the team who published a paper about methedrine use in the *British Medical Journal* in 1969. Of their cohort of 74 regular users, a majority got their drugs from 'a single practice'. This was Dr Swan's practice where Dr Mitcheson went to interview Methedrine users and saw at first-hand what was going on at 8 Queensbridge Road, Hackney. 'He had a terrace house with steps up and step down. Steps up to his consulting room and steps down to a waiting room and where local criminals were giving out prescriptions. Swanny was not prescribing amphetamines; he was writing blank prescriptions onto which the criminals would just fill in the names, usually false.'[19]

Dr Mitcheson, who quietly admits that the whole scene was rather exciting, was there doing interviews when the police raided the surgery. 'They were all over the place. Afterwards I got a call from Bing Spear to say that Inspector X from Scotland Yard was not so unobservant as not to notice the heroin tablets [belonging to the interviewee] you pushed under the telephone.' It is likely that Dr Swan ended up prescribing more Methedrine than Dr Petro simply because he had a regular place to practice and an 'organisation' assisting with distribution. During a court case involving one of his patients, it transpired he had prescribed 3,500 ampoules to one 19-year-old over the course of 6 weeks.

Violence never seemed too far away from what purported to be an ordinary GP surgery. Back in 1968, a teenager named Michael Fagan was heavily into Methedrine supplied by Dr Swan. Fagan's father, also called Michael, broke into the surgery and smashed it up. He didn't try to run from the police but remained there so he could explain why he did it. Apparently, he had intended to kill Dr Swan, but changed his mind. Fagan senior was ordered to pay damages and conditionally discharged. Fagan junior went on to break into Buckingham Palace twice in the early 1980s to engage in conversation with the Queen. He was later charged with a heroin supply offence. Events at Dr Swan's surgery took an even uglier turn.

John Wall was one of two minders employed by Swan to keep order in the surgery, which was often full of drug users wired on amphetamines looking for more supplies. Swan sacked Wall, who began to tell people about what was going on there and so Swan decided that Wall should be taught a lesson. He hired a nightclub bouncer, David Gordon, to do the job, but instead of just beating Wall up, the bouncer stabbed him.

Swan then fell out with Stephen Hartford, employed as Swan's medical secretary, and incited Brian Stevens and John Vaughan to murder Hartford and another man, John White. He also incited John Vaughan to murder George Speller and Mary Rood. She was in the dock charged with being in possession of instruments used in the performance of abortions on two Irish girls.

All this took place between June and August 1968. After various court appearances, finally, at the Old Bailey on 3 January 1969, Dr Swan was found guilty on all the charges – soliciting murder, drug offences, being involved in arranging illegal abortions – oh, and being in receipt of a typewriter he knew to be stolen. The conspiracy to murder seems to have been hatched while Dr Swan was on remand and when he had a mental breakdown.

As a consequence, aged 32, he was sentenced to 15 years in Broadmoor, the hospital for the criminally insane.

Yet again, Dr Tripp took a more magnanimous view of Dr Swan than most, telling Horace Judson, an American journalist who had come to write about 'The British System' that knowing the pressure prescribing doctors were under, she felt much sympathy for Chris Swan. 'He was an unfortunate and ill-used man and when I first met him, he was by no means mad. He explained to me at great length and in great detail why the clinics were going to fail.'[20] Swan himself declared, 'These young people are cracked kids from a cracked society. I see myself as rather like a worker-priest; someone with courage enough to vary out his beliefs in an unorthodox way.'[21]

With both Drs Petro and Swan out of action and the end of retail supplies of Methedrine to pharmacies, the epidemic petered out. And with the clinics up and running, the story of the sixties-type renegade doctor came to an end. However, as so often in this story, an issue that might seem to have been resolved turned out not to be.

8

Masterful Inactivity

As the sixties progressed, the drug scene in London fragmented around the capital, but still focused on the use of cannabis, LSD and pharmaceutical amphetamine, cocaine and heroin. As we enter the seventies, the story becomes more complex, especially in relation to those quite literally at the sharp end of injecting drug use, where a range of different pharmaceutical drugs begin to substitute for the ebb and flow of illicit heroin now coming into the country for the first time from different parts of the world. The widespread use of drugs right across the country such as barbiturates, methaqualone (Mandrax), methylphenidate (Ritalin) and dipipanone (Diconal) constitute Britain's hidden drug history, but which were central to the spread of injecting drug use across the UK.

By the autumn of 1968, there were 39 clinics across England and Wales: 15 in London based at the main teaching hospitals and 24 elsewhere, although to describe what was on offer outside of London as much more than a very basic service would be stretching a point. Even in London, a clinic specifically for treating people with a heroin addiction was regarded by most hospital authorities as their dirty little secret; facilities were often squirreled away out of sight or given anodyne descriptions such as Psychiatric Unit Annexe to hide the true nature of what became known as Drug Dependency Units or DDUs run by consultant psychiatrists with a team including junior doctors, social workers and nurses. Those early days were quite chaotic as Dr Jim Willis explained. They were expected by some to 'solve' the drug problem and by others to 'fail' in equal measure:

> ... it is hard to convey the amount of concern that the 'Drug Menace' had engendered. From day one the psychiatrists in the DDUs were to be watched by the media, by social scientists and criminologists, by the clergy, by an army of the well-meaning and most of all by their colleagues ... who remained lofty and judgemental towards the patients and towards the Drug Doctors, who represented the dirty end of psychiatry as far as they were concerned... It seemed as if everyone was waiting for us to screw up.[1]

In the wake of the recommendations of the Second Brain Report, and with some experience of heroin addiction through his work in two mental hospitals, Dr Willis was appointed as a DDU consultant in 1967, but despite the government memo to hospital boards instructing them to make premises available for the new clinics, Dr Willis spent months battling the medical establishment's stalling and indifference and local resident hostility and threats of violence before finally establishing the DDU at St Giles Hospital in south London.

'It was hard going at first,' he recalled, 'as I started on my own – having been told in no uncertain terms to "get on with it" – and just took on the patients and began a clean-up operation. This was a valuable lesson since I soon found out what a ghastly experience the prescribing general practitioners had endured and that management of addicts by the unsupported is a hopeless task.'

This was brought home by the experience of Dr John Owens, the psychiatrist who ran an early clinic at All Saints Hospital in Birmingham and whose methods became a model for others. Owens' clinic was visited by Home Secretary Roy Jenkins, who came away impressed with the procedures in place for establishing individual addiction status, assessing dosage regimes and avoiding forged or altered prescriptions through a policy of posting prescriptions direct to pharmacists. As he told the American journalist Horace Judson, Jenkins was particularly impressed by the degree to which Owens could demonstrate that the 'clinic approach to controlled prescribing could work'.[2] The clinic also received favourable mentions in Parliament from William Deedes and *The Times* and much later commended by Bing Spear in his book.

There was more to what Owens was doing than just keeping excess heroin off the streets of Birmingham by controlling prescribing. Much of the success of the early years of the clinic came down to treating people as individuals, involving them in decisions about their treatment, and generally taking a pragmatic and flexible approach.

However, there was an unfortunate end to this encouraging story. The clinic became so overwhelmed by patient numbers by 1972 that Dr Owens, trying to cope single-handedly with a huge caseload, became addicted to amphetamines and alcohol. Under pressure, he unwisely gave signed blank prescriptions to a staff member who was handing out prescriptions in exchange for whiskey and cigars. One such incident was witnessed by Dr Martin Mitcheson, who headed the DDU at London's University College Hospital and was the only London addiction psychiatrist to take the trouble to visit the Birmingham clinic. Eventually in 1976, Dr Owens was barred from prescribing controlled drugs, but it was accepted that his actions were foolish, not venal.

In the early 1970s, Dr Mitcheson himself was interviewed by Judson and was honest enough to admit, '"The Psychopathology of the Prescribing Doctor" – that's a paper that will never be written'[3] as he was very much aware that he and his colleagues were on the same prescribing spectrum as the 'script doctors', as the fate of Dr Owens showed.

There was a most unusual dynamic at play between doctor and drug user, unlike any other in the NHS. People go to see their doctor hoping for a diagnosis of their ailment and there is a natural imbalance of power; you are worried about your health and you will usually bow to the superior knowledge of the doctor as to the nature of the problem and what to do about it. At the extreme end, surgeons literally have the power of life and death in their hands. No wonder that such god-like power results in god-like behaviour by many doctors who regard their clinical freedom as sacrosanct and their clinical judgement as inviolable and beyond criticism especially from those they regard as entirely unqualified to question their authority. Then into the surgery or clinic come the heroin users who know everything about their condition, probably more than the doctor and moreover know exactly what drug(s) and dosages they require. Furthermore, they are not backward in coming forward to demand what they view as their 'right' because they have been 'notified' to the Home Office and therefore are 'registered addicts'. Under these circumstances, either the doctor, through fear or greed, or just to be rid of the patient, caves in – or there ensues what Alex Trocchi called in 1966 'a battle of wits' between doctor and patient because while the power balance might appear to be more equal, the user was still reliant on the doctor to write that all-important prescription. As the clinic system bedded in, it was a battle of wits in which the clinic doctor was more likely to prevail due to a growing body of peer support that was not available to the isolated community GP.

Dr Willis for one was very grateful for the support of Dr Mitcheson who was '... great. He arrived on the doorstep at St Giles in search of research material [when he was working at the Addiction Research Unit before taking over at the University College of London's DDU], saw how overloaded I was and just got stuck in. I'll never forget his cheery support and real help. My spirits always rose when he poked his head round the door.'[4]

The name of the game when the DDUs first opened was the competitive prescribing of heroin to undercut any prospective illicit market, but until the end of 1968, they were literally in competition with Drs Petro and Swan. From April 1968, GPs were no longer able to prescribe cocaine and the DDU doctors very quickly agreed that they would not prescribe it either. But the liberal supply of injectable Methedrine was, as Dr Willis described it, 'our worst problem ... The associated behavioural disturbance and the slipping in and out of psychosis made it obvious that this was a practice that had to be stopped ... until methylamphetamine was removed from the scene, there was a constant air of menace that hung around many patients in states of chronic paranoid tension.'[5]

But even those not on Methedrine were in pretty poor shape:

At first, we had a large proportion of patients with major personality disorders ... patients with arms and legs covered in needle tracks, dirty, unkempt and lice-ridden were the norm. There was a general idea, fostered by the media, that many bogus addicts would be taken on and given drugs they did not need, so that they could sell them. My experience was that such phonies were infrequent and easily spotted, including one reporter from a daily newspaper. It may be imagined that the early days were edgy and uncertain.

The situation for those working in the clinics did calm down as 1968 gave way to 1969. There were still confrontations, arguments and the odd violent outburst, but while staff recruitment was never easy – there were no other applicants when Dr Margaret Tripp applied to run the DDU at St Clement's Hospital in East London – some of the staff who were taken on became legendary. Dr Willis hired a porter, a soldier in the Territorial Army, who acted as the clinic 'minder'. 'He had a quiet authority and could calm potential aggression by poking his head around the door and saying, "Everything all right, Dr Willis?" Another of his self-appointed tasks was to get people to tidy themselves up. "Go and get a shave ... Dr Willis is in there in a nice suit ... If he goes to that trouble, so can you. Show respect."

Some patients tried the tricks that possibly worked with the more disreputable doctors. When they were both working at the Addiction Research Unit, Professor Gerry Stimson and Edna Oppenheimer began a 10-year follow-up study of people coming forward to DDUs from 1969 to 1979. One girl aged 18 at the time the clinics opened featured in a TV documentary about the changes on the scene once the clinics took over from the GP. She told the researchers, 'So I went down and I got dressed up ... in a little black chiffon dress and fishnet stockings. And I walked into the clinic and the doctor said, "What are you doing here?" I said, "I've come down to seduce you so that I can have a script."'[6]

Those in the waiting room would ask somebody what mood the doctor was in or leave it as late as possible on a Friday afternoon to ask for 'extras' over the weekend. Early on, the doctors were presented with claims from some patients, especially those who had been seeing Dr Petro, that they received very high doses of heroin. One patient went so far as to obtain a letter from Bing Spear confirming the level of prescription he was obtaining.

As an aside and as an indication of how different the times were, users in search of prescribing doctors would turn up to see Bing in person. He would buy them a cup of tea in the canteen or nearby café in order to learn what was new on the street drug scene. It is hard to imagine a Home Office official now going off with a street heroin user for a latte and a chat in a coffee shop.

As time went on, the doctors and the users came to an accommodation, mainly because the doctors came to a sort of agreement among themselves about DDU prescribing policy. Just as the Home Office had turned to the Rolleston Committee to determine addiction treatment policy, so the renamed Department of Health and Social Security (DHSS) relied on a small group of influential consultant psychiatrists to determine the prescribing policy of the clinics. Stimson and Oppenheimer defined 'The British System' as 'a loose collection of ideas, policies, institutions and activities. There is a legal framework within which clinic doctors and other staff work, but the translation of this into day-to-day practice leaves considerable room for individual initiative and interpretation.'[7]

So, in respect of competitive prescribing, some doctors such as Jim Willis, Dale Beckett and Judith Morgan were more 'liberal' than say Drs Gisela Oppenheimer, Martin Mitcheson and particularly Philip Connell. He refused to believe in the idea of the 'stabilised addict' and with the force of his personality presided over the informal peer pressure brought to bear at the London consultants meetings originally hosted by the DHSS and then (because of car parking problems) at the Home Office. Connell's colleagues welcomed the chance for some peer support – they all agreed not to provide replacement prescriptions for alleged losses, not to see patients from other clinics unless there were special reasons and not to increase doses or provide 'allowances' for holidays and so on (although some did, telling their patients not to tell anybody). It brought a level of consistency and continuity to clinical practice so that one clinic could not be played off against another in this ongoing 'battle of wits'.

However, the more liberally minded doctors resented metaphorically having an arm twisted behind their back. Dr Willis wrote he had 'little time for zealots' and felt that it quickly became a competition to see who could prescribe the least amount of heroin. The same zealots were heavily critical of Dr Willis for providing sterile needles, syringes and water: 'I felt it was the logical thing to do. If we were providing the drug, then we should see to it that the patient injected it dissolved in sterile water, as opposed to the water from the toilets in Piccadilly ... If this was colluding in a destructive process, then all I can say is that the incidence of infections fell away rapidly.'[8]

Some of the clinics also provided what are now called drug consumption rooms for users to inject their prescription, but these too fell out of favour over time. There were some enlightened pharmacists too; Mr Hall who ran Hall's in Shaftesbury Avenue would sell all the paraphernalia for injecting to anybody whereas Boots and John Croyden & Bell restricted sales to those in possession of a script for injectable drugs.

There was an element of rivalry between the leading consultants as government funding became tighter through the decade: Dr Mitcheson said that nobody wanted to miss a government meeting 'in case somebody else got more of the jam'.[9] Patients thought the doctors were under pressure from the government to cut back on prescribing injectable heroin. But the consultants enjoyed a very cosy relationship with officials and there is no evidence that they were pressured to do anything they wouldn't otherwise do. More significantly, the practice of competitive prescribing never sat easy with most of the staff who quickly began to feel they were either quasi-pharmacists or policemen. Not only were they expected to head off an illicit market, but they were also acting as agents of social control to undermine the drug culture itself. So, for example, by sending prescriptions direct to pharmacies and dictating exactly when those prescriptions could be dispensed, they attempted to eliminate the sort of gathering of the clans which had previously existed outside the West End all-night pharmacies at a minute past midnight when those in receipt of large heroin and cocaine prescriptions would be on hand to sell surplus supplies to waiting users. Staff were also spending significant amounts of time controlling user behaviour inside the clinic, taking urine tests, drawing up behaviour contracts, and arguing over reductions in prescriptions for infractions of the rules. Even the act of maintenance prescribing was uncomfortable for some staff, as they were supposed to be 'curing' people. By and large patients simply wanted a script and not, for example, psychological therapies or opportunities for detoxification. In short, many staff felt the work was offering them little in the way of 'therapeutic reward'. They were working in a hospital, employed by the NHS, but could their working environment really warrant the name 'clinic' or the people they were seeing as 'patients? In a way, what was happening called into question the application of a rigid medical model on a situation that was far more complex. There was an acceptance in official reports and among professionals that drug users were not inherently 'bad' simply because they used drugs, so therefore they had to be either sad, mad, or both, and therefore ripe for psychiatric intervention. All the misgivings among the staff about what the clinics were supposed to be doing were reflected in the prescribing statistics. According to the Stimson/ Oppenheimer study, in 1968, 60–80 per cent of the approximately 1,000 patients the new clinics were faced with were in receipt of heroin, only a year later that figure was down to 34 per cent and more than 50 per cent were solely on methadone, and by 1978 less than 10 per cent were on heroin. The switch to methadone was also reflected in the move away from any injectable prescribing, not just to oral methadone for new and returning patients but to reducing doses increasingly becoming time limited. Two additional factors served to reinforce the existing policy.

The first was a study undertaken by Dr Mitcheson and researcher Richard Hartnoll. They conducted a controlled study at University College London (UCL) between 1972 and '75 to see if there was any difference in outcome for those prescribed heroin or oral methadone. There was no clear conclusion to be drawn from the study as to which approach was superior, but it was taken to mean, especially by those psychiatrists who didn't or rarely prescribed heroin anyway, that their way was the right way. The second factor in reducing the availability of injectable heroin was the decision by the manufacturer of the heroin tablets to replace them with freeze-dried ampoules of heroin. Tablet manufacture is relatively cheap, but now the heroin was encased in a glass capsule which was more expensive to produce. What this meant for increasingly cash-strapped clinics in the mid-1970s as the British economy was imploding, was you could maintain 100 patients on methadone for the same price as 6 on the new ampoules.[10]

The relationship between many of the street heroin users of the 1960s and the more notorious of the prescribing doctors could hardly be called therapeutic as users hopped from one doctor to another in search of a script. But strong relationships did build up over years between clinic users, the doctors and other staff. When Dr Mitcheson visited a patient of his in prison and told her he was leaving UCL, she smashed up her cell. Despite all the trials and tribulations of working with a difficult and challenging patient group, and colleagues who could be equally difficult, Dr Willis did feel that among the consultants, 'there was a great amount of goodwill and the feeling that we were all in it together'[11] and that overall,

> despite daily criticism of our failure to solve the problem, sweep it under the carpet, or whatever we were expected to do, I believe our people did their best to set up programmes which evolved gradually and changed radically in the process. It was a brave attempt to tackle a little-understood problem by a group of well-intentioned persons who were not motivated by personal gain beyond their NHS salaries. Furthermore, it was not as has sometimes been represented, an attempt to railroad patients into a coercive system with no regard for anything beyond arguments over prescriptions. A general impression has been created that the system was 'uncaring'... It wasn't like that at all. Caring for patients isn't all about touchy-feeliness and emotional incontinence.

For the patients who were willing to engage, the clinics did their best with limited resources and little general support from the medical profession. However, there were many others who did not want to present to the 'authorities', were sceptical that the Addicts Index of notifications was truly confidential even from the police and, like the Canadians who went home to a more exciting if dangerous life on the streets, some users did not want the constraints of turning up for clinic appointments, giving urine samples and so on. One of the consultant psychiatrists, Dr Thomas Bewley, said he saw it as his job to 'bore' people out of addiction. There was also a significant cohort who did not want methadone, regarded its effects as worse than heroin and felt they were better served by obtaining the illicitly imported heroin which began to appear on London streets as early as the summer of 1967.

A letter from Dr Hawes published in *The Times* on 3 June 1967 warned colleagues that

> the most threatening portent is that addicts are telling me that there is plenty of the stuff even though the source from overprescribing doctors is drying up. [The price of a regular sixth of a grain heroin tablet jumped from £1 to £3]. It looks as if big business, which has been waiting in the wings for so long, has now taken over the stage and is playing the lead. So we may look for an explosion in the teenage addict population as the months go by.

Early imported heroin supplies were known as 'Chinese' heroin, but they did not come from the Chinese mainland, rather from the area known as the Golden Triangle comprising the border regions of Burma, Laos and Thailand but which was controlled by Chinese nationals, the remnants of Chiang Kai-shek's Kuomintang army. The drugs were brought out of the region through transit points such as the Hong Kong New Territories and Malaysia, finding their way to the UK and onwards to London's Chinese community as opium supplies had done, hidden on ships coming in the UK ports, through the post and in airport luggage. The earliest heroin was dirty cream in colour and granular like cat litter and was dubbed 'Heroin No. 3' or 'rice' with a purity of 30–45 per cent, the rest accounted for by caffeine and quinine.

Users could also buy a finer white powder of higher quality called 'Heroin No. 4' or 'elephant' as the packets carried an elephant logo.

The heroin powder scene started off very small; the Chinese who controlled the heroin market from their base in Gerrard Street dealt with white 'go-betweens' who would sell on to London users. One of these runners was 'Jan':

> The guys importing heroin weren't really interested in drugs as such, they just wanted money for gambling. I'd be in one of their clubs where they played Mah-jong, hand over the money and they would just go straight to the tables with it. I'd buy an ounce for say £60 (nearly £1,000 today), meet the contact in the Tottenham Court Road, follow him to Kentish Town, collect the drugs then back to the West End … and of course, there were rip-offs; rice looked like brick dust and a mate of mine sold brick dust to some American tourists imagining he'd never see them again until they cornered him in Gerrard Street and pulled a gun on him. But it was broad daylight in a busy street, so he got away.

Compared to the record 1 ton of herbal cannabis seized at Heathrow and a whopping 3 tons of hash intercepted at Karachi Airport in Pakistan bound for the UK in the early 1970s, heroin seizures were tiny – 1.1 kilos in 1971, which rose to only 4 kilos by 1975. Apparently, some Lebanese dealers had so little success selling their heroin in London that they were caught trying to re-export it to the States.[12] And what little illicit heroin was about in London in the early 1970s was becoming more expensive; 30 milligrams of street heroin sold at £5 in the summer of 1972, and that sum would only get you 15 milligrams a year later with very restricted leakage from the licit market.

Even so, Bing Spear at the Home Office and his boss Peter Beedle were frustrated by the indifference of the police to what they perceived was the beginnings of a serious problem. In 1970, in response to an internal note from Bing Spear in 1969 raising concerns, the Met responded that there was, 'no evidence that the use of Chinese heroin could be an escalating problem among the drug addicts of this country'. Senior Customs management did not seem that bothered either, arguing that whatever slipped through could be picked up by the police, although officers of the Customs Investigative Branch took a different view. In 1970, one of their number briefed a minister whose name he didn't disclose but was probably Home Secretary Reginald Maudling about the potential threat posed to the UK by international traffickers. The minister was alleged to have responded, 'it is not in the British nature to either smuggle, peddle or take illicit drugs. There have been a few seizures of heroin and cocaine. Furthermore, I am advised that the Mafia and Triads are figments of your imagination. Further discussion is pointless.'[13]

Probably the primary reason why the heroin market in the UK was slow to take off, despite the scarcity of pharmaceutical heroin on the streets, was the presence of a range of pharmaceutical drugs to which injecting drug users increasingly turned.

Barbiturates are classed as sedative/hypnotic drugs and, like amphetamines had been before, were freely available from GPs. Under trade names such as Nembutal, Seconal, Amytal and Tuinal they were used to treat insomnia in the general population with some types effective for the treatment of epilepsy. They had a high dependence potential with an equally high risk of accidental overdose because of the very narrow margin between a therapeutic and a lethal dose. Unlike heroin, medically unsupervised barbiturate withdrawal could be fatal. Between 1965 and 1970, doctors in England and Wales wrote 24 million prescriptions for barbiturates – drugs which claimed the lives of more than 12,000 people during the same period. Elderly and vulnerable doctors could be coerced into prescribing; in one case a doctor on house call was held hostage until he signed some scripts.[14] Beyond the prescription pad, thefts from manufacturers and pharmacies were another ready source of supply.

Either by accident or design (swallowing barbiturates washed down with alcohol was a common form of suicide), the drugs infamously took the lives of Marilyn Monroe, Jimi Hendrix, Judy Garland and British comedians Tony Hancock and Kenneth Williams. Even more dangerous than swallowing pills was the practice of crushing the pills to inject them. Users reckoned that you got a better buzz from heroin if you shot up some barbs as well, but the pills were never meant for intravenous injection and would often solidify in veins which, in several cases, led to gangrene and limb amputations. Barb freaks, as they were known, were often seen staggering around the West End or slumped in subways. The newly established clinics were entirely unable to deal with barbiturate users who invariably ended up in a revolving A&E door of overdosing, admittance, then being kicked out onto the streets, only to be readmitted 24 hours later.

Heroin users had been injecting barbiturates from the early 1960s, but it took several years and a reduction in the licit heroin supply for the problem to become acute. In a 1969 study of London heroin users, 80 per cent said they had injected barbiturates. There were talks about including barbiturates in the Misuse of Drugs Act, but there was resistance from the medical profession which didn't want to be restricted in their use for a range of conditions even though barbiturates were being superseded by benzodiazepine tranquillisers such as Valium which, for all the problems they would cause, were at least safer in overdose. Instead doctors started a voluntary scheme to cut back on prescribing under the acronym CURB, but this was largely ineffective.

In 1971, a new voluntary sector agency was founded called the Standing Conference on Drug Abuse (SCODA) whose role was to represent the growing number of voluntary sector street drug agencies which were isolated, poorly funded and with no access to central government. SCODA's early campaign was to urge the setting up of a special short-stay residential facility in London for barbiturate users to try to break the cycle of repeated overdose and hospital admissions. It would take nearly a decade for City Roads to open its doors in 1978, managed not by a psychiatrist but a social worker.[15]

The other sleeping pill in circulation on the street was a methaqualone/ antihistamine combination drug marketed as Mandrax in the UK and

Quaaludes in the USA. Known as mandies, Mandrax induced a drunken-like stupor similar to barbiturates, but which had nothing like the same baleful social impact because the drug became controlled under the Misuse of Drugs Act making availability far more restricted and there was no injecting culture. Quaaludes were a far bigger problem in the States where a condition known as 'luding out' became common especially in rock 'n' roll circles; Keith Richards was caught in possession and the drug was name-checked in songs by Frank Zappa and David Bowie.

Heroin users also latched onto the use of methylphenidate, marketed as Ritalin, as they discovered that injecting the drug as a so-called 'speedball' with heroin (or methadone) reduced the amount of opiate required to get the desired effect and extended the duration of euphoria. 'Jan' says that most GPs didn't have a clue about addiction and could be conned into writing prescriptions by telling them that Ritalin had greatly helped in the fight against alcoholism.

The drug which had most impact on the injecting drug scene across the UK during the 1970s and early 1980s was dipipanone, marketed as Diconal. The drug was developed by Burroughs Wellcome as a painkiller in injectable form, but the formulation induced excessive vomiting and was changed to include an anti-nausea drug called Cyclizine. The formulation was changed again in the early 1960s to a tablet created by Dr Dennis Cahal who ironically went on to become the Senior Principal Medical Officer at the Department of Health responsible for drug dependence issues, who had cause to call his invention 'that confounded preparation'.[16]

Like all pill preparations, Diconal was never meant to be injected. When crushed and mixed with water, it turned into a thick pink paste which produced not only the same sad litany of lost limbs, but also lost lives as the drug caused more overdose deaths than heroin in the 1970s. Yet due to the combination of painkilling and hallucinations caused by injecting Cyclizine, the drug proved very popular and so like all previous drugs of addiction, those doctors prepared to prescribe in large quantities were equally sought after through the very effective user grapevine.

'Jan' recounts the story of one doctor whose activities took some while to come to the notice of the Home Office:

She was a German doctor from north London called Dr A. She was well past it and had a serious drink problem. I was introduced to her by a mate of mine and the deal was always that if somebody put you onto a doctor, you'd give them half the script. I walked into the waiting room and it was like Piccadilly Circus. No other patients in there, just users. She was a private doctor charging £12 for 30 Ritalin and 30 Diconal, but I learned from her surgery 'minder' who I knew well, that if you bought her a bottle of Martini Rosso, that squared it all away. Quite often if you got there late in the evening, she would be pissed and make mistakes writing the prescriptions. There would be a load of screwed up scripts in the bin and her minder would get them, smooth them out, copy her writing, fill in the bits she missed out and then get them filled. She also had some pigeonholes above her desk where she put the money. When her back was turned as she consulted her card index to check when you had the last script, everyone would just take the money back. And even if you had only just got a script, you could always tell her a sob story and get another one.

Eventually the Home Office arrived on her doorstep; she stopped taking on new patients then simply retired. 'Jan' would go all over London to register temporarily with a doctor and walk out with Diconal prescriptions. One doctor would ask patients to bring in their own card from the bureau outside the surgery door. 'Jan' would riffle through the cards to see who was due a script and become that person. He did this on several occasions where remarkably neither the doctor nor the pharmacists realised what was going on despite the ridiculous disguises of hats and scarves. Another scam was to forge prescriptions, take them to a pharmacist who would say he had to phone the doctor to check, but the number was a phone box with an accomplice at the other end. Yet another doctor from south London charged £1 a pill for Diconal as a simple business transaction, writing out a prescription for 'Jan' on Christmas Day. 'Jan' also acted as a dealer for a member of the aristocracy who had a contact at Burroughs Wellcome pumping out Diconal at £2 a tablet, helped another well-to-do user go through their entire inheritance shooting up drugs, and worked with a well-known fashion designer selling methadone to that long-established Chelsea set with 'tons of money and large habits'. But 'Jan' by no means got away scot free; he served time for drug offences, forging prescriptions and other non-drug acquisitive crimes to fund his habit before one day sitting in yet another police cell, deciding enough was enough, and starting on the road to a successful recovery.

His story reveals how fluid the serious end of the London drug scene was in the mid-1970s. There was 'Chinese' heroin, barbiturates, Diconal, Ritalin, Mandrax, some residual pharmaceutical heroin and users ducked and dived depending on what was available and what they could afford. Thai heroin showed up for a short while (users were very suspicious because it was pure white) and 'Jan' sampled some very strong heroin smuggled in from Penang in Malaysia. However, the drug scene was by no means confined to London.

* * *

The scarcity of heroin outside Greater London in the late 1960s and early 1970s and the ready availability of all the aforementioned pharmaceutical drugs from GPs and thefts from retailers and warehouses allowed for injecting drug use to spread across the country in a wave of polydrug use. There was a significant Diconal scene in areas as far apart as Portsmouth, Bristol, Doncaster and Manchester. In the north-west the pharmaceutical drug scene was joined by a revamped drug-driven youth culture for the seventies – Northern Soul.

Northern Soul evolved from the Mod scene of the 1960s, retaining many of its elements, central of which was the use of amphetamines to fuel an all-night dance culture of rare and obscure soul records in places like the Twisted Wheel in Manchester, the Torch in Stoke and most famously the Wigan Casino. One big change was the price of the pills. Back in 1964, before the drug was controlled, a *Sunday Mirror* journalist bought 1,000 amphetamine pills for £18. In 1974, the same quantity cost £150. As pills became harder to obtain through more restrained prescribing and removals from the market by the manufacturers, some users switched to amphetamine-like slimming drugs such as Duromine, Apistate and Tenuate Dospan, known as chalkies, which were controlled as Class C drugs and so not illegal to possess. There was less stringent security at the factories and pills were also imported into the UK. One respondent who talked to Andrew Wilson for his book on Northern Soul said he imported 3,000 tablets every weekend. Another slimming pill imported from abroad was a Spanish drug called Bustaid, which UK rock 'n' rollers from the 1950s knew as Preludin, but those being imported in the early 1970s were analysed as containing a bizarre mixture of methamphetamine and pentobarbital (Nembutal).[17] Old-style amphetamines were still in circulation though; consuming 30 Durophet tablets a night 'was not uncommon'.[18] Another consequence of restrictions on the overall prescribing and manufacture of pharmaceutical amphetamines was the development of home-grown illicit laboratories. Initially these continued manufacturing pills because that's what amphetamine consumers were used to and more likely to accept – blue or yellow tablets sold as backstreets, blueys and dexys. But once the Misuse of Drugs Act came into force in 1973, pharmacists were obliged to keep amphetamines locked away in controlled drug cabinets, further reducing the availability of pills on the street. In response from 1974 onwards, the underground chemists switched to producing high-purity amphetamine sulphate powder: users now had to accept their drug of choice in a different formulation. In his 1976 report, the Chief Inspector of Constabulary reported the discovery of 12 such laboratories.

The changing legal landscape of amphetamines had some serious consequences for the general drug scene. Like the London methamphetamine epidemic of the late 1960s, the appearance of amphetamine powder provided a bridge between speed use and needle culture as some users realised that there were more bangs for bucks in injecting than snorting or swallowing a powder. There were some northern locations that earned reputations as 'amphetamine towns'.

The simple measure of locking amphetamine tablets away located the pills in the same cabinet as powerful painkillers such as Diconal. When a shop was burgled, thieves would just sweep everything out of the cabinet and in the process helped introduce opioid drugs onto northern streets.

Meanwhile down in London in the mid-1970s, the punk scene was emerging, also energised by amphetamine sulphate powder, but where barbiturate use took on a subcultural symbolism of alienation and aggression among both punks and skinheads.[19] And as the decade entered its remaining years, the heroin scene in London changed again, eventually providing another bridge towards injecting drug use.

***

The history of the UK in the seventies was a tale of economic decline: a three-day week, an oil crisis, strikes and the humiliation of the government having to go cap in hand to the International Monetary Fund for a massive hand-out to stabilise the economy. Sixties notions of 'peace and love' went south in the face of IRA terrorism, football violence, attacks by skinheads against those from ethnic communities, clashes between racists and the Anti-Nazi League and Rock Against Racism, and confrontations with police at free festivals and the Notting Hill Carnival. Films such as *A Clockwork Orange* and *Straw Dogs* captured the mood. Margaret Drabble offered this upbeat assessment of the state of the nation in her novel *Ice Age*: 'England, sliding, sinking, shabby, dirty, lazy, inefficient, dangerous, in its death throes, worn out, clapped out and occasionally lashing out.' In 1975, the *Wall Street Journal* said of the land now known as the 'sick man of Europe' as we lurched from one crisis to another, 'Goodbye Great Britain. It was nice to know you.'

Although it was very soon commodified into the mainstream music business, punk epitomised a kind of rage against the machine and the drive that all new generations of youth culture have to spark, shock and disgust society at large. There was back-to-basics rock thrash scorning the over-bloated pretensions of mainstream rock; the disposable bin bag fashions mirroring the rubbish bags piling up in Hyde Park during the dustmen's strike; the spitting, the electric shock Mohicans and the bondage clothes. The razor blades, chains and piercings spoke to a self-harming 'No Future' culture, some of whose iconic figures became mired in the cliché of rebellious rock 'n' roll self-destruction as heroin became for some the chill-out drug from days and nights of no sleep on speed. Downer drugs like barbs, mandies and dikes coupled with a growing heroin scene epitomised the depressed fug that hung over the country, although those on the punk scene itself were actually having a whale of a time.

There was a period when Gerrard Street was virtually an open drug market, dealers sitting on orange boxes taking orders. The police then started intense surveillance with cameras, sending in undercover officers (one of whom bought drugs from 'Jan') ending in some major criminal trials and long sentences. The Chinese networks closed ranks and wouldn't even speak to runners like 'Jan' as white users were prone to give up information in exchange for reduced sentences. Police forces in Germany and the Netherlands were also having success in shutting down Chinese trafficking operations, while the ending of the Vietnam War in 1975 reduced the amount of heroin being smuggled out of the region. Another key development in the early seventies was the break-up of the French Connection by the Americans: the Sicilian Mafia had set up heroin processing laboratories in Marseille for onward shipping to the USA. The picture of global heroin trafficking became more complicated as increasing demand in Europe saw various trafficking groups vying for ascendancy.

In 1972, under intense pressure from the Americans whose president, Richard Nixon, had just declared 'The War On Drugs', Turkey announced an opium poppy ban in exchange for $35 million to help farmers transition to alternative crops. In truth the ban was a sham, as revealed by *The Heroin Trail*, a 1973 Pulitzer Prize-winning article series in *Newsweek*. The ban was formally rescinded in 1974. The end of the French Connection saw a turf war break out between the Sicilian and Corsican mafia for control of the drug trade to the USA. Meanwhile, the brief hiatus of growing meant Turkey lost ground to production in the new heroin processing labs which sprang up in Afghanistan and Pakistan. In response, Turkish crime groups moved from opium production into the wholesale and retail heroin market, moving the heroin from the new processing locations. Using community contacts in north London, Turkish, Turkish/Cypriot and Kurdish traffickers muscled out what remained of the Chinese dealers and took over the heroin trade.

The heroin now coming into the UK was very different from 'Chinese' varieties, not dirty white but brown, chunky and, crucially, smokable. This was the game changer that transformed the UK heroin scene. No longer was it necessary to inject heroin; a user could get almost as strong a hit from simply inhaling the fumes by heating the powder on tinfoil, known as 'chasing the dragon'.

It was estimated that the Turkish share of the heroin market during 1976–77 went from 15 per cent to 85 per cent (Walsh, *Drug War*, p. 250). But the hiatus in Turkish growing allowed opium farmers in Afghanistan to catch up, with the crop refined in both Afghanistan and neighbouring Pakistan. UK customs started seizing heroin imported from Pakistan – some smuggled into the UK on Pakistan Airlines using corrupt cabin crew and baggage handlers. Another route opened up through Iran: there was an influx of Iranian students into the UK, swelling the ranks of one of the largest Iranian communities in the West. Iranian heroin users favoured brown smoking heroin.

The year 1979 proved to be a major tipping point in the history of heroin use in the UK, as the drug became embedded in our society on a scale that has not appreciably receded. On 2 February, as a symbolic harbinger of what was to come, Sid Vicious died of a heroin overdose in a New York hotel bedroom. On 1 April, the Iranian people voted in a referendum to end the reign of the Shah and declare the country an Islamic republic under the leadership of Ayatollah Khomeini. Even during the Shah's reign, there were harsh penalties for traffickers, but 'members of the oligarchy owned vast opium plantations, so the Iranian government subsidised its Establishment opium lords by providing free heroin for 50,000 registered addicts'.[20] But once the Shah was deposed, the trickle of Iranian nationals bringing brown heroin into the UK for their own use turned into a very easy and lucrative way of squirreling assets out of Iran and out of the clutches of the mullahs. On 4 May, Margaret Thatcher became the UK's Prime Minister. In December, the Soviet Union invaded Afghanistan, pushing the heroin refining labs closer to the Afghan/ Iranian border. War and civil unrest are a godsend for smuggling activities in a country such as Afghanistan, already quite lawless, when law and order breaks down even further. What's more, the proceeds from opium and heroin helped fund the fight against the Soviets. The chaos wrought by the Balkan Wars of the early 1990s played a similar role in opening up new opportunities for heroin smuggling.

These seemingly unconnected events collectively played a key role in the drug crisis to come. With all the political, social and economic upheavals of the seventies, it is hardly surprising that there was little that could be called an overarching drug policy. Referring to the 1960s, criminologist David Downes characterised British drug policy as an example of 'masterful inactivity'. Little had changed by the end of the 1970s.

In 1980, a senior Home Office official was quoted in *The Sunday Times* (24 February) calling the whole approach to drug addiction into question in a time of increasing pressure on the public purse. As he saw it, 'the aim has been rehabilitation' [in other words, the work of the clinics] but 'we can't afford this anymore. All we can do is support these people for a time. But once they're hooked, they have effectively passed a death sentence on themselves.'[21]

That year, Social Services Minister Patrick Jenkin gave a speech at the annual general meeting of the Phoenix House therapeutic community saying, 'as with so many health problems, prevention is very much better than cure'. And in tackling drug problems, 'our first and most vital line of defence is obviously the police and customs. They do a magnificent job in limiting the availability of dangerous drugs and without their efforts our drug problems would be infinitely worse.' However, at no time during the 1970s was there any enthusiasm among the senior management of the police or customs for any kind of joined-up enforcement effort despite the evidence that drug problems were becoming a national issue, as they were under no real pressure either from politicians or the media. Yet as Britain entered the early years of the next decade, it became all too clear that the days of masterful inactivity were over.

9

The Dark Side of the Spoon

Doctors at War

The ambition of government advisors and officials to see the clinics act as a brake on the spread of addiction and a barrier to the establishment of an illicit market through competitive prescribing had not been realised. As early as 1973, the Advisory Council on the Misuse of Drugs (ACMD) set up a treatment sub-group to investigate the clinic system. It began work in 1975 and finally in December 1982 published the *Treatment and Rehabilitation Report*, the first of many key ACMD reports on UK drug policy and practice published in the 1980s and '90s. The treatment report was highly significant: a public recognition that drug treatment provision was wholly inadequate, a major catalyst ending the principle of clinical freedom in the treatment of drug addiction and the beginning of the end of prescribing outside the NHS.

The ACMD also recognised that addiction was not just a medical problem, but had legal, economic and social implications for users and coined the term 'problem drug taker' to try to capture this developing perspective and perhaps soften the public image away from pejorative labelling. It followed then that there was a need for a multi-disciplinary approach involving not just doctors. The regional drug-problem teams suggested by the ACMD in the report included social workers, GPs and probation staff, but the teams would still be headed by a consultant psychiatrist. The general view among voluntary sector agencies, given their ongoing antipathy towards the NHS clinics, was that the idea was just 'clinics with knobs on' as one worker put it.[1] But the report did eventually pave the way for an expansion of drug treatment beyond the hospital setting.

However, heavily influenced by the most senior of the London psychiatrists, Drs Connell and Bewley, the report gave inordinate attention to the issue of prescribing as users were increasingly turning to GPs located around the country where few services existed, and also to doctors in private practice through dissatisfaction with clinic regimes in the capital. There was a push to have all opioids subject to licensing – a move rejected by government, concerned that blanket licensing would turn even more GPs away from treating drug users as most didn't want to take on the job in the first place. There was one drug about which the need for licensing was not contested: in April 1984 following widely publicised cases of irresponsible prescribing, Diconal was added to the list of drugs requiring a Home Office licence to prescribe to those with a drug problem.

The ACMD reserved its sternest criticism for those working in private practice and there were serious backstage manoeuvrings to drive the handful of London-based private practitioners (such doctors were virtually unknown anywhere else in the UK) out of business. Going back in time, the Home Office had either managed to quietly warn doctors off or having committed an offence under the Misuse of Drugs Act, doctors were then dealt with by the GMC following media exposure. These doctors never took a stand publicly to defend their own position either individually or collectively let alone criticise NHS drug clinic treatment, although there was plenty of criticism from the few community GPs prepared to prescribe.

Then in 1981 one private doctor emerged who was not prepared to go quietly into the night. Having been expelled from school as a bad influence, Ann Mullins went on to graduate from Oxford and in 1947, was one of the first of three women to enter St Thomas' Medical School in London, where she qualified in 1953 having first met and married a fellow student, psychiatrist Peter Dally. Dr Ann Dally mainly worked in general medicine, obstetrics and gynaecology until 1959; then part-time in general practice, baby clinics, family planning work, medical journalism and broadcasting. She was an ardent campaigner on many aspects of women's rights concerning motherhood, fertility and related subjects. In some respects, her fight can be seen not only in terms of competing notions of drug treatment, but a female doctor's campaign against the male-dominated medical establishment, a battle her friend Dr Wendy Savage would also join at about the same time.

Dr Dally went into private practice with her husband and saw her first drug user in 1979. He was referred to her by his GP after the clinic which had been prescribing him injectable heroin switched him to oral methadone. He topped up with street heroin, lost his job as an electrician and resorted to shoplifting and drug dealing. Other users made their way to her door and eventually, she had 150 patients on her books. This experience made Ann Dally highly critical of the clinic system and she was not shy in making her comments known through the medical press. Quietly encouraged by Bing Spear, who was sympathetic to both responsible private practice and maintenance prescribing, Dr Dally set up the Association of Independent Doctors in Addiction (AIDA) with the intention of writing clinical guidelines and attempting self-regulation.

In September 1981, she wrote a 'personal view' column for the *British Medical Journal* relaying the experience of those patients she was seeing, who regarded the treatment they had received at the clinics as wholly inadequate for their need to live as normal a life as possible while still being an injecting drug user. In her autobiography, *A Doctor's Story* (1990), she cited a whole list of professions constituting her patient group as proof that it was possible to be a 'stable user'. In her *BMJ* article she wrote as a further indictment of the system where 'I have ... been sent patients by doctors who work in drug clinics. They say that under the present system, they cannot prescribe what they believe the patient needs because they think that they must not step out of line and arouse the hostility of colleagues.' This aligns with accounts from some of the more liberal doctors within the system such as Jim Willis who said they received referrals from colleagues citing similar problems. The core of Ann Dally's argument was to support the idea that some, but not all users, could be maintained for an unlimited period in order for them not to have a life that entirely revolved around the acquisition of drugs but instead enable them to hold down regular jobs. No coincidence then that most clinic attendees were unemployed as only this group would in theory be able to fit in with clinic attendance requirements.

The most trenchant opponent of drug treatment in private practice and any notion of long-term maintenance prescribing was Dr Thomas Bewley, in charge of the DDU at Tooting Bec Hospital in south London. His opening salvo in the war of words appeared in the *British Medical Journal* in 1980:

> There are strong economic pressures on addicts to try to obtain controlled drugs on prescription and then to sell some of them; and there are subtle pressures on a doctor who considers prescribing privately to convince him that he will be treating patients rather than selling drugs ... The medical profession should consider whether there is any place for private treatment of addicts where a fee is contingent on a prescription.[2]

And it was this premise, that there could be no ethical therapeutic relationship between a private doctor and drug-using patient where the provision of a prescription relied on a cash transaction especially where there was a risk that part of the script would be sold on, which resulted in every effort being made to prosecute private practitioners. And in this, the GMC was now a very willing partner. Until the 1980s, the GMC had resisted pressure by the Home Office Drugs Branch to discipline doctors who the officials perceived as irresponsible prescribers, unless a doctor had first been convicted of an offence under the Misuse of Drugs Act, such as the cases of Drs Petro and Swan. But the increasing involvement of doctors outside the control of the London psychiatrists was arguably regarded as a threat to their hegemony. Crudely put, they were used to being big fish in a small pond and wanted to keep it that way. Whether the whole issue of cash-driven consultations was a smokescreen for a power struggle is debatable. There is no doubt though that those most opposed not only to private practice but maintenance prescribing in general were in highly influential positions; both Drs Connell and Bewley were on the ACMD of which Dr Connell became Chair in 1982; at different times both were special advisors on drug dependence to the Chief Medical Officer and members of the GMC while Dr Bewley was elected President of the Royal College of Psychiatrists in 1984.

And it was Dr Bewley who apparently reported Dr Dally to the GMC for the first of three appearances she made before it between 1983 and '87. The whole sequence of events and the medico-political power play behind it, is covered in some detail both in Dr Dally's book and by Dr Sarah Mars in her account of the war between the doctors entitled *The Politics of Addiction: Medical Conflict and Drug Dependence in England since the 1960s*. For the interested reader, both books should be read because Dr Dally's account does rather overdo the alleged 'conspiracy' motivations of the London psychiatric 'mafia'. That said, while Dr Mars' book offers a more nuanced and balanced account, she still leaves the reader in no doubt that there was a concerted attempt to end Dr Dally's involvement in drug treatment, which finally succeeded. Dr Dally was never struck off, but after the third hearing, she simply stopped seeing drug-dependent patients, worn out by this war of attrition. However, by way of a taster, what follows is the rough sequence of events leading to that first hearing and the subsequent and critical role that new clinical guidance for the treatment of drug addiction as recommended by the ACMD would have in driving a final nail in the coffin of what passed for the 'British Way of Doing Things'.

Early in 1983 Dr Dally received a formal notification that she would be charged with 'serious professional misconduct' (not just 'professional misconduct') for prescribing Diconal and Ritalin 'otherwise than in the course of bona fide treatment' – a concept which had never been defined and was usually left to individual clinical judgement. The charge related back to 1981 when she had a patient who was later found to have given some of his Diconal to another user suffering withdrawal. Even though the drugs were never directly connected back to Dr Dally, the charge of 'serious professional conduct', for which she was found guilty and 'admonished', seemed to hinge on the degree to which a doctor was responsible for the fate of the drugs prescribed.

Between 1981 and '83, the war of words concerning ethical drug treatment had raged (and would do for many years to come), but three weeks before Dr Dally's first case was due to be heard, the *British Medical Journal* published an article by Dr Bewley and his then junior associate Dr Hamid Ghodse uncompromisingly entitled 'Unacceptable face of private practice: prescription of controlled drugs to addicts'. It was based on a survey of Dr Bewley's NHS patients who were asked about private prescribing doctors even though most of them had never seen a private doctor. It was in effect, a survey of hearsay about what people thought went on in a private surgery. It remains a mystery how it ever passed muster to be published and was roundly criticised by researchers in the Letters pages of the journal. Interviewed later by Sarah Mars, Dr Bewley readily admitted that it 'was not a serious piece of scientific research' but just an exercise in making a point and that the response rate to the questionnaire rendered it 'completely useless'.[3] But it was there in the public domain in the run-up to the case.

Meanwhile, the Department of Health had set up a Medical Working Group chaired by Dr Connell to consider a first in the history of British medicine – a set of clinical guidelines designed to influence medical practice – in this case *Guidelines of Good Practice in the Treatment of Drug Misuse*. There would be four more iterations of the guidelines – in 1991 1999, 2007 and 2017 – and it would be fair to say that at least the next two after the first publication would be marked by a battle royal between the consultant psychiatrists on the one hand and community GPs like Drs Tom Waller, Arthur Banks and Chris Ford who were fighting against the idea that only specialist psychiatrists should be treating drug users and/or if GPs were to be involved they would need to be supervised.

Back in 1984, the guidelines were not evidenced-based, but simply a codification of the clinical practice of Drs Connell and Bewley, who both sat on the Medical Working Group. Moreover, as subsequent doctors hauled up before the GMC found, the guidelines had morphed into a quasi-legal document, contravention of which was enough for disciplinary action to be brought and usually succeed. If Rolleston established the principle of clinical freedom in the treatment of drug addiction, then the creation of guidelines established the narrow parameters of that freedom, especially as their main use initially was to gradually eliminate private practice from the realm of drug treatment.

The pursuit of those in private practice went on well into this century to the point where prescribing to users outside the NHS and voluntary sector treatment agencies has disappeared. Reading all accounts two observations spring to mind. One is that in Dr Dally's case for example, for all the dozens of patients she saw over the years and despite the best will of GMC investigators and the police to find cases to charge her with, they could only come up with a handful of cases against which to pursue a prosecution. And second, those operating within the NHS and voluntary sector clinic system have never been held to account in ways similar to those practising outside the system. When it came to administrative infractions of the Misuse of Drugs Act or Guidelines, some working inside the system admit that practice there might not stand up to too much scrutiny. One wonders how many patients have overdosed due to 'using on top' following insufficient prescribing by a clinic doctor operating a 'one size fits all' regime.

Undoubtedly the creation of guidelines was a significant moment in the history of British drug treatment. They have been interpreted as proof that the State had intervened in clinical practice, except the whole process was driven not by ministers or civil servants, but by consultant psychiatrists keen to impose what they believed was a clinically and morally acceptable drug treatment orthodoxy across the NHS and beyond. Subsequent iterations of the guidelines however have not only been evidence-based but, especially the most recent version, have considered wider viewpoints including service users.

Well before Ann Dally's final appearance before the GMC in 1987, the UK was deep into an existential crisis over what to do about kilos of illegal heroin flooding into the country, which dwarfed the comparative trickle of pharmaceutical drugs – much overplayed by those opposed to private prescribing – that found their way onto the streets. Although journalists enjoyed reporting the cut and thrust of doctors arguing in public and reported it at length both in print and on TV, media attention swiftly turned to what was happening 200 miles up the M1 motorway. Events there and across Britain would ultimately force a complete rethink on national clinic drug policy. But first...

Glue Sniffing: Smells like Teen Spirit

Down the years, there have been several drug-using groups who, despite their small numbers, have been the focus for what Jock Young called a press- and police-driven 'amplification of deviance': from cocaine-selling prostitutes and Chinese opium smokers to West Indian dope sellers, wired-up Mods and acid-crazed hippies. There were two novel aspects of the latest panic: the substances were legal and could be regarded as the cause of Britain's first outbreak of 'legal highs', and those involved were mainly young teenagers.

The term 'glue sniffing' was shorthand for a craze that began in the UK in the early mid-1970s and covered a range of 'volatile solvents' including glue, but also gas lighter fuel, typewriter correcting fluid such as Tippex, hairspray, nail varnish and many other solvent-based domestic products which young people sniffed to release fumes, causing a drunken-like stupor and often hallucinations. The products were cheap and easily available, appealing particularly to those from poorer backgrounds who couldn't get into pubs and had no regular access to drugs. The early days of glue sniffing were associated with punk; one of many punk and alternative fanzines was called *Sniffin' Glue*, named after a song by The Ramones, and selling an impressive 15,000 copies. The link with the punk movement helped establish glue sniffing as something entirely disreputable, but glue sniffing quickly out-stripped its genesis to become a source of general societal handwringing, although 'Mohican aged three. Head says boy sniffed glue' (*Daily Telegraph*, 6 September 1984) kept the punk glue pot boiling.

The first two UK solvent deaths were recorded as early as 1971 but fatalities were still in single figures when the local press in Scotland and north-east England began bringing the subject to their readers' attention. Almost immediately glue sniffing was refracted through the prism of heroin use; sniffers were 'glue addicts'; the *Northern Echo* (18 September 1975) quoted a police source citing glue as 'the new heroin of the teeny bopper'. One edition of the ITV documentary series *This Week* entitled 'On the Glue' featured a glue 'addict' in shadow, claims of glue 'dens' and a parade of experts giving out warning messages, all common features of the heroin documentaries to come.

On the day of the inquest into the death of an 11-year-old Sunderland boy, the local paper denounced glue as 'the demon vapour' and then helpfully explained in some detail how young people sniff (*Sunderland Echo*, 18 September 1975). In tandem with the reporting of tragedies, every act of teenage vandalism appeared to be linked to glue sniffing; headlines such as 'New Peril from High Youths' and 'Glue Sniffing Menace' were commonplace throughout the 1970s and early 1980s. One local Scottish paper sought to shock its readers with 'Glue sniffers used bad language'. And like LSD, 'Glue trip punk in death leap' (*Islington Gazette*, 4 April 1985) collapsed all the tropes into one headline in which the guy thought he was Batman and could fly.

Local press editors ran campaigns to warn parents and to urge shopkeepers not to sell glue to young people. Pressure bore down on manufacturers to add foul-smelling ingredients to put kids off, but there was obvious resistance as this would alienate legitimate customers. Warning labels were rejected as tantamount to advertising the 'good stuff'. The government even tried to recruit the Chemical Defence Establishment at Porton Down to see if they could come up with a solution, but overall government tried to play down the whole phenomenon as just a collection of isolated incidents which could be dealt with by low-key education in schools and youth clubs. It wasn't until 1985 that the government introduced the Intoxicating Substances (Supply) Act making it an offence for a shopkeeper to sell solvent-based products to those under 18 if there was a reasonable suspicion that the product would be misused. Not until 1999 was a ban on sales of butane lighter fuel to those under 18 introduced. Neither ban was particularly effective; just a handful of prosecutions of shopkeepers who were found guilty of deliberately selling 'sniffing kits' comprising glue and bags.

Behind all the overblown headlines about the glue menace sweeping the country and all those horrible sniffers causing mayhem to innocent bus stops, young people were actually dying. At the height of the craze in the 1980s, the rate was two fatalities a week. Overall, solvent sniffing has caused more deaths among teenagers than all the other drugs put together. It wasn't long though before the media lost interest as politicians, the public and the press woke up to the reality of a drug problem that by no means could be called the product of a moral panic.

Powder Keg

In the 1930s Liberal intellectuals led by economists John Maynard Keynes and William Beveridge developed a series of plans that became especially attractive as the wartime coalition government promised a much better post-war Britain. The government signed off on a series of white papers aiming to provide among other societal improvements a National Health Service, the expansion of education and housing, new welfare programmes and the nationalisation of weak industries. In simple terms, there was a broad national consensus on social and economic policy, which also included a commitment to full employment. Apart from the question of nationalisation of some industries, these policies were generally accepted by the three major parties, as well as by industry, the financial community and the labour movement.

However, this loose consensus began to break down in the face of the economic crisis of the 1970s. At its height, even Prime Minister James Callaghan was forced to admit to his own party conference that, 'We used to think that you could spend your way out of a recession and increase employment by cutting taxes and boosting government spending. I tell you in all candour that that option no longer exists.'

This was music to the ears of the shadow Conservative government led by Margaret Thatcher who was influenced by the monetarist economics of Milton Freidman among others. Monetarist policies were more focused on controlling inflation than any commitment to full employment and with inflation peaking at 25 per cent under Labour, coupled with the disastrous 'winter of discontent', it allowed the Conservatives to promise the electorate that they would get the economy under control. On the back of these promises, they swept to power in 1979 with the largest electoral swing since 1945.

With a mandate to control inflation, a belief that the market not government should control the destiny of business and a country fed up with strikes, what became known as Thatcherism delivered a neo-liberal hammer blow affecting mainly working-class people in areas of already ailing manufacturing and heavy industry like shipbuilding, vehicle manufacture, engineering, mining, steel and textiles. Worse still, the labour market was growing, with large numbers of school leavers unable to find work: in 1984, 27 per cent of under-18s were out of work, 26 per cent of those aged 18–19 and 40 per cent were out of work for more than a year.[4] In the mid-1970s, 1.5 million people were out of work; by the mid-1980s, that figure had doubled.

Long-term unemployment or the prospect of leaving school with no prospects at all had a serious impact on individual physical and mental health as the social, psychological and economic benefits of having a regular job became ever more distant. For many, heroin filled the void left by the collapse of the legitimate economy.

All the metrics of heroin use began to rise steeply from 1979 onwards. In 1975, there were about 3,500 heroin users notified to the Home Office. By 1980, the official figure had risen to 5,000 and within four years had shot up to more than 12,000. However, two separate studies, one in London and the other in Newcastle, calculated that for every person notified and in touch with treatment services, there were five users who were not, meaning that the true figure for heroin dependency by the mid-1980s was closer to 60,000. Some drugs workers put the figure closer to 1 in 10. In effect, nobody knew how many heroin users there really were.

The amount of heroin seized rose sharply from less than 50 kilos in 1980 to around 350 kilos by 1984. Again, the officially published statistics concealed a darker truth. A study actually commissioned by the Home Office calculated that the true consumption of heroin in the UK in 1984 could have been as high as 3,800 kilos, which gives some credence to the finger-in-the air estimate from some police and customs officers that only about 10 per cent of the drugs coming into the country are seized. In 1978, it was estimated that 80 per cent of the heroin seized at UK ports of entry was in transit to the USA; by 1981, 80 per cent of seizures were now reckoned to be for UK consumption. Controlled for inflation, the price of heroin dropped by 50 per cent in some areas. In the late 1970s, most heroin was arriving in small packages, for example, smuggled in cars, air travel luggage or through the post. In 1979, just 1 per cent of heroin seizures were from trucks. The Transports Internationaux Routiers (TIR) Convention on International Transport of Goods, which was signed in 1975, facilitated the movement of goods between signatory countries and allowed for sealed containers and minimum checks at intermediate borders. By 1991, Turkish lorries travelling under the TIR's Convention were being intercepted at a rate of one a week.[5] Few major conurbations or manufacturing regions escaped the heroin epidemic. In England, the north-west would be most badly affected, nowhere more so than Merseyside.

Fury 'Cross the Mersey

Just how badly unemployment damaged working people in Liverpool was graphically illustrated by Alan Bleasdale's heartbreaking play and subsequent series *The Boys from the Blackstuff*. In the last episode, Chrissy wheels the ailing ex-docker George in his wheelchair through piles of rubbish on wasteland down to a virtually derelict dock area where George reminisces about the days when the Port of Liverpool was flourishing. There were still 30,00 dockers employed in the early 1960s, but by the mid-1980s the east coast and Channel port rivals, a series of strikes, and automation on the Seaforth dock had reduced the workforce to only 2,000. With some of the worst unemployment rates in the country and long-standing enmity between the police and the black community, the Toxteth area of Liverpool exploded into rioting in July 1981, prompting Margaret Thatcher to secretly urge her ministers to allow Liverpool to fall into 'managed decline'. Fortunately, Minister for the Environment Michael Heseltine strongly disagreed with many aspects of Thatcherism and instead initiated some important regeneration projects for the city. But there seemed little that anybody could do to stifle a major heroin problem once it first took hold in the Wirral, a borough of Merseyside.

While the council was attempting to come to grips with its solvents problem, the police, courts and probation service were observing rising numbers of arrests for heroin possession as concerned parents banded together to form Parents Against Drug Abuse (PADA), which began to command both local and national interest.

It may appear from all that follows that only Merseyside experienced widespread heroin use and that only this region took the then-radical steps to try and save lives. No doubt, the region was more badly affected than most English regions, but in truth, it was the Merseyside outbreak that received the most national and even international attention largely due to a handful of very vocal, media-friendly and charismatic individual drug users, drugs workers and public health officials. Merseyside came to be seen as the front line of the nation's heroin problem; different locations in Liverpool took turns to be dubbed 'Smack City' and as if the problem wasn't bad and sensational enough, the press resorted to nonsense stories such as 'pushers' injecting school milk with heroin to attract 'new customers' (*The Times*, 2 May 1984) while another journalist wrote about an influx of cheap Pakistani cocaine. Among the most outspoken of the Liverpool drugs workers was ex-user turned lay preacher and community worker Allan Parry, who wryly observed at the time that there were more journalists now in Liverpool researching drug stories than there were drug users.

In 1986, researchers from Liverpool University undertook an intensive project detailing the genesis and subsequent story of heroin use in the Wirral, interviewing many users, both known and unknown, to the treatment services. They submitted a report to the Wirral Drugs Committee in 1986 and subsequently turned their findings into a book, *Living with Heroin*, published in 1988.

London's post-war 'non-therapeutic' heroin scene was given a boost in the early 1950s when 'Mark' started dealing the drugs he stole from his former hospital employer. The Wirral researchers discovered, much to their surprise, that the borough's heroin problem was also probably initiated by an individual who moved into one of the Wirral's more affluent locales and began dealing 1 ounce and ½ ounce weights of brown heroin to existing users who had been scoring large amounts of Diconal and another opiate painkiller, Palfium, from local GPs. Other early customers included those who had been injecting amphetamine on the Northern Soul dance scene.

As the researchers discovered, the Wirral heroin user was very different from the bohemian-style, anti-establishment rebel user of sixties London. Typically, he (there was always about a 2:1 to 3:1 male/female user ratio) was much younger, in his late teens, unemployed having left school with no educational qualifications, living at home with his parents and having to find £20–£35 a week to support his heroin habit, which he did by adding to the soaring rates of acquisitive crime on Merseyside. Reported domestic burglaries on the Wirral went from 2,824 in 1979 to 10,238 in 1986.[6] The average young male heroin user had no punk or other subcultural affiliations; it was just what you did. As one user put it: 'Why not? There's nothing to do anyway except spend all day watching the telly.'[7]

Perversely, maintaining a regular heroin habit took some organisation and actually got people out of the house. As another user told the Liverpool researchers, 'I was that busy, y'know, getting up, going out to score, having a toot, going out again to score.' This individual coyly left out the bit about how he got the money, but apart from shoplifting and housebreaking, many street users were also dealing. High unemployment rates saw a rise in organised crime as those out of work joined the ranks of the foot soldiers needed to supply the labour for the burgeoning heroin dealing operations.

From the early 'single operative' heroin dealers supplying existing users, heroin use quickly spread through family and friend networks until 1983 when, after months of surveillance, customs broke up a crew running heroin through the Liverpool and Dover docks. Liverpool had a long history of smuggling, theft and corruption among dock workers and officials, so Liverpool's established white criminal networks were ahead of the game compared to traditional white gangs elsewhere in the UK in realising the huge profits to be made from heroin trafficking. This co-existed alongside the long-embedded cannabis trade whose organisation was largely in the hands of Toxteth's black dealing fraternity. Many of Liverpool's older white gangsters had come from these same tough streets and after the Toxteth riots found a sort of common cause with the black community in their hatred and distrust of the police and a mutual interest in working with local black cannabis dealers to together import and distribute cannabis. Between 1981 and '84, police and customs seized 8.5 tons of cannabis, prompting DCI Peter Deary to tell the 1984 conference of Chief Police Officers that his patch was the UK centre for cannabis importation.[8]

Referring to the white criminals, there was talk of a Liverpool 'mafia' among police and journalists, but this was never structured along 'Italian family' lines, more a loose association of gangsters who cooperated with each other when it suited them, even while remaining bitter rivals. Local gangsters like Tommy Comerford made connections with overseas cartels and suppliers in the whole menu of illegal drugs. Much of the heroin came from Pakistan, into Liverpool docks and on through a region-wide dealing network which became increasingly violent as both the market expanded and the profits escalated. At £40 a gram, Merseyside had some of the cheapest heroin in the UK, so much so that dealers would come from Ireland to buy heroin in Liverpool for resale at £140 a gram in Dublin. So what options were there for those heroin users who wanted to get off this dangerous carousel ride of thieving, scoring and using? The answer was precious little.

The first port of call would usually be the GP. Users would often go with their mums seeking help, showing how different the scene was from London. But they would get turned away by receptionists who said that the surgery didn't see heroin users, or the GP would refuse to prescribe methadone, even though they did not need a licence to do so, and instead send the user away with large prescriptions of Valium. The withdrawal from that drug could be fatal if not conducted under medical supervision. There was at least a 3-month waiting list to be seen at the Regional Drug Dependency Unit in Chester. Even if a user secured an appointment, facing him or her would be Dr Spencer Madden, an ardent abstentionist who refused to prescribe anything but a time-limited reducing dose of methadone. There was also a drug detoxification unit which left users to their own devices once they had been detoxified: most relapsed as there was no reason not to go back to using heroin. The inherent dangers for injecting drug users soon became dramatically worse.

Scotland was also experiencing some serious heroin problems; scarcity of the drug across a country with no ready port access meant for economic reasons, users there were injecting rather than smoking heroin. In the early days of HIV recognition in the USA, it was assumed the virus was only transmitted through men having sex with men. Then in 1985 in Edinburgh, scene of some of the worst heroin problems in Scotland, GP Dr Roy Robertson and Dr Ray Brettle from the Infectious Disease Unit of Edinburgh's City hospital identified the virus in around half the city's injecting drug users. Further investigation revealed the virus could have been present in the drug injecting community since 1982. They concluded the virus could be spread by sharing injecting equipment, which was common practice due to the decision by Lothian police to confiscate injecting equipment when apprehending users.

In September 1985, Professor John Ashton and Howard Seymour from the Merseyside Regional Health Authority (MRHA) and community worker Allan Parry attended a WHO health education conference in Dublin. While there, they met with Glen Margo, Director of Health Promotion for San Francisco. Glen, who would himself die of AIDS, was a key figure fostering AIDS awareness among the gay community. Professor Ashton recalls, 'We asked him what he would have done back in 1980 that didn't happen. The answer was needle exchange.' At the time, there were no recorded cases of drug-related HIV in Liverpool or anywhere else in England, so it made sense to try to get ahead of the game. Glen Margo was invited to Liverpool for a week of intensive lectures to educate health professionals on the risk of injecting drug users acquiring HIV.

As heroin use among young people in Liverpool gathered pace, there was little help or information available other than for those getting treatment from the newly opened drug dependency clinic in Hope Street, right in the city centre. But many didn't want to attend there due to a general fear and mistrust of authority. With the help of John Ashton and Howard Seymour, Allan Parry set up a drug information centre, the Merseyside Drug Training and Information Centre (MDTIC). It provided a more informal, user-friendly and non-threatening environment for drug users to get help and advice and in October 1986, the workers were instrumental in establishing the needle exchange scheme – in an adjacent toilet. Around the same time, similar facilities opened in Peterborough, Cambridge, Swindon, and at the Kaleidoscope Project in south London, while Boots the Chemist began operating the first pharmacy exchange in Sheffield.

What was happening in Liverpool and elsewhere might be termed 'guerrilla public health'. On paper, providing injecting equipment to drug users was illegal under the Misuse of Drugs Act. But Liverpool drugs worker Alan Matthews explains:

Peter Deary was a very forward-thinking head of the drugs squad who said they wouldn't arrest people carrying works, and we also got the support of the *Liverpool Echo*. We asked them not to run 'needles for junkies' stories, but to give us six weeks to see what happens and then we would give them the story as an exclusive.

It was all word of mouth, no advertising, and we saw about 300 people in those first few weeks who had never been near a drug service. We had a guy come down from Glasgow, another from Manchester, and one day this steroid user turned up. We were operating out of this little toilet, so you didn't even have to go into the information centre. Suddenly everything went dark and there is this big beefy guy filling the doorframe. We never asked questions of anybody: they could give a false name, but we logged post code and gender just to collect some basic statistics. But I said to this guy, who looked nothing like a heroin user, 'Do you mind me asking what you're injecting?' 'Steroids,' he said. 'Oh, does that happen a lot then?' He said all the guys down the gym were injecting and they all shared. 'Have you heard about AIDS?' 'Yes,' he said, 'but you only get that from using heroin not steroids.' So, I told him about AIDS and injecting, and he became an outreach worker at the gym.

Another guy ran a shooting gallery and one day he came with a few syringes to exchange. We asked him if he had anymore. 'Oh, yes, loads.' 'Well, bring 'em in.' 'Oh, I thought it was just for personal use.' Next day he turns up with three bin bags full of works, needles sticking out and everything. We gave him sharps boxes and everything, and he became an unofficial outreach worker too.

While the controversial needle exchange was operating under the radar, the prescribing practice at the new clinic, while not illegal, was both symbolically and literally miles away from the standard operating procedure of the London psychiatrists who masterminded the clinical guidelines. The first incumbent of the clinic was Dr John Marks, a general psychiatrist working in Widnes where he first came across injecting drug users. 'We had to have a speciality and as I was the new boy I was given the drug users by Bert Kier Brooker, ex-RAF and Atlantic Survey who taught me what little practical knowledge I have about psychiatry – and he was prescribing heroin in the old Rolleston style well before I was.'[9]

Dr Marks agreed to be seconded to the Hope Street clinic as the Regional Health Authority wanted somebody in post quickly because of the rising panic about AIDS. Dr Marks' first spell at the clinic spanned 1985–1987 when Dr Jim Willis, recently returned from working in the Middle East, took on the job permanently. However, following a train accident in which he was seriously injured, Dr Willis retired, and others stepped into the breach until Dr Marks returned on a temporary contract basis from 1988 to 1990 because nobody else wanted the job. Subsequent history has forgotten (or never knew) that like Dr Brooker, Dr Willis too carried on prescribing heroin as he had done back at the St Giles clinic in 1968, again predating what became Dr Marks' 'infamous' prescribing practices.

It is worth mentioning at this point that over in Manchester another psychiatrist, Dr John Strang, was also prescribing heroin. He began his career in London and was at one time a senior registrar under Philip Connell, although he also worked with Jim Willis and another compassionate and forward-thinking psychiatrist, Peter Chapple. Dr Strang then moved to Manchester for five years before returning to London and the Maudsley Hospital where he was associated (I think unfairly) with the zealotry of the 'Maudsley Mafia'. I say unfairly because although now Professor Sir John Strang was always uneasy about private prescribing, he did become a senior government advisor and strongly supported opiate substitute therapy to the extent much later of running a UK heroin prescribing trial.

But to return to Dr Marks who was not only prescribing in the spirit of Rolleston, but like Dr Dally, was not about to stay quiet concerning his criticisms of the UK drug treatment system and the refusal to accept the basic principles of Rolleston. He was a defence witness for Ann Dally, gave advice to legal counsel relating to similar subsequent prosecutions, wrote articles, sent letters to the medical press and was a willing media interviewee.

Drs Willis and Marks and those involved with the needle exchange and the information centre, police and public health officials were all making their contribution aimed at preventing Liverpool and the surrounding area becoming an HIV hotspot. Collectively, these public health interventions became known as harm reduction, the idea being that when people are engaging in risky behaviour such as unsafe sex or injecting drugs, rather than relying on 'just say no' messages which do nothing but put at further risk the lives of those people who for whatever reason continue to take risks, it's better to find a way of keeping people alive. Either give them more of an opportunity to make changes in their lives – or at least reduce the risk of dying. Nobody can recover if they are dead.

As a medical or public health intervention, you could trace the idea of harm reduction right back to the Rolleston idea of the 'stabilised addict' who could best function with a small regular dose of their drug of addiction.

The term also applied to a solvents leaflet aimed at teachers, youth workers and other professionals dealing with young people called *Teaching About A Volatile Situation,* written by ISDD's Research Director Nicholas Dorn and published by ISDD in 1980. The deaths of many young people from solvent use came from inhaling glue in large plastic bags covering their face, from which they suffocated. This leaflet caused a storm of media protest and worried calls to the ISDD Director Jasper Woodcock from the Department of Health, which cast a brief shadow over ISDD's government funding as it suggested (correctly) that if young people sniffed from something else such as crisp packets instead, many lives could be saved. The leaflet also warned that panic over glue sniffing prompted young people to sniff in secluded places such as on canal banks and in derelict buildings, where accidents could happen without help arriving in time.

In fact, any accident-prevention intervention such as seat belts could be called harm reduction. No one proposes banning cars because there are accidents, so instead the aim is to help prevent accidents and road deaths. But harm reduction became, and remains, more than just either a medical- or health-and-safety intervention. Instead the idea was closely linked with those groups suffering marginalisation and discrimination such as gay men or injecting drug users trying to take control of their own health through community and grassroots activity. Dutch drug users first took the initiative to start handing out clean 'works' (the equipment to inject a drug) to deal with a pre-HIV outbreak of hepatitis B. HIV and drug harm reduction became social and quasi-political movements which grew around the world as more and more user groups formed and campaigned for the universal right to health symbolised by interventions geared to keeping them alive. Drug-user activists and their supporters faced huge opposition from anti-drug campaigning groups, governments and international agencies that accused them of not only condoning drug use but also opening a back door to legalisation. Even today, while the WHO endorses harm reduction interventions, you would struggle to find the phrase in official UN documents. Back in January 1987, it was one of the Wirral drug researchers, Dr Russell Newcombe, who gave voice to the contemporary interpretation of harm reduction with an article written for the ISDD magazine *Druglink – High Time for Harm Reduction –* broadening the concept beyond the safety of injecting drug users to that of all drug users.

In Liverpool where Dr Newcombe and colleagues had conducted much of their research, a volatile atmosphere around drugs was stoked by one group who exploited the desperate drug situation as a means of leveraging power in the city council. During the early years of the 1980s, a far-left group called the Militant Tendency, or Militant for short, became influential on the Labour-controlled Liverpool City Council way out of proportion to the number of their elected councillors. Given the state of a city with some of the poorest housing stock in Europe and suffering under the weight of unemployment, Militant's populist anti-Conservative rhetoric found general approval among the voting public. However, they sought to solidify their power base by exploiting the fears and anger among local communities about the drug problem. Militant were vehemently anti-drugs, believing that opium really was the opium of the people; drugged-up youth were hardly in a fit state to advance the coming socialist revolution. In his account of Militant, Michael Crick wrote:

> Militant has a very puritanical outlook and requires a strict lifestyle from its members. Short hair and ties are common. At Militant and Labour Party Young Socialist summer camps and conferences, Militant members are expected to go to bed early and comrades sleeping together is frowned upon. Indulging in drugs is one of the worst crimes in Militant's eyes, since these are liable to 'corrupt' working class people and to 'numb their consciousness'. In the past, Militant members have even been expelled for smoking cannabis.[10]

Militant took its anti-drugs stance beyond the ranks of its membership. They seized control of the council's drug portfolio and created their own drug administration in competition with the Regional Health Authority facilities, doing everything they could to undermine harm reduction efforts in the area, including bullying and physically threatening those involved. They organised anti-drug marches, vigilante groups to attack alleged dealers and published their own ludicrous drug education pack for schools. They even backed the introduction of neuro-electric therapy as a treatment. This was the famous 'black box' treatment undergone by Eric Clapton and Pete Townsend. Electrodes were attached to the patient's ears sending mild electrical impulses to the brain, stimulating the body's natural opioids and so lessen the impact of heroin withdrawal. However, like all detoxification methods, the treatment did nothing to address all the reasons why the person became addicted in the first place. Clapton said it was a waste of time.

Where Militant came unstuck on the drugs issue was over their promise to drive out the dealers. Such promises sounded very hollow, especially in the aftermath of the 1985 death of 14-year-old Jason Fitzsimmons who died of a heroin and methadone overdose having bought the drugs from a local dealer. Jason's uncle Tony Murray, already a career criminal, launched his own anti-drug campaign only to be sentenced to 13 years in jail in 2005 for heroin trafficking. (*Liverpool Echo*, 15 March)

Enraged residents shouted down the Militant officials who had arranged community meetings on the worst affected estates to try to whip up local support. But paradoxically, Militant also tried to block police attempts to track down dealers by refusing to allow officers access to council house tenant lists until the police threatened to go to the press.

Ultimately, Militant failed in its attempt to capture the anti-drug high ground and derail the efforts of local drug agencies – as it failed in everything else – but it was an interesting episode in the history of the UK drug scene as the first and only example of the drugs issue being front and centre of local politics.

John Marks carried on until an interview in 1992 given to an American news programme signalled the beginning of the end of his work in the UK treatment system. He caused consternation in high places by correctly stating that heroin prescribing was lawful UK medical practice. The news report then showed heroin and cocaine cigarettes made up for Dr Marks to prescribe to patients by local pharmacist Jeremy Clitherow as part of the policy to give drug injectors a less dangerous option. All this was highly embarrassing for the UK government.

In April 1985, under the 'Just Say No' slogan, Nancy Regan hosted a First Ladies Conference on Drug Abuse at the White House to which Margaret Thatcher was invited. The UK PM in turn raised the issue at a G7 summit meeting in Bonn the following month, getting an agreement on more anti-trafficking cooperation, and went on to address a meeting of the American Bar Association on the 'evils of drug addiction and abuse'.[11] In 1988, the UK was a signatory to the UN Convention against Traffic in Narcotic Drugs and Psychotropic Substances. The convention was the third of the three major UN anti-drug treaties; the first was the Single Convention covering plant drugs; the second covered pharmaceutical drugs such as amphetamines, sleeping pills and tranquillisers, and was signed in 1971. The 1988 convention was a reaction to the explosion in the global drug trade, clearly immune to all efforts at control, let alone elimination. Built into this new convention was an attempt to control the availability of the chemicals needed to produce illicit drugs – known as precursors – and to 'follow the money' with enhanced political ambition to tackle money laundering. Thatcher also hosted a World Ministerial Drugs Summit in 1990.

All this activity meant the UK government was acutely aware of the anomalous position they appeared to inhabit over drug treatment and went so far as to produce a pamphlet called *The Medical Use of Opioids in the UK* to try to dispel the myth abroad – and especially to American officials – that heroin here was on tap so long as you were 'registered'. Nevertheless, the Americans (probably in shape of the drug czar of the day Bob Martinez) were deeply unimpressed by the interview with Dr Marks and apparently expressions of concern found their way to senior levels in Whitehall.

Although it sounded as if Dr Marks was handing out controlled drugs like Smarties, at least the statistics of his time at the city-centre clinic from 1985 to 1987 tell a different story. Another Liverpool University researcher, Cindy Fazey, was commissioned to conduct an evaluation of the service and found that of the 1,000 patients seen during that time only 6 per cent were given intravenous drugs and less than 20 per cent were on an oral maintenance methadone script. More than half were sent on a 4-week detoxification course. Seen by ISDD at the time, parts of the unpublished report were redacted when patients complained of having to wait for ages to be seen, caused mainly by what Dr Fazey regarded as woeful management by the health authority resulting in chronic understaffing. And generally, former patients and drugs workers say the Hope Street clinic was only unique in the nature of the prescribing; otherwise the procedures in place and the power play between doctor and patients was little different from the experience of those attending clinics in London. For example, patients had to submit to urine tests and if the test showed they had been using on top, the script could be forfeited.

Yet despite the publicity giving to his prescribing practices and in the light of the Clinical Guidelines, Dr Marks never found himself in front of the GMC for prescribing outside the realms of 'bona fide treatment'. His reading of that was not for the want of trying by the Home Office and others, but says, 'as a Fellow of the Royal College of Psychiatrists (RCP) and having been a founder member of the addiction section of the RCP and a member of its executive committee at that time, they may have thought it would be politically too embarrassing to haul me up before the GMC'.[12] Until his retirement through ill-health in 1986, Bing Spear could be relied upon to back Dr Marks so long as he stayed within the law. Spear's successors took a different view, but John Marks' career as a UK addiction psychiatrist ended not through disciplinary measures, but through the 'reorganisation' of his local NHS region. He returned to the Widnes Clinic which then lost its contract to a more politically acceptable provider, although at the time local health officials claimed that the health authority could no longer afford to prescribe heroin.

The Kraken Wakes

Flash back to the mid-1980s and what steps were the government taking at the centre to combat a double whammy of unprecedented heroin use and a virus which threatened the whole country? Well, according to Conservative MP Bernard Brain (no relation to Russell Brain), not much at all by 1984. He fronted a debate in the Commons on 13 April 1984 where he began by reminding MPs that back in 1979, he had warned of a coming crisis, yet

> there appears to be little understanding or even concern, in this place or in the country as a whole, of the immediate or even the long-term effects of what can only be described as a grave illness and a terrifying social evil encouraged by ruthless criminals who import and distribute illicit drugs

He then went on to point out the still poor state of NHS drug treatment services '... in many parts of the country there are no treatment centres whatsoever. Even when treatment centres are available there is almost always a long delay sometimes up to two months before even an initial assessment ...' He made specific mention of 16 English counties with no service provision at all, and the fact that many London boroughs were outside the catchment areas of the 15 specialist London services.

This was one criticism of the ACMD treatment report, that while the content was a damning indictment of the 1974 reorganisation of the NHS, the report only appeared to recommend central funding 'possibly by way of pump-priming grants', putting the onus on Regional and District Health Authorities to stump up for drug treatment services once the money ran out (something they told the Department of Health in a 1984 survey they were not prepared to do). This appeared to play to the Government's 'get out of jail free card' of local authorities being best placed to assess local needs and allocate resources. By taking this approach, there was a strong feeling that the ACMD had acquiesced with the Conservative commitment to 'small' government and a tight grip on public spending. Even so, in response to the ACMD report, in December 1982, Health and Social Services Secretary

Norman Fowler announced a Central Funding Initiative (CFI), initially £6 million over 3 years. Fears over the AIDS epidemic pushed up the sum to £17m over six years to 1989 and provided the platform for the growth of voluntary sector drug treatment services. Nearly half the funds were allocated to new community-based walk-in centres, a marked shift away from entirely hospital-based services and by 1989 approximately 70 per cent of the drug services in England had been established in just over five years.[13]

But the CFI needed to be understood not simply as a response to a growing public health crisis but more broadly in terms of how the State perceived its role in the funding of social policy. CFI money ended just before the establishment of the NHS internal market through the NHS Care and Community Act 1990. Now instead of government providing long-term funding, instead it might provide start-up or pump priming funds, leaving the local authorities to 'purchase' ongoing services from local 'providers' who might be other statutory services or, increasingly in treatment, providers from the voluntary sector. But there was a paradox here: CFI-type arrangements were introduced by the Thatcher government across a range of policy areas not just drugs which didn't really chime with the political zeitgeist of 'rolling back the State'. However, the government could not swerve around the political imperative to act centrally in support of efforts to stem a national drugs crisis.

As the evidence of the scale of the problem began to build in the mid-1980s, the government came under yet more pressure to demonstrate how it was responding. In 1984, stung by parliamentary criticism and increasingly irked that the Labour Party was scoring law and order political points over the announcement of huge cuts to customs staff, the government set up an inter-ministerial group chaired by David Mellor, the junior Home Office minister in charge of drugs, to avoid even more grief from its own party at the annual autumn conference.

In 1985, the Home Office produced *Tackling Drug Misuse: a summary of government's strategy* quoting the Home Secretary Leon Brittan whose words signalled the belief now in government that despite being the party of law and order, enforcement could not do the job on its own. 'Drug abuse is a disease from which no country and no section of modern society seems immune ... Stamping it out will be slow and painful. It requires cooperation between Governments, law enforcement agencies, professionals, schools and families. The rewards are great if we succeed – and the price of ultimate failure unthinkable.'

Notwithstanding this admission that the UK could not police its way out of the problem, the focus of new initiatives in the strategy (and its further two editions), aside from increases in central funding for treatment, was on enforcement. This covered overseas funding of UN anti-drug efforts, appointing the first Drug Liaison Officers to work overseas in producer countries, creating the National Drugs Intelligence Unit, increasing drug enforcement capacity in all the 43 Constabularies and the Regional Crime Squads, raising the maximum sentence for trafficking in Class A drugs to life, introducing the Drug Trafficking Offences Act aimed at seizing assets and reinstating some of the previously axed customs capacity. However, from a political point of view all these developments would be largely hidden from public view; one developing problem the government would definitely want hidden from public view was the growing territorial tensions over drugs enforcement between police and customs.

To repeat, through the 1970s the drug problem was not regarded as particularly serious either by police or customs at senior management level. With a few notable cannabis exceptions, seizures were mainly from small criminal networks or hippy adventurers on the way back from Morocco in the ubiquitous VW van. Customs officers on the ground, however, had a very different view of the developing scene and came to regard the drug turf as their own.

Then as the political temperature on drugs rose, the government considerably ramped up police resources and now police senior management had to demonstrate they were worth all the additional investment at a time of public sector spending restraint. With the police now seen to be muscling in on their patch, customs tended to pull up the drawbridge, refusing to share information – a somewhat justified tactic as there had been a number of very public Metropolitan Police drug-related corruption scandals involving collusion with gangsters. In fact, part of the reason why police officers were often wary of working on drug (and 'vice') cases at all was precisely for fear of being tainted by the spectre of corruption. One officer quipped about handling files with gloves on.[14]

Although rare, customs had their own occasional rotten apples. In July 1982, a Heathrow-based customs officer, Bhupinder Singh Seran, was sentenced to 9 years for heroin smuggling.

Individual officers often worked well together, but there were lots of structural differences that made police and customs relations difficult. The ranking structure and regulations concerning overtime were different; the legislation under which customs and police operated was different. Methods of working could be very different; if customs were following up on a case, they might start banging on doors on a council estate without informing the local police, who not only would be more in tune with local sensitivities – especially after the riots across the UK and the murder of PC Blakelock on the Broadwater Farm Estate in north London in 1985 – but would go to the trouble of getting a search warrant. If a suspect had been arrested, then Section 18 of the Police and Criminal Evidence Act allowed for a search without a warrant. This was the preferred option by customs as they would otherwise have to wait for a magistrate to issue the warrant. But to have customs banging on the door without any paperwork, even if legal, could only inflame already very volatile community relations.

Often it became all about grabbing the headlines for the big seizures. To perhaps oversimplify some complex professional relations, what it boiled down to operationally was this: when there was intelligence of drugs coming in, customs might in some cases want to make the seizure and arrest at the border to make sure of not losing the consignment while the police often favoured letting the couriers in to find out what happens next, and of course depending on where the drugs are seized would be where the press would highlight who did the seizing. A Regional Crime Squad might have put huge time and resources into tracking an in-country gang and then discovered they were involved in trafficking – or might even know they were trafficking from the get-go but withhold the information from customs.

The hostility between police and customs rarely surfaced in public, but in 1986, a story leaked to the press by an infuriated customs officer centred on a case in which customs wanted to arrest two drug mules coming from France in to Heathrow whereas the police wanted to let them run. When it became clear customs had no intention of letting the couriers into the country, the police phoned the French police who arrested the smugglers at Charles De Gaulle airport with 5 kilos of cocaine, thus depriving UK customs of the arrest.

To compound the problems, trafficking was becoming vastly more complex; no longer gentleman smugglers, but well-organised cartels who in the producer countries had embedded themselves in governments right up to the highest levels and included police, customs and secret service operatives, making overseas intelligence work by UK drug liaison officers immeasurably harder.

A high-level ministerial meeting in May 1986 failed to reach a compromise on the issue of who had authority over drug enforcement operations with neither Home Secretary Douglas Hurd nor Chancellor Nigel Lawson, who held the purse strings, willing to force the matter despite the public spat being another source of government embarrassment over the drugs issue.[15] It was left to the Deputy Chair of Customs and Excise, Valerie Strachan, and her counterpart at the Home Office, John Chilcot (who would later head the inquiry into the Iraq War), to draw up a joint memorandum of understanding which stated the obvious, that the police were responsible for domestic distribution while customs dealt with trafficking. But it didn't resolve the issue – in fact according to one senior customs officer, relations worsened. Heroin might have been screwing up relations between police and customs, but it was also screwing up the lives of thousands of people.

Heroin Screws You Up

In 1984, the ACMD published its *Prevention* report defining three levels of prevention: stopping young people from trying drugs in the first place (primary); reduce the numbers currently using drugs (secondary); and mitigate the harmful effects of drug use through treatment, rehabilitation and social integration (tertiary). The ACMD acknowledged there were several ways of delivering on all three aims but didn't think that national campaigns aimed at reducing drug use had any evidence base nor did the use of scare tactics. Back in the 1970s, for example, there was one British charity who used posed photos of kids on mortuary slabs to get its anti-drug messages across in schools.

The government didn't go down that road, but Norman Fowler felt he needed to respond to the intense media interest in the heroin situation with a very public demonstration of some tangible proof that the government was 'doing something'. This would not be the last time that a government needed publicly to prove it was taking positive action over drugs and itself became an indicator of the degree to which drugs became highly politicised over the next two decades.

Articles, features and interviews filled the pages of the national and local press; prime-time TV documentaries solidified the drug documentary trope first glimpsed around glue sniffing – the bereaved parent; the user and/or dealer in shadow; the professional analysis of why this is happening and what we should do about it. TV personalities such as Michael Parkinson and Esther Rantzen hosted campaign/awareness shows while TV dramas like *Brookside, EastEnders* and *Grange Hill* grasped the social responsibility nettle with drug-related stories concerning schoolkid Zammo and the highly stereotypical figure of 'Nasty' Nick Cotton. Musicians took to the stage in anti-heroin benefit gigs for treatment services as drugs took its toll on many in the industry. Boy George was arrested for drug possession, Topper Headon was sacked from The Clash for his drug use; Culture Club and The Pretenders both lost members to drug overdoses. Drug tragedies were brought right into the heart of government: in 1986 Olivia Channon, daughter of Trade and Industry Secretary Paul Channon, overdosed on heroin and alcohol at Oxford. Having suffered from anorexia aged 14, Mary Parkinson, eldest daughter of Cabinet Minister Cecil Parkinson, began a long and destructive relationship with drugs at university in the early 1980s.

The nationwide anti-heroin campaign was aimed squarely at young people with two TV commercials, advertisements in the youth press and street billboard advertisements. There were also booklets about drugs in general for parents. Under the headline 'Heroin Screws You Up', the key message was that heroin leads to degradation; boys lose control, girls lose their looks. The images majored on spots, yellowing skin, sunken eyes, messy hair, the thin and wasted body. The government commissioned some post-campaign evaluation which essentially concluded that anti-heroin feelings among non-users were reinforced while there was little or no impact on existing users.[16] Crucially though, there was no evidence that expressing hypothetical anti-drug sentiments would mean that a drug offer would invariably be refused. Writing in *Druglink,* Nicholas Dorn, who was a member of the ACMD Prevention group, quoted the market research agency Cragg, Ross and Dawson who, based on their own work surveying young people and drugs, observed, 'It is our impression that convictions about how evil/ stupid/destructive heroin is fall away with surprising ease when apparently contradicted by the example of a friend. A friendly offer and easy accessibility seem to cut heroin down to size and the dangers with it.'[17] There were also anecdotal reports of the posters disappearing from school walls to reappear on the bedroom walls of those who thought the wasted teenager looked cool.

Don't Inject AIDS

Norman Fowler had no problems getting the green light from colleagues and Margaret Thatcher about launching an anti-heroin campaign. A campaign to alert the nation about HIV/AIDS proved significantly more problematic;

he managed to get approval for some newspaper ads in March and July 1986, but he felt more was needed. He wanted every house in the country to receive a warning leaflet. It needed to be sexually explicit about how the virus was transmitted but was blocked by objections from Margaret Thatcher who was horrified at the thought of such material dropping through the letterbox of every household where children could read it. The text of the 'Don't Die of Ignorance' campaign went backwards and forwards for weeks. Eventually it was suggested to set up a special sub-committee of Cabinet just to focus on AIDS. Norman Fowler's concern, however, was that the PM would want to chair the committee and the campaign would still be blocked. In his book *AIDS: Don't Die of Prejudice* Norman Fowler recalls that the Cabinet Secretary and head of the civil service Sir Robert Armstrong came to his rescue by persuading Thatcher that she didn't have the time or need to chair the committee; instead her deputy William Whitelaw would be more suitable.

Fowler's hope that the AIDS committee could work faster especially if the PM stayed out of it proved correct. The committee had its first meeting on 11 November 1986 and by January the leaflets were going through letterboxes nationwide. Then they had to consider the injecting drugs angle. Two months previously in September, the Scottish Committee on HIV and Injecting Drug Misuse published what became known as the McClelland Report, which stated that the Lothian police policy of confiscating needles and syringes from users was encouraging sharing and helping to spread HIV. Furthermore, they controversially recommended establishing needle exchange schemes.

Interviewed for this book, Lord Fowler recalled that the existence of the committee smoothed the way for him to get his AIDS work endorsed, although it was a close call: 'It could have gone either way, but I had a very close working relationship with Willie Whitelaw who summed it all up in our favour.' (Norman Fowler recalls Douglas Hurd and Tom King among others being on his side.)

Meanwhile up in Liverpool as the needle exchange began its work in October 1986, John Ashton was looking for political cover from the top of Merseyside Regional Health Authority. He had a good relationship with the Chair, Sir Donald Wilson, who John describes as 'an unusual, eccentric character, an old-fashioned paternalistic Tory who was on first name terms with Margaret Thatcher'. John also knew Sir Donald Acheson, the Chief Medical Officer, who in turn sold the idea of needle exchange to Norman Fowler. Having a special group also worked in the health secretary's favour regarding needle exchange, although as he recalled, 'it was the Scottish ministers who were most opposed'. However, on 18 December 1986, barely a month after the committee's first meeting, Norman Fowler announced in Parliament that firstly, there would be another AIDS campaign, this one specifically aimed at drug users – launched in September 1987 under the banners 'Don't Inject AIDS' and 'Smack Isn't Worth It' – and secondly, the establishment of needle exchange pilot schemes that would be formally evaluated, taking into account those already up and running. The government response was typically British. In the run-up to Norman Fowler's announcement, there had been meetings at the Department of Health to decide what to do about the technically illegal needle exchanges already operating. They could have shut them down or they could have formally endorsed and funded them. Instead they simply let them carry on but dressed up the decision as an evaluated pilot project. If it was a disaster, government could distance itself; if not the decision to evaluate first would be vindicated.

In May 1987, the ACMD began considering what to do about AIDS in relation to drug use. Eventually it published another landmark report in March 1988, *AIDS and Drug Misuse Part 1* (with *Part 2* in 1989 and *Update* in 1993), whose primary conclusion was that 'HIV is a greater threat to public and individual health than drug misuse'. The report shied away from endorsing long-term maintenance prescribing, emphasising instead that abstinence was the 'ultimate goal'. But it was clear that the advent of HIV would mean a shake-up in clinic prescribing policy and a move away from the holy writ of the short-term reducing dose of oral methadone if there was to be any hope of encouraging people into treatment and away from injecting. In a meeting with leading consultant psychiatrists, the Department of Health quietly urged they take a 'flexible' approach to prescribing. Decisions about drug prescribing taken in light of concerns about AIDS would spark another prescribing row 20 years down the line.

Sitting alongside the ACMD report in 1988, the government-funded research project conducted by Gerry Stimson and colleagues at Goldsmith College reported that the existing schemes had succeeded in drawing more people into services but enumerated many ways in which services had to be improved to build on the gains achieved. All of which made the government response to the ACMD report in the words of Dave Turner from the Standing Conference on Drug Abuse 'extraordinarily disappointing'.

The government declared that there would be no new money to enhance drug service capability to deal with AIDS, nor would be it be funding more needle exchange schemes because in the words of Health Minister Tony Newton, 'We do not consider that we yet have sufficient evidence to recommend an expansion of schemes in England.' But by then Norman Fowler had been replaced by John Moore, who was much closer to Margaret Thatcher and likely to take a less liberal view of how to tackle HIV among drug users. Tony Newton was simply relaying his master's voice; he would take a far more positive role in developing drug policies in later years under John Major.

However, the statistics could not be denied: the upshot of the concerted harm reduction effort was to head off a major HIV epidemic among drug users and deliver some of the lowest HIV rates among injecting drug users in Europe. Norman Fowler admitted that if it could have been proved that injecting drug users could not pass on HIV to the wider community, convincing colleagues about the need for harm reduction would have been even harder.

The provision of needles and syringes was specifically exempted from Section 9A of the Misuse of Drugs Act and Section 34 of the new Drug Trafficking Offences Act which outlawed the provision of any implements which could be used for drug-taking. The new provision also targeted 'head shops' selling pipes, bongs and scales. As harm reduction became further embedded in the treatment system and as the imperative to attract drug injectors into treatment was always a priority, more and more items were being dispensed by both needle exchanges and pharmacists including citric acid to dissolve heroin (smokable brown heroin needed to be dissolved before injecting) and sterile water. Rather than simply repeal Section 9A, over the years, the government just kept adding exemptions through a tortuous process of seeking the advice of the ACMD and then taking months (or in one case years) to respond. Throughout, those engaged in distribution would seek so-called 'Letters of Comfort' from the local police which would give a green light on the promise that users would not be arrested or harassed going to and from a needle exchange. The police invariably took a very pragmatic view of harm reduction and treatment generally as it became clear through later research that those who engaged in treatment were far less likely to engage in criminal activity.

If there is one thing certain about the drug scene, you never know what's coming around the corner. While a senor customs officer was briefing Home Office Minister David Mellor in private on what he believed was an impending cocaine explosion, the head of the National Drug Intelligence Unit, Colin Hewett, was writing an article in the March/April 1987 issue of *Druglink* explaining why he thought it wouldn't happen. He was right to suggest that just because a drug takes off in America does not mean it will gain traction in the UK, a good example being phencyclidine, or Angel Dust, which caused many problems for US enforcement and health professionals in the 1970s. He thought that cheap amphetamines would undermine attempts to flood the UK with cocaine without appreciating that cocaine would be targeting a very different market. In fairness to both views, customs and police would have very different perspectives and intelligence. With their overseas contacts, especially the DEA, customs would have been very aware that the multi-ton shipments were arriving in the States through Florida and heeding US warnings that at some point the US market would reach saturation point. From his point of view, Colin Hewett would see very little cocaine seized in the UK, although he overestimated the capacity of UK drug law enforcement to counteract the activities of well-motivated, sophisticated drug traffickers with unlimited resources.

10

Smoke and Mirrors

Pharmaceutical-grade cocaine had been circulating in Soho since the 'panic' of the First World War years; initially it was bought over the counter and then, as controls tightened, mainly as a result of excess prescriptions being sold on, there were some wholesale thefts and a few examples of pharmaceutical cocaine being smuggled in from Europe.

Through the 1920s and 1930s American production of cocaine as a key ingredient in patent medicines for respiratory conditions such as asthma and hay fever using Peruvian coca leaves had been shut down. The coca plant itself was subject to international narcotics control and its centuries-old indigenous use in Peru demonised by US state officials, all of which meant that otherwise impoverished Peruvian coca farmers had no legitimate outlet for their product. Eventually they threw in their lot with a new and ultimately highly lucrative consumer base.

Cuba was the back door that would eventually open the floodgates for cocaine into America. Less than an hour's flight from mainland America, Cuba had long been a bolthole for gangsters and bootleggers. In 1952, Fulgencio Batista took over the country and immediately struck deals with Mafia top dogs Bugsy Siegel and Meyer Lansky who invested heavily in the island's tourist industry. Their other business interests included drugs. Lansky had been the brains behind the French Connection running heroin through Cuba on its way to the States. But heroin was not a drug for the island of fun. Reflecting the image of glamour, mystery and expense that surrounded the silent movie stars' use of the drug in the 1920s, cocaine became the perfect party drug for rich Americans on holiday. Lansky knew the plant grew in Peru and Bolivia but where to refine it for convenient transport to Cuba? The answer was Chile, where the government helpfully ordered the army to assist the Mafia to transport cocaine to Cuba.

Batista and his mobster cronies were thrown out by Castro in 1959. The now-exiled anti-Communist Cubans living in Florida received CIA training to help them plot the overthrow of Castro in return for the proverbial blind eye being turned to increasing smuggling of all kinds, including cocaine. Despite the drug war rhetoric, elements of US foreign policy have been based on the idea that being anti-Communist was far more important than being anti-drugs. If you needed help on the drugs front to strengthen your economy (or line your pockets) and increase the robustness of your anti-Communist stance – so be it.[1]

In 1973, Augusto Pinochet overthrew the Chilean socialist government of Salvador Allende; the CIA had backed the coup in exchange for which Pinochet brought Chile's role as the point country for cocaine distribution to an abrupt end. With the French Connection also a busted flush, the Mafia needed new partners and chose Colombia, a country undergoing an economic depression and one steeped in smuggling history. So began the oft-told bloody tale of the rise of the Colombian drug cartels.

Cocaine began to creep back into the USA in the late sixties; an expensive luxury, it was immediately taken up by the 'new aristocrats' of the music and film industries. In the very early days, *Easy Rider*-types would arrive in Colombia looking to take a few kilos back to the USA. They didn't last long when the Colombians realised just how much money could be made from a white powder comprising mashed-up coca leaves and a few chemicals. A kilo costing $3,500–4,000 at the farm gate could be turned into a $300,000 profit per kilo, depending on how much it was cut.[2]

For an illegal drug, cocaine had an incredibly benign image: it looked clean – white, sparkly, fluffy and pharmaceutical and no need for needles. In 1970, *Rolling Stone* dubbed cocaine 'drug of the year'. *Esquire* magazine put a gold coke spoon on its front cover; in 1971, *Newsweek* described cocaine as 'the status symbol of the American middle-class pothead'. *The New York Times* magazine heralded 'cocaine: the champagne of drugs ... speed kills, but coke heightens all your senses ... orgasms go better with coke'. In the same article, an officer from Chicago's Bureau of Narcotics said in contrast to heroin, 'you get a good high with coke and you don't get hooked'. *High Times* magazine carried adverts for sterling silver cocaine accessories while patrons of the Beverly Hills head shop could pay in excess of $2,000 for a coke spoon. There was a famous scene in Woody Allen's *Annie Hall* where the guy reverentially chops the coke, tells Allen the coke costs $2,000 an ounce, who then proceeds to sneeze the whole lot up in the air. Robin Williams among others was quoted as saying, 'Cocaine is God's way of telling you you have too much money.' At the 1981 Oscars ceremony, host Johnny Carson quipped, 'The biggest money-maker in Hollywood last year was Columbia. Not the studio, the country.'[3]

The socio-demographic user profile in the UK was similar. At £75–£100 a gram, it was only likely to find its way in any quantity to the gilded palaces of the rich and infamous, the new wave of louche aristos and the entertainment spangle babies, where cocaine was seen as the essential weapon in the self-protecting armoury of proving you were super-confident and ahead of the game 24/7. That many a fragile temperament became paranoid snow monsters manifested itself in the blizzard of 'my cocaine hell' stories that became the cliché of later rock star confessionals.

Richard Wingfield was a typical early seventies lone dealer. Failed medical student, former Grenadier Guard and a member of the Chelsea set, he was sentenced to 7 years in July 1973 for smuggling in 3 kilos of cocaine. The next year, customs seized 4 kilos of coke in the luggage of a well-dressed mature English woman who arrived from Bogota via Zurich. This case alerted UK customs that Colombian traffickers were already beginning to wise-up from using obvious people and obvious routes. Yes, this woman was caught, but it would be a common ploy to sacrifice small-time mules in the expectation of smuggling in much larger consignments undetected. Pablo Escobar, by the way, was simply regarded as a 'worthless drug mule' by Colombian police in the mid-1970s.[4]

As the seventies gave way to the eighties, cocaine became increasingly favoured over hash by traffickers because it was more valuable and easier to transport in commercial weights. Most cocaine came into the UK in small amounts through the post. However, British criminals hiding out in Spain – such as Eddie Richardson who with his brother Charlie led the 1960s south London Richardson gang, Great Train Robbers Charlie Wilson, Gordon Goody and Jimmy Hussey, and others of the armed robbery fraternity – began rubbing shoulders with cartel bosses. They in turn were looking to use the language connection with Spain as the most convenient way of establishing a distribution chain in Europe. Even these hardened criminals though were unprepared for the violence associated with cocaine. They had been peacefully smuggling tons of cannabis for years; the wake-up call was the drug-related murder of Charlie Wilson in Marbella in April 1990.

Cocaine became equally attractive to the new breed of young traders working in the world of finance where you needed to demonstrate that in that testosterone-drenched environment you had the biggest balls on the Stock Exchange floor. The stereotypical image of the 1980s City Boy was red braces, a mobile phone the size of a brick and, in the words of Harry Enfield's song 'Loadsamoney', with access to unlimited amounts of champagne and cocaine.

However, the undeniable presence of cocaine in the UK did present something of a mystery. The amount seized rose inexorably from 1975 to 1991, but it was relatively small. In 1992, writing for a book on cocaine and crack edited by criminologist Philip Bean, I looked at some of the cocaine statistics and contacted several treatment facilities, both NHS and private. Only 2 per cent of those notified to the Home Office in the early 1990s sought treatment for a primary cocaine problem, while the community drug treatment services told me that cocaine users only constituted about the same percentage of their caseload. I assumed, therefore, that as cocaine was so expensive those with a problem would seek private treatment. Yet the major private residential rehabilitation facilities said they too saw very few people with just a cocaine problem – usually alcohol and tranquillisers were in the mix too. There were about 1,000 people notified to the Home Office in 1990 with a primary cocaine problem who typically would be using cocaine in binges, around 3 grams a day on a 4-day run before taking a break and starting again. A typical heavy user could therefore consume approximately 600 grams a year or roughly a ½ kilo. So, the whole notified group could consume 600 kilos between them, around 10 per cent more than was seized and that's just a group of hardcore users. On the basis that far more cocaine was entering the country than was seized (as with most drugs), what was happening to it?

It seemed reasonable to assume (and still does) that those who used the drug only occasionally or maybe as a weekend treat, did not come to any great harm and certainly did not need treatment. No less a body than the WHO came to the same conclusion in 1995 in a global cocaine survey it published with the UN Crime and Justice Research Institute (UNICRI). The press briefing stated: 'Few experts describe cocaine as invariably harmful to health. Cocaine-related problems are widely perceived to be more common and more severe for intensive, high-dosage users and very rare and much less severe for occasional, low-dosage users.'[5] The WHO's American paymasters were furious; in threatening to pull funding, they widened their attack on the WHO for supporting harm reduction and for its 'association with organizations who support the legalization of drugs'.[6]

By and large then, cocaine users were not visible to UK police because they were not hanging around the streets, nor to community drug treatment services because most of them did not have a problem and the few that did squirreled themselves away in private treatment. Nor was there much media clamour. That was possibly because Fleet Street itself was hardly a coke-free zone. However, certain celebrity downfalls made the news such as the 1998 sacking of *Blue Peter* presenter Richard Bacon for snorting cocaine, the 1999 shot of Liverpool striker Robbie Fowler alluding to usage by 'snorting' along the white goal line during a game, or in 2000, the photos revealing that *EastEnders* star Danniella Westbrook's cocaine habit had destroyed her nasal septum. Cocaine retained a champagne-lifestyle image most associated with the rich and famous and so was seemingly out of the reach of ordinary people. It was way down the political agenda of drug problems that needed to be addressed. And then came crack.

* * *

For centuries, coca leaves mixed with lime were chewed by indigenous populations in Peru and Bolivia. Once the medicinal properties of the cocaine molecule were identified, cocaine hydrochloride powder was produced for its anaesthetic properties and for various conditions affecting the nasal membranes. There were production steps along the way between green leaves and pure white powder, the early stages of which involved turning the leaves into an off-white sludgy paste called *pasta basica*, more commonly known as *pasta*, *bazuko* or *basé*. Those processing the leaves discovered the paste could be rolled up as cigarettes and smoked to produce a very intense high. For many years though, this was a trade secret known only to those working the fields of Peru and Bolivia. Exactly how coca paste smoking became more widely known is something of a mystery, but cocaine expert Professor Ron Siegel offered a credible narrative. Interviewed by Dominic Streatfeild for his book on cocaine history, Siegel reckoned that a white American trafficker travelled to Peru in the early seventies looking for supplies and found the local workers smoking what they called *basé*.

The trafficker smoked it, was most impressed by the effects and tried to replicate this back in the States. He thought they were smoking the finished article, so when he tried to smoke cocaine it didn't work. He asked a chemist friend to work out how to do it; research revealed that cocaine was cocaine hydrochloride, which was a salt. They reasoned that if you took the salt out, you would be left with the 'base'. They added a strong alkali, dissolved the result in ether, allowed it to crystallise and freed the 'base' from its salt, giving 'freebase'. But this was not what the Peruvian workers were smoking. They called it *basé*, which was Spanish for 'foundation', not the chemical meaning of the word 'base'. Their smokable paste was a mixture of crude cocaine sulphate molecules. What the Americans created, nobody had ever smoked before and its impact among the cocaine cognoscenti was immediate. And like *basé*, it remained a secret known only to relatively few until 1980 when Richard Pryor managed to blow himself up trying to make freebase, although most of his burns came from setting his nylon shirt on fire with a cigarette having spilt high-proof rum down himself while in a freebase haze.

But the story on the streets was that freebase caused the explosion, so freebasers looked for alternative chemicals. They tried ammonia, then discovered all you needed to do was boil up street cocaine, add baking soda and let it dry out. What remained were hard crystals of smokable cocaine which became known as crack, named for the sound heard when it is lit. The result was a very intense, but very short-lived high, making crack extremely moreish with a very high dependency potential.

During the 1980s, the US drug scene exploded in much the same way as it did in the UK, in the same type of inner-city locales and for the similar reasons. Cocaine production rose dramatically along with a rise in purity and a fall in the wholesale kilo price. The total acreage devoted to coca leaf growing in Peru, Bolivia and Columbia rose from 220,000 acres in 1980 to more than 500,000 acres by 1988; cocaine purity in the USA increased from 30 per cent in 1980 to 80 per cent by 1991; the wholesale kilo price went through the floor from $50,000 in 1980 to $12,000 in 1992 while US seizures rose from 50 tons in 1979 to 200 tons in 1989.[7] Producers needed to find a whole new market for cocaine; crack was the answer. Chip off bits of cocaine rock, sell it for between $2 and $20 for a hit the size of a raisin and thousands of poor people, mainly black, get an all-access areas pass to the world of cocaine at a time when unemployment was soaring and public services and welfare benefits were being cut. The UK had Thatcherism; the USA had Reaganomics. Their similar social policy was based on the same ethos that those with the worst problems were causing the worst problems.

The US crack epidemic began in South Central Los Angeles supposedly with a young cocaine dealer called Ricky Donnell Ross who started out selling powder, then switched to crack after some of his customers wanted ready-made freebase without having to go to the bother of cooking it up themselves. His Ready Rock product took off; the area market for powder cocaine collapsed. At his height in 1982/83 Ross was making crack in industrial quantities, shifting 15 kilos a week as the crack boom took off all up the West Coast.[8]

The *Los Angeles Times* was first out of the gate with a crack story in November 1984; it took another year for the first national reference in a *New York Times* article and then media coverage soared in 1986 with the sort of press and TV coverage mirrored in the UK with heroin. Probably the most enduring mythology about crack was the revelation about 'crack babies' who were allegedly dying in their hundreds solely because their mothers had smoked crack during pregnancy. The babies filmed by CBS, which 'broke' the story, had actually been born needing to be weaned off heroin, not cocaine, and those babies who had supposedly died just because their mothers had smoked crack were actually the victims of their mothers' poly-drug use and a deep and enduring impoverished lifestyle.[9] But it wasn't just the tabloid media caught up in the crack frenzy. It may come as a surprise to some people that scientific and clinical publishing is not so evidence-based and objective as you might hope. Apart from babies dying a crack-related death, it was also claimed that those who survived suffered long-term damage. In 1989, *The Lancet* published a paper that demonstrated that those studies which purported to show long-term damage were more likely to be published that those which did not, even if the methodology of the latter was more robust.[10]

And in the UK, it was the usually more sober and thoughtful *Observer* which started the crack crisis ball rolling in February 1987, dramatically telling its readers that crack was so potent, 'a single dose can lead to addiction … this drug is a killer. And Britain could be its next target.' US-style freebase and crack had been around in the UK since 1986; there were pockets of use in most metropolitan inner-city areas including London, Merseyside (where a study found regular use among sex workers), Nottingham, Cardiff, Newcastle and Manchester. In March 1989, Interpol identified a new cocaine route from Jamaica to Europe. The Caribbean was a transit region for cocaine coming from South America into the USA and some of the very earliest reports of crack use had been in the Bahamas in 1984.

But it was the arrival in the UK of soon-to-retire DEA agent Robert Stutman to speak at the April 1989 drug conference of the Association of Chief Police Officers (ACPO) which created a crescendo of political and media alarm. Stutman told of 10-year-old crack addicts and the instant and incurable ravages of crack addiction, announcing that a study to be published shortly after his talk would prove that 75 per cent of all those who try crack will be physically addicted after their third hit. Heroin he said 'was not in the same ballpark' as crack when it came to addiction potential. Crack use had generated such violence, he said, that all DEA agents had been issued with submachine guns. Given that the worst of crack problems were occurring in black and minority ethnic parts of major inner-city areas, this ramping up of ordnance had echoes of southern state police being issued with higher-calibre guns back at the turn of the twentieth century to take down 'cocaine-crazed negroes'. He ended his speech by saying that if the UK did not get on top of the problem immediately, 'I will guarantee you the following: three years from today you will invite me back because you will be looking back on the good old days of 1989 and that won't be pleasant.'

Straight out of the Anslinger playbook, Stutman had form on using the media to push political buttons; in his 1992 autobiography *Dead on Delivery* he said, 'There was no doubt in my mind that crack was on its way to becoming a national problem. But to speed up the process of convincing Washington, I needed to make it a national issue and quickly. I began a lobbying effort and I used the media. Reporters were only too willing to cooperate because as far as the New York media was concerned, crack was the hottest reporting to come along since the end of the Vietnam War.'[11] In 1986, within two months of Stutman starting his campaign, the New York press alone had published 200 articles on crack with Stutman taking reporters to crack house busts and was 'helped' in this by the cocaine-related death of basketball legend Len Bias.

The political and press reaction to Stutman's speech was as incendiary as Stutman's manner of delivery. Home Secretary Douglas Hurd told the *Daily Mail* that crack could be the worst health disaster to hit the UK since the Black Death. Under the headline 'Crack Crazy; evil gangs spread drug through Britain', *The Sun* famously ran with the 'three hits can get you hooked' claim. Not to be outdone, the Scottish press weighed in with 'Warning on crack reaching Scotland' (*Glasgow Herald*, 30 June 1989) and 'Cops wait as evil drug creeps north' (*Glasgow Daily Record*, 26 December 1989), although somebody wasn't paying attention because back on 21 September 1986, *The Sunday Post* declared, 'Now crack spreads to Scotland'.

Tim Eggar, the Parliamentary Under-Secretary of State for Foreign Affairs, told a Home Office meeting that 'crack is by far the single greatest threat that faces the United Kingdom. It is worse in its social implications than the threat posed by any known disease.'[12] Ministers went on a fact-finding mission to the USA and came back both stirred and shaken, not least by the instruction not to leave the hotel unescorted for fear of attacks by crack-crazed teenagers. The Home Affairs Committee's subsequent report rushed out on 27 June following their US visit repeated the 'three hits and you're hooked' mantra' in bold type and recommended an all-out national anti-crack campaign along the lines of 'Heroin Screws You Up'.

There was an interdepartmental split over the idea of a national campaign, with the Home Office and Foreign Office in favour, while the Departments of Health and Education urged a more local and targeted approach, fearing that spreading the word about a drug that was hardly present in the UK would simply stimulate interest. As ISDD later found out, our *Crack Briefing* which was sent to the Home Office and Department of Health setting out the landscape of the published evidence on the drug, was aiding officials in their ability to persuade ministers to hold back on potentially stoking interest in crack. ISDD publications had already received a mention in despatches when on 27 June the Labour spokesman on Home Affairs, Robin Corbett, asked Home Office minister Douglas Hogg to list all his sources of information about crack, to which the minister replied that he had taken his information from ISDD's *Drug misuse: a basic briefing*, a copy of which he had been placed in the Commons Library.

The notion that crack was essentially a black problem caused by black drug dealers generated concerns among local community workers that crack would be another drug-related excuse for some police to harass young black youths. Whether it was a case of rotten apples or whole orchards, relations between the police and the African-Caribbean community had been especially toxic in London going back as far as the Notting Hill riot of 1958. Black youths hanging around the streets and in cafés became easy targets for a Metropolitan Police force which, as the McPherson Report into the death of Stephen Lawrence concluded, was institutionally racist and, when it came to drugs, sometimes corrupt. The Bristol riot of 1980 followed a drug raid on the Black and White café in the St Paul's area of the city. In Brixton, one of the subtexts of the unrest was the alleged favouring by the police of some drug dealers over others in order to keep the drug problem under control. Some dealers appeared to be operating with impunity in exchange for informing on others. There were allegations too that seized cannabis seemed to find its way back onto the streets.

Community fears of a new era of conflict appeared confirmed on 23 May 1989 when 120 police mounted a drugs raid on a pub in the Heath district of Wolverhampton. The ensuing fracas saw a large crowd gather with both black and white youths fighting it out for 2 hours with 250 police in riot gear. The drug haul was 14 wraps of crack worth about £140 (*The Times*, 25 May 1989). Douglas Hurd told the *Daily Mail* (2 June 1989) that the incident confirmed in his mind that 'drug trafficking leads to violence'.

In September, Dr Reed Tuckson, Commissioner of Public Health in Washington, told another UK Chief Police Officers' meeting that the UK's better health and welfare system would not protect us from the predicted societal meltdown.

However, doubts were beginning to grow about Stutman's credibility as the study he announced to the ACPO delegates with the 75 per cent figure duly reported in the media as if the study had already been published, failed to appear. The *Grimsby Evening Telegraph* (2 August 1989) even attributed the report to the Home Office. In October, at the City of London's high-profile crack conference, Stutman and Dr Mark Gold, who had set up a cocaine hotline in the States, traded insults with UK speakers about their attempt to graft the US crack experience onto the UK. Bing Spear's successor Peter Spurgeon did a quiet but thorough de-escalation job on the impending crack crisis while Dr Andrew Johns simply poured cold water on the biochemical doomsday tone of the American speakers about cocaine's ability to hijack the human mind irrespective of the socio-economic circumstances of the individual, especially as it related to those animal experiments where rats and monkeys obsessively self-administered cocaine in entirely artificial laboratory environments. On 10 April 1990, BBC's *File on Four* programme concluded that Stutman's address was 'littered with misinformation'. And ACPO never did invite him to return.

Despite the frantic aftermath of Stut-speak, the Home Office was dissuaded against both a national crack campaign and a cocaine/crack specific helpline along US lines. It also dialled back on another parliamentary recommendation: the idea of parachuting 'crack teams' into local hotspots. What these teams were meant to do where few professionals had any experience of the drug remained unclear. Instead, the proposal was replaced in October 1989 by a more generic Drug Prevention Initiative (DPI) aimed at helping local communities tackle drug problems whatever their nature. The crack campaign became a more generic anti-drug campaign in 1990 while the helpline idea was the seed which eventually grew into FRANK, the still current national drugs helpline.

In the same month as the DPI was announced, the Metropolitan Police formed two units; one had a very definite enforcement role, while the other looked more to the community response to crack. The first unit had in its sights the arrival into the UK of so-called 'Yardies', Jamaican gangsters who were importing small amounts of cocaine into the UK, usually carried by female drug mules, for conversion to crack. Using their UK connections, Jamaican criminals embedded themselves in parts of London and elsewhere and, given the violent gun-related background of Jamaican politics, they certainly did bring a new level of crime into the UK drug scene and caused many problems in local areas as they were also engaged in other criminal activities such as prostitution. But the amounts of drug they had smuggled in were relatively small, which didn't prevent a tendency in the media to attribute every crime in the African-Caribbean community to these exciting and dangerous gangsters.

The other police unit was more concerned with the local impact of crack across London and for the first time, the police were officially tasked with talking to, for example, drug treatment agencies about crack clients. Lorraine Hewitt ran the Stockwell Project in south London, and she told the police who visited about the inordinate difficulty of encouraging African-Caribbean users to come into the service. Unlike for heroin clients, there was nothing that the services could offer by way of a substitute drug for crack; black users especially were very suspicious of attending white services, fearing a subsequent knock on the door – and as crack users, the effects of the drug itself would often render the user paranoid. Crack users tended to hit a crisis point and want help immediately, even in the middle of the night when no service was open. So rather than crack users being 'hard to reach', they were 'under-served'.

The issue of service provision for black users later caused something of a controversy among those campaigning for community-specific services; some believing in separate services for ethnic minority groups while others believed this simply let white mainstream services off the hook allowing them to employ a token black or minority ethnic worker to deal with anybody who wasn't white, so that service managers could tick the 'diversity' box.

The crack problem did not explode in the UK; instead it crept up on us, becoming entrenched primarily where serious heroin problems already existed. The drug certainly had nothing like the devastating impact on African-Caribbean communities here as it did in the USA. In fact, studies revealed that contrary to popular belief most UK crack users were white, often existing heroin users and already deeply immersed in the drug scene.

Through the 1990s, heroin and crack use developed in tandem where dealers would often sell 'brown and white' together and those mainly using crack often became dependent on heroin as they had used the drug to come down from the high intensity effects of crack. This was contrary to Stutman's view that heroin addiction wasn't in the same 'ballpark' as crack; it was often the other way around, with crack users finding it much harder to break the heroin habit. I recall speaking to one drug worker who said that in his experience, if you could get a person's heroin problem under control, then it helped mitigate or resolve other problems in their life including crack use.

As officials and ministers were tussling over responses to crack which were both visible and proportionate, a whole new drug culture was bubbling under, one that was very different from the depressed, poverty-stricken world of glue, heroin and crack. This one came with a smiley face. At first.

11

When Britain Ruled the Raves

In 1985, journalist Peter Nasmyth was researching a feature for *The Face*, a London-based music, fashion and culture magazine founded in 1980 by ex-*New Musical Express* editor Nick Logan. The article focused on a new drug capturing the attention of both the latest iteration of the Soho's irregular community and a 1980s creation, 'yuppies' (young urban professionals), in well-paid jobs who were well up Maslow's hierarchy of needs.

The drug was 3,4-methylenedioxymethamphetamine, aka MDMA, Adam, XTC or just plain ecstasy, virtually unknown in the UK outside of this cultural and professional elite, and they wanted to keep it that way. They didn't want Nasmyth to write about it and so the whole article was based on MDMA's American story and even then, Nasmyth couldn't get an interview with the main man who did not want to be heralded as ecstasy's Timothy Leary – Alexander 'Sasha' Shulgin.

MDMA is one of the many children of the parent drug MDA, all of which fall along a continuum between hallucinogen and stimulant. The drug was first synthesised by the German pharmaceutical company Merck in 1912 and patented in 1914. Merck briefly resurrected MDMA in 1921 but there is no documented evidence they had any use for the drug in mind. It is possible that MDMA was just an accidental by-product of a process or simply a failed idea, but even so companies usually patent any compounds created in its laboratories to secure ownership in case some use is found later. MDMA languished on the shelf until the 1950s when the CIA added it to the list of candidates for the elusive 'truth' drug. No luck there either.

Alexander Shulgin was a research chemist working for Dow Chemicals in California where he developed Zectran, the first biodegradable insecticide. Zectran proved highly profitable for Dow; as a reward, they allowed Shulgin to set up his own laboratory and conduct research into whatever interested him – which, having experimented with mescaline – turned out to be psychedelic drugs. In 1965, when they found out what he was doing, Dow and Shulgin quietly parted company. Albert Hoffnman and Gordon Alles had personally tried out their own compounds; Shulgin took this to a whole new level, introducing himself and a select band of friends to an enormous range of compounds. Shulgin and his wife eventually wrote up their experiments in two massive tomes published in 1991 and 1997, which extensively described their work and personal experience with two classes of psychoactive drugs. The first book was entitled *PIKHKAL (Phenethylamines I Have Known and Loved)* – a broad category including both hallucinogenic drugs such as mescaline and amphetamine-based compounds including MDA and MDMA. The second was TIHKAL, all about tryptamines, including psilocybin, the magic chemical in magic mushrooms and DMT, the powerful hallucinogen found in Amazonian ayahuasca.

For many years, he had a DEA 'licence to pill'. Agents would come to him with compounds to test, while in the UK (and elsewhere), Shulgin's books full of chemical formulae and 'recipes' were pored over by forensic chemists and enforcement agencies trying not only to identify new compounds, but attempting to second-guess what might be the next big thing. Those underground chemists on the other side of the legal wall were equally enamoured.

Eventually the whole DEA/Shulgin love-in became an official embarrassment and in 1994 Sasha's badge-wearing buddies raided his lab, charging him with a violation of his DEA licence. Undeterred, he continued beavering away at new compounds right up to the point when ill health brought an end to his work.

Having first re-synthesised MDA in the mid-1960s and then MDMA in the early 1970s, through self-experimentation Shulgin discovered the unique selling point of MDMA – its ability to induce empathy in users. Through his networks, therapists began to use the drug in marital therapy, giving the warring parties a controlled dose of MDMA before the session. Meanwhile the drug began to appear on the streets, courtesy of underground chemists based in Boston who, like the early acid protagonists, wanted the world to realise the unique potential of MDMA as a catalyst for peace and understanding. A new pharmacological descriptor was created – 'empathogen' – to describe the effects of this class of drugs and ecstasy was marketed particularly through the urban gay club scenes of Chicago and New York. One of the Boston chemists hooked up with a posse of interested cocaine dealers who between them opened another MDMA gateway in Texas where the drug was sold in bottles labelled 'sassyfras' to try to fool the law that this was a health food product. But the federal authorities were not fooled for long. There was a genuine scare about 'designer drugs', those drugs deliberately formulated or designed to sit outside the law, when some underground chemists accidentally produced an analogue of the opioid drug fentanyl, causing a spike in overdoses while some users exhibited irreversible symptoms of Parkinson's disease. Coupled with some research claiming MDMA caused brain damage in rats, in July 1985 MDMA becoming a Schedule 1 controlled drug in the USA attracting the toughest penalties for possession, supply and manufacture. Therapists, already appalled that MDMA had become just another street drug, launched an unsuccessful attempt to have the drug controlled under the less draconian Schedule III, which only served to increase publicity about ecstasy while closing the door on clinical research and use.

Even while American therapists were beginning to trial the drug in their work under a cloak of secrecy, the UK had already banned it. In 1975, the West Midlands Drug Squad raided an amphetamine lab and seized samples of a drug they couldn't identify. Tests results came back as MDMA. There was no evidence that anybody was using the drug here but in 1977, MDMA was brought under the Misuse of Drugs Act as a Class A drug because of its chemical link to other phenethylamines like mescaline and a powerful hallucinogen called DOM, known on the US scene as STP (Serenity, Tranquillity and Peace – another Shulgin invention) that were already Class A drugs, but very different in their effects from MDMA.

The first British news story about MDMA appeared in the *Daily Express* in April 1985 under the headline 'How The Evil of Ecstasy Hit The Streets', which picked up on a 15 April *Newsweek* article from the USA headlined far less dramatically, 'Getting High on "Ecstasy"', which focused entirely on the therapeutic potential with just a one-line mention of some bad reactions to recreational use. And in a predictable rerun of Stutman, a DEA agent came to warn an ACPO conference about MDMA, reported in the *Daily Telegraph* (1 May) under the headline 'Ecstasy – The New Narcotic Menace'. Then Nasmyth's article appeared in October followed by another *Daily Express* scoop on 17 March 1986 that Scotland Yard were 'standing by' 'As New Ecstasy Arrives in Britain', although MDMA didn't really 'arrive' in the UK until towards the end of 1987/early 1988.

Ecstasy was slipped into the UK, albeit in very small quantities by travellers coming back from the USA. Nasmyth called his article the 'Yuppie way of knowledge'; its first iteration here was more to do with spiritual investigation than all-night dancing, although supplies reached mid-1980s London clubs such as Taboo and the Hug Club. One of these very early clubs hosting the decadent androgyny of the New Romantic scene gave away a free E tab with every entry.

On 18 January 1986, under the headline 'Calling Card of a Deadly Salesman', a strange item appeared in the *South Wales Echo*:

South Wales is at the front line of the battle to beat the threat of deadly so-called 'designer drugs' from the United States. Only a handful of seizures of the perversely named ecstasy have been made in Britain. 'We have got to stamp this out' said Detective Inspector John Wake of the South Wales drugs squad. 'Nobody knows the full extent of the damage this can do. We believe it can lead to death.' One club goer told the *South Wales Echo* how calling cards and pamphlets were handed out to youngsters in one city centre club. 'We have seen drug pushers before but nobody quite like this. He was wearing a dark pinstripe suit as he walked around handing out his leaflets. He was aged about 45 to 50 and had receding hair. He said he didn't have the drug on him but wanted us to read the leaflets. He would come back later if anyone wanted any. The 22-page booklet contains articles from United States magazines on the use of ecstasy, guides to its abuse and hippie-like verbiage. One nonsense quote read: 'You are in a pure space of non-thinking … this is the Nirvana all masters and saints talk about.'

The real action though was happening on a Spanish island in the Balearic Sea. Ibiza had been a hippy hideaway since the early 1960s. But in the early 1980s, the beginnings of cheap air travel took hordes of new tourists to the island, including many young people from the UK and all over Europe, attracted too by the cheap food, drink and accommodation. Clubs like Amnesia, Pacha and Ku opened to attract the new young tourists, playing a new sound derived from American throbbing four-to-the floor urban House dance music where DJs, not musicians, were the stars.

With the new music came the new drug from an unlikely source, the Orange People, followers of Osho, aka Bhagwan Shree Rajneesh, on the run from their Oregon enclave. Potential new recruits were given ecstasy prior to their acceptance interview, which presumably also made them more amenable to parting with all their worldly goods to help maintain Osho's fleet of Rolls-Royces. The drug was being manufactured in Holland (and not banned until 1988) and so great was demand from the Orange brigade arriving from the USA that production was stepped up and as cult members gravitated to the natural chill-out island, they brought quantities of MDMA with them.

Among the island visitors for the summer holidays of 1987 were London DJs Danny Rampling, Paul Oakenfold, Johnny Walker, Trevor Fung and Ian St Paul. What they found would profoundly change the UK music and drug scene for years to come. Not only did they soak up the sun and sangria, but the combination of MDMA and its hug drug qualities in the atmosphere of revolutionary banging dance music, created a determination to bring the E-biza vibe back to the UK to revive a sterile club scene.

What happened over the next four years, from 1988 to 1992, can best be plotted by the size of the events hosting the new drug/dance culture that swept through the UK. It started with what was called acid house music in London; there was Shroom near London Bridge and Future, hosted for one night at Richard Branson's Heaven club in the West End. Both venues quickly became too popular; as word spread and the queues got longer, there was clearly a need for these events to find a new home. Larger venues opened such as Spectrum (also at Heaven), RIP and The Trip, signalling a transition from small club acid house to full-on rave.

Increasing in size came the outdoor, unlicensed pay party where hundreds and then thousands of people would gather in any space big enough to house a thumping sound system. The word went out through flyers and pirate radio; hordes of those wishing to attend would gather at a motorway service station awaiting instructions as to where the party would be. As venues, personalities and laws changed and basic house music balkanised into genres and sub-genres, one consistent element throughout this time was the drugs, resulting in the dramatic growth in the market.

In the early days of acid house, the house drug was LSD; what little MDMA was around cost £25 a pill whereas LSD was more like £2–3 a dose. At first Danny and Jenny Rampling at Shoom did have that 1960s ethos in mind as to what the club atmosphere and its clientele should aspire to. It was important though that the press (and police) should not equate the new music with drugs, so as press interest grew, the party line was to assert that 'acid' referred to black urban club slang for 'theft', derived from the technique of sampling sounds.

During 1988, the press appeared confused as to what was going on. In September, Richard Branson banned acid house from his Heaven club after *The Sun* revealed that LSD was being sold to 'hippie-style kids'. However, on 15 October, the paper was advertising at £3.50 'our Acid House T-Shirt', which apparently was 'groovy and cool'. Yet on the same page, their resident doctor Vernon Coleman was giving readers the '10 reasons to say no to evil LSD'. Just shy of two weeks later, on 28 October, Janet Mayes became the first publicised MDMA death: the brief love-in between the hacks and the 'hippie-style kids' was over. 'Shoot These Evil Acid House Barons' was *The Sun's* response and from then on, every MDMA death made front-page news.

In the decade 1988–1998, hundreds of thousands of young people enjoyed the atmosphere of fun and freedom that typified rave culture however you define it. They shed responsibilities and reverted to the symbols of childhood: dummies, lollipops, Andy Pandy suits and bouncy castles. Few came to any real harm and many looked back with fond memories to the time they were allowed go well off the rails. Many later said the confidence and sociability that MDMA inspired stayed with them long after they stopped using the drug. Gloomy predictions of permanent brain damage and a generation of depressed post-rave people whose 'happy' brain chemical serotonin had been depleted by the drug never materialised. MDMA went in lockstep with the *zeitgeist* – a stimulant drug to get you raving until dawn and loving everyone around you as you danced cheek by jowl. No less with LSD and cannabis in the sixties, rave culture could not have developed in the way it did or maybe even at all, if it hadn't throbbed to the beat of ecstasy.

The scene was very egalitarian; as one female raver commented, 'Acid House was probably the most liberating invention since the pill. As anyone who last[ed] the night knew, acid house bred a legion of spectacularly intrepid, red-blooded young ladies. House fans were not dippy pictures of femininity, washing their hair in waterfalls. While the official British female was at home comparing whites and grateful for the right to make gravy for her ugly bald husband ... the ladies of acid house were climbing on the roof of a car doing ninety.'[1]

There was a brief period when it was argued the use of MDMA helped reduce football violence. Opinions differ on this. In his account of MDMA and acid house, Matthew Collin thought the link was overplayed, citing other reasons for fewer arrests such as the establishment of the National Football Intelligence Unit and a general distaste for hooliganism in the wake of football tragedies at Heysel, Bradford and Hillsborough.[2]

Interviewed by Push Silcott for *The Book of E*, Bill Brewster, then co-editor of football magazine *When Saturday Comes* from 1990 to 1993 and a writer for *Mixmag*, which covered music, dance events, festivals and club nights, for much of the '90s, said 'I think it's all bollocks. I don't doubt all the stories of football crews going to acid house clubs like Spectrum, dropping Es and stroking their Millwall tattoos, but I don't believe there are any knock-on effects to the terraces. In around 1992 or 1993 I was in a cab on my way to Ministry of Sound with a guy who was a serious Tottenham hooligan. At one point this guy says to me, "Have you ever had a fight while on E?" Then he said, "It's fucking great. I love fighting on E." I remember thinking,

"Hmmm, he appears to have missed the whole peace and love point of it all but some people didn't get that side of it, some people saw it as just another drug, just another way of getting off their heads.'[3]

But Mark Gilman, former drugs worker with the Manchester-based service Lifeline, had another view. Talking to Nicholas Saunders for his book *Ecstasy and the Dance Culture*, Mark reported on a study he was conducting into a possible link between football and MDMA, both as a participant observer and speaking to fans. During the 1989/90 season there was some serious violence between Manchester City and United supporters. The next season was a bit quieter but come the start of the following season 'many of the hard-core lads from both United and City had spent most of the summer dancing the weekends away to the sounds of house music at raves fuelled by the drug ecstasy. They had done this together!' Mark relates how the night before the first derby game of the new season, two groups of fans found themselves in the same pub with the expectation that a fight would break out. One of the City fans came over to the group of United fans and everybody held their breath but then he said, 'Well who would have thought that we would be stood side-by-side the night before a derby game and there's no trouble. It's weird innit?' And apparently some United and City fans gathered in one of their houses after the match to share some cannabis. Said one fan, 'I went home to bed about 5 a.m. and as I lay there waiting to get to sleep and couldn't stop thinking how right he was. This could never have happened before E.' However, hostilities resumed as the quality of MDMA diminished, the large commercial venues started selling alcohol and the sound of cocaine chopping could be heard coming from every toilet and flat surface. The more organised football gangs such as West Ham's Inter-City Firm became deeply involved in the increasingly darker side of ecstasy and the rave culture.

The culture rapidly became a business – and an illegal one at that – unlicensed venues swarming with people using and dealing drugs. The more enterprising started clubs, made T-shirts, created flyers and fashions, built sound systems, organised parties and dealt drugs. Anybody could be a drug dealer, and anything could be passed off as E: dog worming and fish tank tablets or headache pills shaved down to remove the markings. A pill is a pill is a pill. There was, incidentally, a strong right-wing libertarian streak among those campaigning against any legislation aimed at curbing the freedom to party. How would the police respond?

On 5 November 1988, Ted and Margaret Mayes built a bonfire but it wasn't to celebrate Guy Fawkes' night. Instead they were burning the T-shirt and fluorescent jumpers which belonged to their daughter Janet, who died taking ecstasy during an acid house party at the Jolly Boatman pub in Hampton Court, Surrey. Less than an hour before the 21-year-old collapsed, the venue had been surrounded by nearly 100 police officers awaiting orders to raid the party. The police had launched several operations in and around London during the previous few weeks, including Operation Echo targeting east London parties, one in Stepney and another on the Isle of Dogs. The raid on the Jolly Boatman was projected to be the biggest raid yet but was called off when the news filtered through that somebody had collapsed inside.

Instead, following an investigation, Janet's friend David Butler was initially charged with unlawful killing, but this was reduced when he admitted to a supply offence.

One of the most dramatic raids was carried out under Operation Seagull targeting a party on the *Viscountess,* a Thames pleasure boat moored at Greenwich Pier. The boat was the sister ship of the *Marchioness,* which sank in the summer of 1989 with a loss of 51 lives. The party was infiltrated by several undercover detectives and the boat was surrounded by police launches with police frogmen in the water in case anybody fell in. Officers swarmed aboard, arresting 18 people, including the promoters Robert Darby and Lesley Thomas, who were subsequently sent to prison for 10 and 5 years respectively for managing premises in which drugs were supplied. This raid went off peacefully. Others didn't.

Police raided a large derelict house in Sevenoaks, Kent. As they entered the house, a section of the 250-strong crowd turned hostile and a pitched battle ensued. The disturbance spilled out onto the street taking more than 60 officers 2 hours to bring it under control. There were 13 people arrested on public order charges rather than drug-related offences.

In 1989, up in the north west, as police were regularly raiding events in Liverpool and Manchester, the scene moved to Blackburn – attracting partygoers from as far away as Glasgow. The town was overwhelmed. On one night the police got wind of a rave and when the convoy arrived, a running battle broke out causing several injuries on both sides.

As well as busting parties, the police were also attempting to hit ecstasy supplies. In January 1989, several thousand pills were found during a raid on a house in Birmingham. Staffordshire police uncovered a large consignment of ecstasy which led to 67 arrests, while in a separate incident, police raided a house in Wembley where they found what they believed to be Britain's first ecstasy factory.

Police were successfully raiding indoor parties and the events themselves were outgrowing the physical space offered by the capital; in response, organisers began moving outdoors and out of London to escape detection. One of the first events was organised by Sunrise in June 1989 in an aircraft hangar at White Waltham in Berkshire. Called *A Midsummer Night's Dream,* it was the brainchild of Sunrise founder Tony Colston-Hayter, a gaming machine entrepreneur turned professional gambler, already dubbed by the *Daily Mirror* as the 'Acid House King'. *The Sun* reported this event under the headline 'Spaced out', claiming the event was attended by 11,000 'drug crazed kids – some as young as 12' who, according to *The Mirror,* took to 'biting the heads off pigeons' and when the party was over reporters claimed they saw 'thousands of empty ecstasy wrappers littering the floor'. Even the police remarked they thought this reporting was way over the top, while the youth and music press noted that nobody sold MDMA in wrappers nor was it much impressed by the description of the drug as 'an opium concentrate which can boost sex drive with side effects of paranoia'.

Inspired by the White Waltham event, Sunrise rivals held several large-scale gatherings in the south east during the second half of 1989, in fields, chalk pits, hangars, and forest clearings, mostly close to the newly opened

M25 orbital around London. Colston-Hayter and his business rivals got the word out through pirate radio stations and flyers in record shops. No location would be specified, only a meeting place, usually a motorway service station. Organisers used the BT Voice Bank system which allowed several lines into one answering service and facilitated changing the message if the location needed to be changed at the last minute. Once the would-be revellers got the message, off they went.

The constabulary bearing the brunt of this latest iteration of the rave scene was Kent, and particularly the area of the county which straddled the M25, commanded by Chief Superintendent Ken Tappenden. He established an incident room at Dartford police station to investigate the acid house phenomenon and it wasn't long before he was being flooded with calls from other stations all over the country wondering, like him, what on earth to do about it.

In the autumn of 1989, the team transferred to Gravesend to set up the Pay Party Unit, which rapidly grew from an initial complement of 6 officers to 250 officers, with satellite squads across southern England and East Anglia.

By his own admission, Tappenden hadn't realised the degree to which drugs were fuelling these parties or the risks that young people were taking. His surveillance team started filming the parties 'and then we knew we had a dreadful problem. We saw dealers bringing in drugs in barrows and security firms taking pills off people to recycle them to sell on again. We saw people collapsing and security men throw them over the fence, so they were outside the perimeter of the parties. There was no care for them. Then there was the aftermath. From lunchtime onwards on Sundays, youngsters would be taken to police stations or the village doctors by local residents who found them wandering around the countryside in a senseless state.'[4]

Tappenden was a pragmatist: he knew that even if he deployed all his officers to one party of 10,000 ravers, there was no way to arrest everyone who was taking drugs. Instead the tactic was to try to stop the events happening in the first place. What transpired was a cat and mouse game between the police and the promoters. The Pay Party Unit monitored the pirate radio airwaves and underground press: undercover officers were sent into clubs and record shops to collect flyers. If they discovered somebody had agreed to hire out their land or property to a party organiser, the police would seek an injunction against them, although some of the smarter promoters got wise to that and arranged convenient holidays for landowners so they could not be served with the necessary legal paperwork. From midweek onwards, police helicopters would be on the lookout for fairground rides and steamrollers on the move, used to flatten sites. Tappenden also pulled a few stunts that sailed over the line, such as threatening any company who hired a party organiser with a conspiracy charge that he knew would never stand up in court.

If a party got underway, roadblocks would be set up at strategic points, convoys would be directed towards an empty site, officers would literally dig up road signs so that people couldn't find where the venue was or police would feed false information to the pirate radio stations. The Kent police had their own technological assistance in data-gathering capacity, the HOLMES computer system, which came into operation in 1986 as a counter-terrorism tool for the Metropolitan Police. The impetus for HOLMES was the botched investigation into the Yorkshire Ripper, whose crimes crossed seven different police force areas with no mechanism for collating information. Tappenden was using HOLMES for the first time for drugs investigations. The Unit started 20 major investigations, held more than 5,000 names and monitored over 4,000 phone calls.

However, despite spending substantial police time and resources to put the party promoters not only out of business but behind bars if necessary, Tappenden had a grudging admiration for some of them. In 1990 *Melody Maker* hosted a debate about rave attended by Energy promoter Jeremy Taylor and Commander Tappenden who said,

> all the promoters had was a bank of mobile phones yet they could still move 10,000 people around on a Saturday night and still get a fairground attraction in place without me knowing and still start the music up before I got to them and still run it for the next 20 hours. I had to admire that: we were used to planning big operations, but I don't think a top police or military team could have done what those lads did Saturday after Saturday. They were masters at it. They weren't real villains either, they had simply seen an opening, the way to fill their pockets.

Jeremy Taylor's father was a judge who told his son what he could legally get away with.[5] One promoter tried to persuade the Commander to work for him after he retired. He declined the offer.

As well as technology, Tappenden also used whatever public order, environmental, and health and safety legislation he could muster. He made this important point to Matthew Collin:

> If you took it as a hard issue on drugs, I don't think you'd have got the support of the other authorities. Health and safety means a lot to local authority, drugs don't. Health and safety took on board every conceivable public authority we could get involved. The Fire Brigade came on board and all the district councils. Why health and safety? Why emergency lighting? Why noise? Because it was easy, drugs were difficult without thousands and thousands of men.

Licensing was another weapon in the war against raves. In January 1990, Graham Bright MP put forward a Private Members Bill which in July became the Entertainment (Increased Penalties) Act, raising the fines for organising an unlicensed event from £2,000 to £20,000 and a risk of 6 months in jail. The police wasted no time in acting on it: in the early hours of 22 July, police raided a warehouse party outside Leeds. Many officers taking part wore riot gear and arrived on horseback. Several thousand pounds of drugs were confiscated after a pitched battle in which bottles and bricks were thrown. Nearly 900 people were taken into custody, at the time one of the largest mass arrests in UK policing history with the detainees being held overnight in 20 different police stations across West Yorkshire. Most were released after a few hours and subsequently the police were sued on several counts of wrongful arrest and assault.

Former MP and *Times* editor William Deedes, the defender of Mick Jagger in 1967 and by 1990 in his late seventies, had this to say about Bright's Bill: 'What troubles me most about this Bill is the smell of moral outrage attached to it. A politician is safer when he is slightly tipsy and accompanied by a prostitute than when he is under the influence of moral outrage.'

Given how lucrative the rave business had become, it is debatable how effective the Bright Act was, but police were cracking down on raves all over the country, especially in the north-west. Tappenden's operation was closed to make way for similar units elsewhere like the West Midlands, but rave activity fell off significantly in the south as BT stopped hiring out their phone system to organisers. There was also more of a carrot and stick approach to partying with some clubs allowed to stay open beyond the normal 3 a.m. shut down.

The end of the large-scale unlicensed open-air scene saw the advent of the licensed super clubs such as Ministry of Sound in London and Cream in Liverpool, but the massive outdoor rave wasn't quite over yet. Alongside the growing band of urban ravers came the New Age Travellers in their trucks, vans and hefty sound systems. The two groups mingled in very large crowds, which culminated in a 40,000-strong event at Castlemorton, near Malvern in Worcestershire, lasting from 22 to 29 May 1992 after which legislation killed the unlicensed event and rave culture merged into the commercial entertainment business. Illegal events still took place: warehouse parties where a sound system and an audience would appear in a disused commercial building and disappear next morning. Later, a resurgent illegal rave scene attracted a much younger audience, too young and too poor to be admitted to expensive over-18 venues with tight door security.

As far as Ken Tappenden was concerned, the real nail in the coffin of the unlicensed outdoor rave was the involvement of criminal gangs taking advantage of a business based on illegality and operating under cover of darkness. Wayne Anthony of the Genesis organisation told how he was kidnapped twice – once by a gang of former Falklands war veterans who demanded half of all takings in return for security services. Bound and gagged with a gun to his head Anthony had little choice but to comply. As Tappenden observed, 'the criminal element which infiltrated the raves were more sinister than anyone at government level ever wanted to know and more sinister than the public ever perceived'. The HOLMES system threw up many names already well known to the police as serial villains.

Record shops in the East End of London were getting smashed up three or four times a month as a warning not to run parties without them. Some people got seriously hurt: the message was 'you don't want to look like him'. It's hard for policemen to admit to being frightened, but I got frightened lots of times. I got frightened for my officers. I got frightened for the youngsters at the parties. We recovered four sawn-off shot guns in one night at a rave in Ockenden in Essex.

The police filmed security men urging Rottweilers to attack people at a rave in Reigate in Surrey, putting 16 in hospital and saw the guards walking around with CS gas canisters. 'I thought we would have mass slaughter with the gangs. I talked about the danger of a Hillsborough-type disaster if it suddenly went off at a crowded party. It did never happen but it's no exaggeration to say we are often on the brink of this.'[6]As if to underline the reality that the amateur dealer and college boy rave organiser were now way out of their depth, on 6 December 1995, three men with long histories of serious crimes and known links to MDMA importation and distribution were gunned down in a professional hit while they waited in a Range Rover deep in the Essex countryside. The triple murder generated huge media interest including books and films.

Housing events indoors, however large, saw many of the public order and health and safety issues associated with the outdoors resolved because of the demands made of the promoters by the granting of licences. The use and supply of drugs now became a key factor in whether a venue would keep its licence when it came up for renewal. But the drugs market seemed completely impervious to any attempts to stifle it. In 1989, police seized 39,000 doses of MDMA; by 1998 that figure stood at 10 million doses and if the 10 per cent seizure figure was remotely correct, around 100 million doses could have been in circulation that year suggesting a weekly consumption of some 2 million tablets. As Commander Tappenden observed, neither the press, the public nor the politicians had much insight into the depth of criminalisation of the rave scene, but what nobody could escape was the mounting casualty rate, which takes us to the enduring and unresolved mystery of the ecstasy death.

***

The Hacienda in Whitworth Street, Manchester, opened its doors in 1982 financed by Factory Records boss Tony Wilson and the label's top band New Order. In 1986, The Hacienda was one of the first UK clubs to play House music, which turned the fortunes of the club around within a year from loss-making to rammed to the rafters every night of the week. Although the idea of 'Madchester' wasn't born at the Hacienda, it certainly took its inspiration from the Hacienda vibe and music which saw bands like Stone Roses, Inspiral Carpets and the Happy Mondays rise to a more traditional rock 'n' roll fame and notoriety.

The Hacienda had its own share of notoriety around the fast-developing drug scene and the attendant criminality which affected most rave venues. On 7 July 1989, Claire Leighton, a 16-year-old who had just finished her GCSEs, set off from Cannock in Staffordshire. At around 10 p.m. inside the Hacienda, Claire swallowed a single MDMA tablet. She collapsed shortly after midnight and died in hospital three days later. The story didn't even make the local news. According to journalist Gibby Zobel, writing years later for *Druglink* magazine, 'A few days later, DJ Dave Haslam, who did Thursday's Temperance nights at the Hacienda told me, "You're a journalist, you should write something about this. A girl died in there after taking E last week and they're not talking about it and I don't think it's right."

I checked out the story and called the nationals. The following day it was front page of every tabloid, a frowning "Smiley" face to illustrate the scary reality.'[7] To show how little publicity there was at the time, the coroner at Claire's inquest stated that this was the first such death, 'but regrettably it is not likely to be the last'.

In fact, there has been three previous deaths; the first recorded death was Ian Larcombe in June 1988, who swallowed 18 tablets and died of a heart attack having been stopped by police on the way to a rave. Janet Mayes only swallowed two tablets but still died, and Ian Hazelden consumed four tablets and had three heart attacks before he died on 4 June 1989. Claire had only swallowed one. According to one account, Janet had more MDMA in her body from two tablets than Ian Larcombe had from swallowing nine times that amount.[8] Subsequent deaths appeared to be similarly random. Among those who died, some were supposedly first-time users, others not. Some had consumed one or two tablets, others several more. The cause of death was not always the same; some died of heart attack, others died of the symptoms of heatstroke – the body rises to dangerously high levels and internal bleeding occurs, causing the blood to clot where it shouldn't. Some had organ failure; Collette McCarthy died in August 1989, 16 days after taking MDMA at a warehouse party in south London and following a liver transplant that failed to save her. Coroners readily identified the cause of death, but nobody could identify why these individuals has succumbed in the context of the millions of doses in circulation. As rave became more popular and more venues opened, so the death toll rose from 3 in 1988 to 15 in 1992.

Clubbers blamed the pill manufacturers and it remains true that there is no quality control on the illicit drug market. But the MDMA deaths and Accident & Emergency admissions (for which we have no data) generated messages (usually from the police) about 'rogue' pills or batches of drugs which suggested there was such a thing as a 'safe' MDMA tablet. There is much concern these days about very high-dosage MDMA tablets, but Claire Leighton died from a 28mg tablet with no other drugs present in her body while Brian Moss consumed 70mg when the 'normal' dose was judged to be 75–100mg.

As far as the pills themselves were concerned, there was a bewildering array of shapes, colours, and sizes, which were often reflected in the brand names, some of which were associated with the 'freedom of childhood' aesthetic: rhubarb and custard, banana split and Dennis the Menace. There were the early white doves, flat brown disco burgers, triple-deckers, Mitsubishis – pill types that came and went, some found in very localised clusters, others created for specific events. The pill contents could vary enormously; some were mainly MDMA or mixed with drugs in the same family such as MDEA or MDA. Other frequent additives which changed over time included amphetamine, caffeine, LSD, ketamine, ephedrine as well as inert substances like lactose and the material used to bind the pills together. The same type of pill from the same batch could contain entirely different drugs or the same drugs in different concentrations. The main problem with the tablets for most people was that the experience itself would be very unpredictable;

if the pill included a significant quantity of MDA, this would result in a more amphetamine-like experience without the MDMA empathy.

Another aspect of the lack of quality control meant there was no way to judge how quickly a pill would work. This is known as a drug's bioavailability or how efficiently the drug is absorbed into the body. If the pill releases its psychoactive content slowly, the danger is that the user will think the pill hasn't worked and so take more pills. This is not necessarily related to the amount of MDMA in the pill: one containing 250mg of MDMA (not unusual these days) might release the drug more slowly than one containing only 100mg. How slowly the drug is absorbed will be determined on existing stomach content. Mention of this has only recently appeared in the scientific press[9] but back in 2000, the magazine *Mixmag* conducted its first drug-user survey and reported on a drug 4-methylthioamphetamine or 4MTA, known as flatliners, which it said had claimed five lives including that of Stephen Evans who died in November 1998. The drug was deemed particularly dangerous not only for its potency but its slow-release action.

The history of drug use has seen journalists getting their information spectacularly wrong largely through not being part of the scene themselves and instead printing rumour and speculation – the more dangerous sounding, the better. There is a regular trope about powdered drugs being cut with strychnine and rat poison. Not only are these substances rarely found when heroin, amphetamine or cocaine are tested, it makes no commercial sense to have your customers dropping dead. Such incidents can happen when there is a dispute between a dealer and a user/dealer and the latter is sold a 'hotshot', although this is more likely to be a deliberately high-purity bag of heroin.

Confusion and misinformation were rampant even among publications which should have been better informed. Quoting *The Face*, *The Independent* wrote that white doves, which invariably contained MDMA and/or drugs in the same family, were an unlikely mixture of methadone and amphetamine (*The Independent*, 28 September 1981). Some drugs probably never existed such as the aptly named 'fantasy', a mixture of whatever dance drug you cared to name. There were claims that substances like strychnine were mixed into MDMA, which baffled Dr John Ramsey, an eminent toxicologist with an encyclopaedic knowledge of the nature of illicit drugs. As he told *The Guardian* (28 June 2001), 'The whole issue of contamination of ecstasy is a myth.' His team at St George's Hospital routinely collected samples of drugs from venues to see what they contained: 'And there is no evidence of widespread contamination.' Aside from the 'fillers' such as lactose which bulk up the pills, 'all the tablets we ever see contain nothing but drugs'.

Even though nobody could explain why just a few individuals had died, one thing was obvious. The majority had died while dancing for hours on end inside a hot, overcrowded venue with no air conditioning and no access to free drinking water. In the spirit of Russell Newcombe's 1987 *Druglink* article in which he said there was no reason why harm reduction interventions should not be applied across the drug scene, drugs workers in Liverpool and Manchester, home to some of the north-west's main dance venues including Quadrant Park and The Hacienda, considered what they might do to help stem the rising tide of MDMA deaths. What people needed was accurate, realistic and non-judgemental information, which acknowledged that people took drugs at raves, but which was not presented in a worthy looking, government-approved style, carrying stern messages.

In 1991, the Mersey Drug Training and Information Centre published *Chill Out – A Raver's Guide,* produced to look like a club flyer giving brief but potentially life-saving information to those who might have taken drugs as well as to their friends as to what best to do (and not do). The press response was explosive. *The Daily Star* was especially incensed, urging readers to pop down to the agency offices and chuck Director Pat O'Hare into the River Mersey. Over at the Manchester's Lifeline Project, Michael Linnell, an outstanding cartoonist with a bone-dry sense of humour, had created 'Peanut Pete', the first of many characters presented in a style reminiscent of Gilbert Shelton's Fabulous Furry Freak Brothers. This was in-your-face health education; rude and hilarious in equal measure playing directly to the audience. Naturally, 'right-thinking people' were outraged but the local authority backed Lifeline, which went on to provide a whole range of audience-relevant information about drugs. In 1992, Pete tackled the issue of overheating with recommendations about the need not to dance until you drop, sip liquids and chill out every so often. This kind of advice began to appear in the medical press and was central to the Manchester City Council-backed Safer Dancing Campaign, and the Home Office-backed Safer Dancing Campaign in London. Some venues had been in the habit of turning off the drinking water so they could overcharge for a bottle of water, but in the light of drug deaths and the obvious threat to their licence, most (but not all) responded by providing free water and allowing drugs workers onto the premises to offer help and assistance where needed.

Sadly though, the advice to drink water was taken by some to mean that drinking lots of water would of itself protect you from the effects of MDMA. On 22 February 1995, Andy Naylor from Derby drank 26 pints of water after taking one MDMA tablet and died. This very unusual death hardly warranted any media attention at all. The next time it happened though, the response was very different.

In the early hours of 12 November 1995, 18-year-old Leah Betts, at home in the Essex village of Latchingdon celebrating her 18th birthday party, suddenly felt very ill. She collapsed into a coma and was rushed to hospital where she stayed in intensive care as her parents made the agonising decision to switch off her life-support machine four days later. In the intervening days, press interest in the case intensified. Leah Betts was by no means the first teenager apparently to succumb to the effects of MDMA. The difference here was that her parents allowed a photo of her in intensive care to be shown on the front pages of every national newspaper and a video of her funeral to be distributed around schools. They also endorsed a national billboard campaign paid for by an advertising agency showing a smiling chubby-faced Leah stamped with the single word slogan 'Sorted'.

It was determined that Leah Betts, like Andy Naylor, died of dilutional hyponatremia caused by drinking too much water. The brain acts like a sponge, soaking up the water. It then swells, putting undue pressure on the body's vital organs, like lung function, which ultimately fail. Leah's death went down in subsequent retellings as related solely to excessive water, but in fact MDMA did play its part. The drug releases an anti-diuretic hormone called vasopressin, high levels of which can cause a fluid imbalance implicated in the build-up of water in the brain.

Leah Betts' death remains the most well-remembered of all ecstasy-related drug deaths. The very public display allowed by her parents brought home the fact that drug use could no longer be regarded as simply the activity of the mad, bad or sad heroin injector, crack smoker or glue sniffer living on some sink council estate. This could happen to anybody's child whatever the family background, however bright, intelligent and full of promise the teenager might be. Paul Betts was an ex-policeman. The father of Claire Pierce, who died from a cocktail of MDMA, vodka and painkillers in May 1996, was a police superintendent in the Nottinghamshire Constabulary.

Another myth that was blown away was that the only teenagers who used drugs were those who were lacking in self-esteem, unhappy or wanting to follow the crowd; in other words, victims of archetypal peer pressure. Subsequent research showed that those kids who were most comfortable in their skin were more likely to take risks, at least when it came to drugs like ecstasy that were hardly regarded as drugs at all. They were simply coloured pills, which looked very similar to the ones found in any domestic medicine cupboard or in packets of sweets.

The media used Leah's death to review many of the previous deaths and issue the stark warnings about the dangers of drugs, but her passing appeared to have little impact on the rave scene itself. Only a week after her death, *Daily Mail* journalists went to Raquel's in Basildon, Essex, where Leah had bought her ecstasy tablets. Mingling with the crowd, the journalists reported drug dealing (including making a buy themselves), drug using and security guards confiscating empty plastic bottles so they couldn't be refilled from taps, allowing the venue to charge £1.50 for a tiny bottle of water. Apparently, Leah had taken an ecstasy tablet with an apple motif. A criminologist conducting research amongst young people in the north-east revealed that demand for that particular brand of ecstasy soared in the wake of Leah's death and that the £2 million poster campaign was largely ridiculed on the basis that few believed you could die just by taking one tablet; however, some switched to drugs they regarded as safer.

In 1997 during the first week of Channel 5, I went with a camera crew to the 3,500-capacity Sanctuary in Milton Keynes to interview people about their drug experiences and what impact Leah Betts' death had on their drug use. It was obvious that they regarded Leah as just one of the unlucky ones, and statistically, in relation to amount of drugs in circulation and the numbers of users, that was true. It certainly didn't deter them from drug use, although some did say that they had switched away from MDMA to amphetamine and LSD. For their part Janet and Paul Betts began touring schools to deliver anti-drug talks. Other grief-stricken parents subsequently went down a similar path, setting up small charities and foundations to educate young people. It's impossible to know how many young people decided not to use drugs as a result of all the anti-drug publicity surrounding Leah's death and subsequent tragedies. But for their part, the Betts felt that they were banging their heads against a brick wall and stopped their drug prevention activities.

In February 1997, Brian Harvey was sacked from boy band East 17 after admitting he took ecstasy. Noel Gallagher came to his defence saying that taking drugs was as normal as drinking tea. After the usual flurries of press and political apoplexy, the *Daily Mirror* conducted a readers' poll and found a majority who voted supported his view. And he was right; although most young people didn't use drugs, even at the height of use during this late 1990s period, among the many thousands who did it was not seen as something deviant and unusual. And MDMA was really the tipping point in terms of drug acceptance among those in the 16–24 age range, the peak drug-using years. MDMA was seen as just a pill, very few people knew anybody who came to serious harm and as a result it gave 'permission' to try a range of other drugs – the old ones – cannabis, LSD and amphetamine – and the new ones like poppers (amyl nitrite), GHB and ketamine.

The vibe of MDMA infused itself beyond the club and into popular culture. The Shamen had a Number 1 hit with 'Ebeneezer Goode'; a film about the heroin scene in 1980s Edinburgh was played out to a banging techno soundtrack. Heroin use itself seemed to take on a 'cool' look as the fashion industry were accused of promoting 'heroin chic', using wasted-looking ultra-thin and pale models such as Kate Moss. In the early days, Miss Selfridge and Topshop put the smiley logo on their fashions. This enthusiasm among retailers waned briefly, but the relentless pulse of rave culture, and the sales revenue it promised, proved irresistible. Television and cinema screens throbbed to the beat of hyperreal advertisements for soft drinks – another indication of how well-publicised health and safety aspects of drug use in clubs permeated commercial consciousness.

While the debate over musicians' use of drugs raged on, Britain had a general election. In May 1997, it was goodbye John Major, hello Tony Blair. How would the new government deal with what was perceived as a drug situation that was out of control?

12

Things Can Only Get Better

Until now, this book has concentrated on the rapid ebb and flow of the drug scene itself as there was very little sustained strategic activity at a national government level – those years of 'masterful inactivity'. What next? On 2 May 1997, to the tune of 'Things can only get better' after '18 years of Tory misrule', Tony Blair and New Labour swept to power on the back of the largest parliamentary majority since Stanley Baldwin's 1935 National Government. For the next 10 years, there were no significant changes to the drug scene itself in terms of major new drugs; however, new political imperatives to tackle the drug problem generated an unprecedented torrent of government initiatives – mainly in drug treatment. Things certainly got better for drug treatment, but politically they got a whole lot messier and revealed the chasm between the aspiration inherent in that well-worn public sector phrase 'multi-agency working' and the grim reality of politics, agendas and territory.

Tony Blair was convinced that the key to addressing the social exclusion that helped ferment the civil unrest of the Thatcher years was to try to fix broken communities riven by urban decay, unemployment and lack of hope. The philosophical underpinning came from Blair's belief in 'communitarianism', a doctrine espoused by John MacMurray, a Scottish Communist turned Christian theologian (which also chimed with Blair's Christian values), and, more forcefully, by the German-born American sociologist Amitai Etzioni and the American political scientist Robert Putnam. In the early 1990s this was a reaction against the 'individualism' of the 1980s, best expressed in the UK by Thatcher's declaration that 'there is no society'. The general counterargument was that human beings are fundamentally social creatures with responsibilities to the community in which they live, and if they act against the best interests of the community (albeit a vague and woolly term in itself) then the community has the right to curb individual freedoms. To the incoming government, those who were clearly not acting in the best interests of the community were criminals, including drug dealers and drug users.

Elected in 1983, Blair had been MP for Sedgefield in Country Durham. The first wave of the heroin epidemic centred mainly in the north-west of

England and parts of Scotland, but from the early 1990s, many other parts of the country became affected including the north-east, Yorkshire and south Wales. Blair could see first-hand from his local surgeries the impact of drugs among his constituents – not just the toll of death and addiction affecting families, but all the associated low-level crime such as burglary, shoplifting and what became known as antisocial behaviour, which had a corrosive and invidious effect on perceptions of community safety.

Blair's commitment to home affairs saw him elevated to shadow Home Secretary from 1992 to 1994 when he became leader of the party leaving him to believe he was the best Home Secretary the UK never had.[1] He often locked horns with Michael Howard, Home Secretary under John Major, as to who was toughest on crime: an abiding mantra of Tony Blair and New Labour in office was 'tough on crime, tough on the causes of crime'. New Labour also came in on a promise to enact evidence-based policies. Taking cues from UK and American research-based evidence showing a strong link between drugs and crime, breaking that link became one of Tony Blair's top political priorities. The issue of drugs was also personal for Tony Blair: he was the first modern-day PM to bring up a young family at No. 10, and when asked by pollsters, drugs were invariably high up on the list of parental concerns.

Blair was not working from a clean policy slate. The HIV/AIDS crisis and the early days of the heroin epidemic had seen the creation of an inter-ministerial group, which produced three editions of a drug strategy 1985–88, although these were little more than iterations of individual departmental responsibilities and activities. The two strategic aims were to reduce supply by essentially doing more of the same enforcement measures, while 'demand for drugs is being tackled by discouraging those who are not misusing drugs from doing so [and] helping those who are already misusing to stop doing so' – vague to the point of meaningless. No wonder then as shadow Home Secretary, Tony Blair found fertile ground attacking the law and order party in government for purveying a strategy now several years out of date and largely ineffective, there being no attempt to recognise that the drugs problem needed political leadership.

Dialling back to the 1970s, there were the very beginnings of a realisation within government that you couldn't deliver public services such as health or social services just by relying on one set of professional actors. It became clear, for example, that just relying on consultant psychiatrists to stop the spread of addiction and the development of an illegal market was not working. One arena that was ripe for collaborative effort was crime prevention, increasingly seen as a whole community issue needing a whole community response.

In 1991, the Home Office published the Morgan Report. It investigated the options for local delivery of crime prevention strategies and made recommendations about community safety and crime reduction, giving local authorities statutory responsibility to bring together key agencies in local partnerships. However, the report came out in the dog days of the Thatcher government; Thatcher hated local authorities, not least because many cities were Labour controlled. She was determined to curb their authority and influence by drawing as much power to the centre as possible while hobbling their room for manoeuvre through, for example, rate capping and demanding that 'right to buy' income – the policy allowing people to buy their own council house – went to the Treasury. The Morgan Report gathered dust.

The vacuum in drug policy delivery at local level opened a window of opportunity for local authorities to try and re-generate the policy flexibility they had in the 1970s. The Association of Metropolitan Authorities, the Association of District Councils and the Association of County Councils came together to form the Local Government Drug Forum (LGDF). One of the recommendations of the 1982 ACMD Treatment Report was to set up District Drug Advisory Committees, but the LGDF concluded these were no more than talk shops that did little. Now under John Major, the Department of Health (DH) commissioned a report by a consultant Roger Howard (later CEO of SCODA and DrugScope) to investigate the evidence of good practice in local collaboration.

A draft of Roger Howard's report *Across the Divide: Building Community Partnership to Tackle Drug Misuse* was delivered in January 1993, but the DH was not happy that the report also identified a lack of strategic coordination at the centre and ordered deletions and redrafting. Civil servants at DH feared that should an idea of national as well as local coordination gain traction, the Home Office, as the department that led on drug policy, would simply take it over. This showed the tension between the two departments over drug policy, which went back to the creation of the Ministry of Health in 1919.

Civil servants were also peeved that Tony Blair leaked those bits of the draft report containing criticism of lack of national leadership before they were deleted. This was a foretaste of the interdepartmental battle that would break out over control of the drugs agenda, a new skirmish in the drug war.

So it was credit to Tony Newton, by then Leader of the House of Commons and President of the Privy Council, that he was able to bring potential warring departmental factions together and push through an agreement that the government should establish a Central Drugs Coordinating Unit (CDCU) to coordinate a new drug strategy to be produced under the leadership of two highly effective civil servants: Sue Street and Stephen Rimmer.

The creation of the CDCU linked to the Privy Council kick-started a political process underpinned by the assertion that while drugs were everybody's problem, they were also everybody's responsibility. What probably helped the process was that the CDCU would not impinge on central departmental powers or budgets as it would be coordinating action at a local level. Roger Howard's report, eventually published in 1994, recommended the creation of 'drug misuse community partnerships' comprising senior figures from local authority, health and criminal justice agencies.

In 1995 two national drug strategies were published, one for England, *Tackling Drugs Together* (TDT), and one for Scotland, *Drugs in Scotland*. There would be later strategies for Wales and Northern Ireland. TDT and its Scottish equivalent had many similar elements built around three obvious pillars – treatment, preventing young people using drugs and enforcement – but with some important differences in emphasis. Because TDT was geared to responding to law and order concerns, it made the jaw-dropping observation that poverty and deprivation as primary risk factors for drug problems were 'a matter of conjecture' set alongside individual pathology and inclination, thus swerving around any notion that Conservative policies in the 1980s played a part in creating the heroin epidemic.[2] So, the focus was on criminal justice interventions to tackle drug problems, prompting one ACMD member and service manager to remark, 'I'm not in the crime prevention business.' This comment reflected a view that the ACMD had marginalised itself because, as one ex-civil servant put it, the council was perceived (perhaps unfairly) at this point of being too medically oriented and out of touch with the increasing politicisation of drugs and the drift towards penal responses.[3]

The key strategic innovation in TDT was to implement Howard's recommendation of creating local partnerships. They were named in the strategy as Drug Action Teams (DATs) with a DAT coordinator in post to bring the key players to the table. There was criticism that the DAT excluded drug treatment providers, but this was the early days of a rethink on how drug services would be commissioned, so the government wanted decision makers, not providers, around the table. Drug treatment services and users served instead on Drug Reference Groups of other interested parties convened to advise the DAT on the local landscape. TDT came into being with very little money; approximately £8 million was allocated for the establishment of local DATs, but no money was to be spent on doing anything. However, some DATs were able to pull together bits of money for needs assessments to gauge the extent of local problems and, in the early days, DAT coordinators enjoyed a good relationship with the centre as the CDCU civil servant visits offered support and guidance on how to deliver the strategy at a local level. Unfortunately, benign central support would not last.

Alongside the creation of the CDCU and the drafting of TDT in 1994, Health Minister Dr Brian Mawhinney ordered a review into the effectiveness of drug treatment. The broader concern was simply the rising numbers of people notified to the Home Office's 'Addicts Index' coupled with a belief that because of the drive to tackle drug-related HIV infection, abstinence treatment had been side-lined. TDT fudged the whole harm reduction issue, stating that the objective of treatment was to get users to a 'drug-free state' while acknowledging that there had to be action to stop the spread of disease.

Mawhinney was a deeply religious man from Belfast, a leading member of the Conservative Christian Fellowship and the General Synod. Disliked by his civil servants and the drug sector for his abrasive manner, he wanted a review that would prioritise abstinence which, in an era of government cutbacks in public-sector spending (as the UK plunged into recession in 1992) would also be far cheaper than paying for harm reduction interventions. He had the support of Home Secretary Michael Howard who announced that 'prison works' at the 1993 Conservative Party Conference and was in turn no lover of harm reduction. Mawhinney chose Sir John Polkinghorne to chair the review. A Cambridge science don who would certainly give scrupulous attention to the evidence base, Polkinghorne was also a theologian and Anglican priest, which probably meant the Health Minister hoped Sir John's views were in line with his own. But no sooner had Dr Mawhinney commissioned the review in April 1994 than he was shuffled to Transport in July.

Whatever the political subtext of the review, the DH did stump up £1 million to commission research for the review and gave Sir John two years to deliver his report. There had been an expectation that with the word 'effectiveness' in the title, the treatment review would actually come to some conclusions as to which was the most effective treatment. But this was (and remains) an impossible task. There is an underlying assumption that people with a heroin problem, for example, are a homogenous group for whom one type of treatment is better than all others. But heroin addiction is not like diabetes where insulin is the gold standard treatment for all. While one person might respond well to a methadone detox and counselling, another might need longer-term prescribing while a third does best in residential rehabilitation. And many heroin users will try all the treatment options more than once while others become drug-free outside the treatment sector, either with the help of friends and family or a peer support group such as Narcotics Anonymous (NA). Moreover, as one study discovered, often it doesn't matter what the treatment is, what really matters is the quality of the empathy shown by the health professional. For users living a life of isolation, humiliation and danger, simply having somebody care about their well-being can be transformative.[4]

The Effectiveness Review made it clear that treatment needed to fit the client's need with services providing the full range of help and support, including outreach, needle exchange, self-help networks, counselling, opioid detox and both methadone maintenance and reduction programmes as well as residential rehab. Moreover, it identified service users as 'stakeholders' with rights including the right to be involved in the formulation and delivery of services, the very first time that the notion of 'service user involvement' was raised in an official document. As Sir John said, 'On joining the Task Force, I found myself on a steep learning curve. It was soon clear that the drug scene was one of great complexity in which it would not be possible to lay down a single procedure that could be universally relied upon or a simple goal that could be universally attained.'[5]

Most of the £1 million was allocated to funding a National Treatment Outcomes Research Study (NTORS). Run by Dr Michael Gossop at the Institute of Psychiatry, NTORS was a long-term follow-up study of over 1,000 service users which continued beyond the life of the Task Force. NTORS delivered preliminary findings in October 1995 and was able to demonstrate that being in treatment of itself reduced frequency and quantity of drug use, reduced injecting behaviour, but critically from a political standpoint the headline finding revealed that just being in treatment reduced crime and that for every £1 spent on treatment, there was a saving to the public purse of £3. The calculations changed and have since been endlessly argued over, but as a challenge to 'prison works', services could declare 'treatment works' and NTORS had a huge impact on New Labour's belief in treatment as the pathway to break the link between drugs and crime and the Treasury's willingness to pay for it. The treatment service purchasing guidelines issued to Health Authorities by DH in April 1997 put harm reduction firmly in the mix of interventions.

So, by the time Tony Blair took office, the start of an overarching drug strategy was in place, the beginnings of acceptance that the drug problem needed a coordination facility all underpinned by an evidence base supportive of a drugs–crime agenda. This too has antecedence. Back in the mid-1980s, the London borough of Southwark started a police referral scheme, the idea for which, local drugs worker Jud Barker said came from an episode of *Hill Street Blues,* 'There's this episode, cop walks in with a junkie and he says, "You can go to that desk and get help or you can come to my desk and I'm gonna book you" and that seemed such a neat idea.'[6] This eventually morphed into the Southwark Arrest Referral Pilot Scheme. Around the same time, the Demonstration Unit of Inner London Probation Service led by senior manager Paul Hayes looked at the options for developing a service-wide response to working with drug-using offenders.

In 1991 the Criminal Justice Act had introduced a provision allowing a drug treatment requirement to be attached to a Probation Order, the first legal attempt to integrate health and criminal justice responses. The problem was that the Home Office hadn't quite cottoned onto the consequences of the emerging purchaser/provider split in the NHS and automatically (and wrongly) assumed that the NHS would simply foot the bill for court-mandated treatment. Nobody wanted to pay for it, so few orders were made.

In the intervening period, 1991–1997, the evidence was building that made the links between drugs and crime. The ACMD produced three reports on drugs and the criminal justice system, and all three included recommendations about creating effective pathways for offenders into treatment either from police cells or prison. Both Paul Hayes and Mike Trace, then Director of the Parole Release Scheme, sat on the ACMD Criminal Justice Working Group. Both would figure significantly in the drug treatment story to come.

The Home Office through the Drug Prevention Initiative were coming on board with the idea of arrest referral and funded an expansion of the Southwark pilot scheme to surrounding London boroughs and it contributed to schemes in Derby and Salford. Social policy academic Professor Mike Hough wrote a literature review for the Home Office in 1995, demonstrating that many drug users do commit low-level acquisitive crime to fund their drug use.

Much of the evidence came from the USA: when Justin Russell was working with Ruth Runciman at the Mental Health Foundation, he travelled to the States on a Harkness Fellowship and returned convinced of the evidence; he wrote his findings in *Substance Misuse and Crime – Some Lessons from America* (1994). On his return, Russell was appointed to a Home Office advisory post for the Labour Party and from there his star rose, first as special advisor to shadow Home Secretary Jack Straw in the run-up to the General Election – and from there he was appointed special advisor to Tony Blair. He became very influential behind the scenes, persuading the politicians to invest in drug treatment to reap a crime reduction dividend.

From his experience in the States, Russell met with Roger Howard, Mike Trace and Paul Hayes to see what interventions might translate to an English criminal justice system. From this emerged the idea of Drug Treatment and Testing Orders (DTTOs), one of the provisions of the Crime and Disorder Act 1998 whose other main legislative innovations were the Anti-Social Behaviour Order (ASBO) and the creation of Crime and Disorder Reduction Partnerships (CDRPs), the responsibility of local authorities. The DTTO required offenders to submit to regular drug testing, to attend treatment programmes and to have their progress reviewed regularly by the courts. As DTTOs rolled out, so did the problems in making the system work, but DTTOs were a political recognition that if you were going to break the link between drugs and crime, then all the evidence pointed to the central role of drug treatment.

That said, the early days of drug policy under Tony Blair were still wide-ranging and diffuse as money remained tight. In the heady honeymoon period after election, there were celebrity receptions at No. 10 Downing Street (Harold Wilson had invited The Beatles) which included Noel Gallagher on the guest list despite his comments about the normality of drug use, probably because back in February, in a *Daily Mirror* poll, 87 per cent of readers agreed with him. He was briefly a flag waver for 'Cool Britannia' and the new broom 'Call me Tony' regime. No. 10 as a celebrity hangout didn't last too long though and PM receptions rapidly became much 'safer' affairs as the business of government kicked in.

Knowing he would probably face resistance from civil servants and his own ministers, Blair instituted a very different sort of UK government to drive through the policies on his hit list. An unprecedented number of Special Advisors (Spads) were appointed who became the PM's delivery attack dogs. Spads (originally known as irregulars in Victorian times) were brought in by governments to supply advice in areas when civil servants either lacked experience – such as in issues relating to industry and commerce – or because the Civil Service had to remain politically neutral. Spads had a role during the two World Wars but were dispensed with at the end of each conflict. They re-emerged under Harold Wilson and by 2005, under Tony Blair, peaked at 85. The Miliband brothers and Ed Balls were all initially spads, but two of the most influential during the Blair years were Alastair Campbell and Jonathan Powell. Between them they created a powerful and well-resourced communications and delivery machinery. Tony Blair changed the law giving his two lieutenants power over civil servants and anointing them with *West Wing*-style job titles – Director of Communications and Chief of Staff. Reference to 'The Administration' also betrayed some of the many influences the Clinton Administration had on Tony Blair's premiership. Jonathan Powell's appointment caused problems for the Cabinet Secretary who literally sat next to the PM as his 'right-hand man' taking minutes at cabinet meetings. From the inception of the post in 1916, there had been just 12 Cabinet Secretaries. From 1997 to 2007, there were four. As journalist Adam Boulton noted in his book on the Blair government, 'Tony Blair oversaw changes which took power out of the hands of elected politicians and career civil servants and made them share it with others. He multiplied vastly the number of special advisers with a role in policy-making.'[7]

While Blair was PM, the internal political pressures that would bear down on both central and local government officials were matched by external media pressures on politicians. This increased dramatically with the launch of the 24/7 Sky News in February 1989, but even more significantly for the UK government with the arrival of the BBC News 24 service in November 1997. Talking to journalist turned academic Jon Silverman in 2008, former Home Secretary Douglas Hurd recalled an observation by Edward Heath that 'the first account of anything is always wrong – 48 hours later it will look different. Well, today you haven't got 48 hours.'[8] To counteract this new development and not only stay on top of the ever-churning news cycle but to try to dictate what was news and what wasn't (from a government point of view), Campbell substantially tightened an existing internal government tool called the news grid. If a minster wanted to make an announcement, it had to go through Campbell's office to ensure it didn't conflict with something else going on that day and that it followed the government's line. So how did this micro-management of policy and communications play out regarding drug issues?

Tony Blair had been highly critical of existing drug policy, so while basic structures would be maintained and enhanced, politically he still needed a new angle to signal change. Again, taking his cue from Bill Clinton, one of Blair's first actions was to appoint a UK Anti-Drugs Coordinator, quickly known as the drug czar. The man chosen for the job was Keith Hellawell, Chief Constable of West Yorkshire and previously Cleveland. By his own account in an autobiography titled *The Outsider* (2003), Hellawell grew up in a dysfunctional, abusive family then spent five years as a coal miner before joining the police, so he was well acquainted with the scourge of deprivation and dislocation both from his own background and in the communities he served as an officer. Despite the post being officially advertised in *The Daily Telegraph* in the summer of 1997, he appeared to be a shoo-in for the job. During his time as Chief Constable of Cleveland he addressed a Labour Party meeting in Middleborough and caught the attention of the local MP Peter Mandelson, who suggested he meet an unknown party figure, Tony Blair. Increasingly concerned about the drug problem in his region, Hellawell was involved in the creation of the drugs sub-committee of the Association of Chief Police Officers (ACPO) and through that role began raising the issue of drugs more publicly in the early mid-nineties. He appeared in the BBC *Panorama* programme *Needle Park*. In the run-up to the 1997 election, he said he was contacted by a Blair aide (probably Liz Lloyd) and told that the Labour leader was making a speech on drugs on 25 March at the Dyce Academy in Aberdeen. 'What would be your response to the appointment of a drug czar?', the aide asked, simply floating the idea without any sense of what a job description would look like. The idea of announcing this in Aberdeen may also have been partly influenced by Grampian's outspoken hard-line Chief Constable, Ian Oliver, who did apparently apply for the job.

Within weeks of the election, Hellawell said, with a group of others, he was invited to see Ann Taylor who succeeded Tony Newton as Leader of the House of Commons and Privy Council President to sound him out again on the question of a US-style drug czar. It was on the cards that the government would appoint a senior policeman to the role, but they also appointed Mike Trace with drug sector experience, albeit also from a criminal justice background, as Hellawell's deputy. The interview panel of Taylor, Home Secretary Jack Straw and Health Secretary Frank Dobson had concluded as the interview progressed that while Hellawell would make the ideal man to front drug policy, they needed somebody more versed in the technical details such as what should a treatment strategy look like and does prevention work?

Hellawell started work in January 1998 despite, he said, warnings from friends that the job was a poisoned chalice, drug problems were insoluble, any success would be claimed by ministers while he would shoulder the blame for any failures. He was also taken aback by the cynical attitude of journalists at his inaugural press conference, but they too were prescient in their comments: 'It's all spin and no substance', 'Aren't you a tiger without teeth?', 'You won't get any power or funding'.[9] Hellawell must have also been aware that the first US drug czar, William Bennett, quit after only a year in the job, citing similar problems to those Hellawell would face. In the USA, the czar was something of a political pawn whose presence variously benefited the White House, the Legislature and the Judiciary but who was essentially a front man – the four-star general who would get tough on drugs and sort it all out. Bennett suffered a lack of direct authority, inability to dispense grants, and a relatively small staff. In Hellawell, however, we had a top policeman with many years of front-line experience brought in to tackle what politicians, the press and the public all agreed was one of the most pressing social problems of the day. What could possibly go wrong?

From the get-go, Hellawell made the nature of their respective roles clear to Trace; Hellawell was the high-profile point man who would be out and about meeting and greeting, making the speeches, cutting the ribbons, doing the interviews and putting a public face on the new impetus to deal with the UK's drug problem. Every DAT chair got a visit showing relations with the centre were still good. Trace also had many a cup of coffee in local cafés; 'there was a real feel in the sector that something was happening around drugs with the Blair government; it became very high profile and masses of people were coming to see us.' And he says he was perfectly happy in his role behind the scenes and was quite impressed with Hellawell. As a Chief Constable, he was known in the sector around 1996–97. 'He knew there were no quick wins for government around drugs; he was not keen on big legislative change, but he was keen, in effect, on "support don't punish"'.[10] In his book, Hellawell says that the problems faced by drug users were 'exacerbated' by the criminal justice system.[11]

The 'dream team', as they were dubbed, also needed to hit the ground running. There was, in effect, a parallel process with Hellawell fronting the strategy while Trace worked with Steve Rimmer, now heading the renamed UK Anti-Drugs Coordinating Unit (UKADCU), to devise the detail of a new 10-year drug strategy. Immediately, there was a problem trying to find out how much money was currently being spent on drugs.

Eventually, they managed to ascertain that the government was spending about 60 per cent of the budget on police, probation, court and enforcement agencies, with the balance split roughly evenly between treatment, prevention and education and international work. But they had no reliable figures for how many people were in treatment, how many were not in treatment, what quantity of drugs were coming into the country and only a rough idea of the extent of drug use itself. Part of the problem was a basic lack of data; when *Tackling Drugs to Build a Better Britain* was published in April 1998, it was more about action than TDT which was primarily aimed at developing structures. Even so, it was of necessity a rushed job and full of ambitions constructed in a policy zone devoid of clear definitions and baselines; for example, reduce proportion of people under 25 reporting use of illegal drugs in the last month and previous year; increase participation of problem drug misusers, including prisoners, in drug treatment programmes; and reduce access to drugs among 5–16-year-olds. The real nub of the problem that the UKADCU and particularly Hellawell faced was the resentment felt by civil servants and ministers toward the idea of a cross-cutting department sitting above them and, worse still, lorded over by a non-civil servant.

As political and public concerns about drugs heightened during the 1990s, TDT acknowledged that it would be impossible to begin tackling drugs at a local level without some mechanism for bringing the police and criminal justice agencies around the table with health and social care. This was the role of the DATs and they were successful at least in establishing dialogue.

Centrally, the CDCU had greatly assisted in that process. Now it made sense to replicate that coordinating role at the heart of government – exactly what the Howard report had suggested. To do that meant after nearly 80 years at the helm of drug policy, the Home Office was now expected to cede control to the UKADCU. Other departments too, specifically Health and Education, were also expected to cooperate. However, at a senior level, Health and Education were never really that engaged with the drugs agenda, seeing it as a very small part of their overall work, concerned with the NHS and the National Curriculum respectively. Not so the Home Office; newly installed Home Secretary Jack Straw did his utmost to wrest back control. Government departments and even units within departments were very resistant to ceding power and money. Added to that, although the drugs issue was always a highly toxic and tricky area for ministers – a so-called third-rail issue (touch it and you get fried), it was perennially in the media spotlight, offering ministers many opportunities for high-profile interviews. This meant departmental civil servants and spads were protective of their own bailiwicks and eager to push their ministers into the media spotlight – even if it was only to reiterate parts of the strategy or announce spending previously announced.

Hellawell, of course, had no experience of the workings of Whitehall; he genuinely believed he was brought in with the support of the PM to devise and deliver a cross-departmental national drug strategy and then oversee progress. Ministers would report to him; he in turn would have regular meetings with the PM to relay that progress. That wasn't the name of the game. As a later head of the UKADCU Julian Critchley explains, 'Hellawell failed to understand what drug policy was. As far as No. 10 and ministers were concerned – he *was* the drug policy. Czar appointed – job done. The ministers' view absolutely was that his job was to exist, so that any time somebody said, "What are you doing about drugs?" "Oh well, we've appointed a czar." It was entirely presentational.' At one point, Alastair Campbell said, 'Drugs needs a brand, you're the brand' and when Hellawell's first annual progress report was published, Campbell was pushing for some headline-grabbing results only for Hellawell to tell him that government had to be honest with the public and tell them there were no quick wins, only hard slog. It was not what anyone wanted to hear.

Hellawell wrote that he was warmly welcomed by Tony Blair and Gordon Brown but his relations across Whitehall were pretty toxic, partly due to a misreading of his role and because he was used to being a powerful and influential Chief Constable in a highly hierarchical police structure where he only had to cough for people to jump. Ministers regarded Hellawell as an irritant, imposed upon them by the PM; one Secretary of State literally squared up to him at the end of a meeting, witnessed by an official who said, 'It was one of those moments where you are just about to leave the room and decide to stay'. Another turned to the czar during a Cabinet committee meeting and shouted, 'Get your tanks off my fucking lawn.'

Relations with the civil servants were no better. Hellawell says he was less than impressed with the attitude of the head of Civil Service, Sir Richard Wilson, who at their first meeting rather patronisingly observed that the czar might have got an easier ride had the civil service had a role in his appointment. There was another eyebrow-raising moment when he attended a meeting hosted by former Civil Service chief Sir Robert Armstrong; Hellawell expressed a view about government departments working together. 'What a charming idea,' was the classic *Yes Minister* Sir Humphrey response.

Hellawell didn't appoint his own staff; they were civil servants seconded from other departments, so they owed their primary loyalties to their home departments' line managers and resented taking orders from an outsider. Some of his team tried to steer a fine line between being a loyal Cabinet Office official and a departmental secondee, which caused at least one official to break down under a tongue lashing from the czar, born of years spent in the abrasive canteen culture of the police. Others of his staff were there simply to report back to their own departments about what was going on.

Nor was there a hug-fest between Hellawell and his own Cabinet Office ministers. Siting the coordination of drug policy above individual departments meant putting it in the Cabinet Office, which in theory gave it a direct line to the PM. However, it only had coordinating functions with no legislative powers and so the Cabinet Office minister was always at a political disadvantage when faced with more powerful ministerial colleagues such as the Home Secretary. Yet at the level of civil servants, the UKADCU did have a direct line to No. 10 which other departments did not – another cause for general resentment.

Those ministers assigned to run the Cabinet Office were often in the twilight of their ministerial careers. In 1998, David Clark was replaced by

Jack Cunningham from the Ministry of Agriculture and Fisheries. Officials and Hellawell all say Cunningham came with no great interest in drugs, but as it was the only item in his portfolio with any media profile, he tussled with Hellawell over who would front the drug strategy. Cunningham got more publicity than he would have wanted when he presented Hellawell's second National Plan to the House of Commons in May 1999. Already known in the media as 'Junket Jack', both the *Daily Mail* and *The Independent* took pleasure in rubbishing the targets set in the new plan. For example, a 50 per cent reduction in young peoples' drug use by 2008 when Cunningham was forced to admit to the House that although there were now published target figures, there were still no baselines. Hellawell would also have to publicly admit that the targets were 'aspirational'. Behind the scenes, ministers were trying to distance themselves from the shifting sands of credible target setting, but it was Jack Cunningham who took the brunt of media scorn, although Hellawell had an uncomfortable time facing Jeremy Paxman on BBC's *Newsnight*. Hellawell was also gaff prone, making mistakes in public statements the more knowledgeable Trace would have avoided; for example, the czar said that doctors could not prescribe heroin (yes, they could, with a licence). *Guardian* journalist Malcolm Dean recalled a meeting with Hellawell in his office in early 2000. 'It was a sad and embarrassing occasion. He looked absolutely lost and was in a desperate search for allies in an increasingly hostile world that was questioning his pay, effectiveness and various U-turns' [12] – for example swinging from supporting a harsh response to cannabis as a gateway drug and then urging police to lay off cannabis and concentrate on heroin and crack.

On 6 February 2000, he had told the *Sunday Observer*, 'We need to discriminate between different drugs and the relative harm caused and then talk openly about the difference we can make. The focus is going to be on the drugs that cause the major harm.' He said too many people were being convicted for the possession of small amounts of cannabis to hit the drug–crime targets. 'By far the greater proportion of arrests are for cannabis and I am looking for a change on that. I am looking for a shift towards those dealing in heroin and cocaine.'

Regarding drug law enforcement, there were continuing deep divisions between police and customs, which also served to undermine the UKADCU and attempts to coordinate activity through the creation of the Concerted Inter-Agency Drug Action Group (CIDA). Customs were chairing CIDA, much to the chagrin of the National Criminal Intelligence Service (NCIS), which saw HMCE as nothing more than a revenue-collecting agency. Hellawell sat on CIDA but the police had little time for him either. As senior customs manager Terry Byrne told me, 'The police never recognised any authority for CIDA and essentially sneered at Hellawell and did nothing to recognise or respect his role or status.'

Cunningham was succeeded by Mo Mowlam in October 1999. She was very aggrieved at being moved from the Northern Ireland office. Again, as drugs were the only attention-grabbing item on the Cabinet Office agenda, Mo wanted to be seen out and about, especially when it came to overseas work. According to Hellawell, she suggested that they split the international work between Colombia (Mo) and Afghanistan (Keith). She seemed to think her experience in Northern Ireland could help broker peace between the left-wing FARC rebels who were heavily involved in cocaine production and the Colombian government. In relation to opium, Hellawell believed one solution would be to buy the crop from the farmers. He was annoyed at being quoted as saying the West should buy from the Taliban – but purchasing opium from the farmers was equally unsustainable. According to one official Mo 'hated his guts' probably because, backed by Blair and Campbell, Hellawell suggested she should desist from pushing the PM on drug legalisation and definitely stop people smoking cannabis at her ministerial residence.

To a degree, the attempts to launch a palace coup to oust the czar were something of a political sideshow. This period did produce the first coherent and long-term national strategy, accompanied by funding boosts in several areas, and the beginning of a focus on the drugs that caused the greatest harm. This led to a more proportionate (if short-lived) view of cannabis. As Tony Blair was increasingly focused on Northern Ireland and the fall-out from unpopular welfare reforms, the UKADCU was left to get on with the day-to-day business without, as Mike Trace puts it, 'some 12-year-old coming over from No. 10 saying, "I've got an idea about this drug thing."'

Having more political and diplomatic smarts than Hellawell, it was Trace who was the power behind the throne. That first year, 1998, was a honeymoon period for the UKADCU with Trace spending months convincing spads and the Treasury that the treatment investment would save money and play well politically. Then towards the end of the year, came the negotiations over Labour's first Comprehensive Spending Review (CSR). A committee was established to look at drug treatment. This kind of spending review was normally owned and managed by civil servants, so DH was less than happy not only to have Mike Trace, who chaired the sessions, in the room but to also have Roger Howard and Noel Towe from the LGDF at the table. By his own admission, Roger Howard came up with a fag-packet calculation for how much investment would be needed in drug treatment, but more detailed papers were submitted by the UKCDCU, which almost caused a corporate coronary among DH civil servants who were only mollified by a guarantee that their core priorities would also be met in the spending calculations.

By the time of the next CSR, the purse strings had been significantly loosened, but the fight continued. In relation to the Department of Education and Employment (DfEE), as one ex-UKADCU official told me,

> There was a recognition that treatment was one thing, but you needed to help people out of treatment into meaningful lives and that meant jobs. At the time there was no UK literature as to what that might look like, and some stuff from America. We asked DfEE to bid for a pretty small amount of money for employment service support workers to help people coming out of treatment. But the resistance was absolute, it was like 'Well, if you give us everything we are asking for, like class sizes of six, then we might support this ludicrous and unevidenced proposal.' The whole CSR was a game of poker – who was going to blink first.

Yet when the money flowed in 2000, it flowed; that same official said,

> It was really odd – after the bids were closed, I was asked at 10 a.m. to
> knock together a bid before midday and it came to about £10 million.
> I rang it through and 10 minutes later the Treasury rang back, 'You've got
> £17 million.' The Chancellor was very keen to throw money at this, like
> his £300 million Community Against Drugs Initiative, mainly to be spent
> on disrupting local drug markets and reduce drug-related crime which sat
> outside normal departmental silos. I'd be sitting in Treasury meetings and
> they'd be saying about drug treatment 'Can't you be more ambitious?' How
> quickly can you grow this?'

Once the money was secured, how would it reach treatment agencies,
especially those in the voluntary sector? Realistically it had to go down a
health route, but there was a recognition that there were many departments
with an interest in the outcomes of drug treatment, so the budgets, objectives
and accountabilities needed to be cross-cutting. Trace and others also had
concerns that not only would it get swallowed up in the behemoth of NHS
bureaucracy, but there was a lack of trust that the money would really be
spent on treatment. The answer was to set up a Special Health Authority,
which would technically be the guardians of the cash with a line management
responsibility to the DH, but in effect it would be the Home Office boots on
the ground to deliver the criminal justice dividend. In 2000, it was Home
Secretary Jack Straw not Health Secretary Alan Milburn, nor significantly
Keith Hellawell, who announced the formation of the National Treatment
Agency (NTA) whose job it was to grow the treatment system and have some
oversight on the treatment budget pooled from the Home Office, Department
of Health and local authorities.

The idea of a pooled treatment budget developed from an idea in a report
published in January 2000 by No. 10's Performance and Innovation Unit
(later the Strategy Unit) of the Cabinet Office called *Wiring it up: Whitehall's
Management of Cross-cutting Policies and Services*. It is likely the report was
prompted by the problems faced by the UKADCU (and the Social Exclusion
Unit launched in 1997) attempting to build bridges across departmental
silos. On finances, the report said, 'Further changes to Treasury's budgetary
rules should be considered to make it easier for departments to move money
between years, organisations and budgets to promote cross-cutting working,
and more use should be made of pooled or cross-cutting budgets where
this makes sense.' Together Mike Trace and Justin Russell pushed for the
pooled treatment budget, emphasising that accountability should be cross-
departmental involving prisons and probation, although in the end, health
interests dominated on the NTA Board.

There was strong political ambition and action to pump serious money
into tackling the drugs problem, but while these negotiations were coming
to a head, much of the political enthusiasm for a drug czar and the office of
the UKADCU was dribbling away. No. 10 was backing off, Hellawell was
not getting his PM meetings and the Whitehall waves were beginning to close
over him. Julian Critchley had some sympathy for his boss:

A drug action day was planned where all the ministers who had their fingers in the drug pie would all make an announcement on the same day to demonstrate coordinated action. We planned the timing, what the announcements would be – all meant to be a big PR exercise.

The day came but Health, Education and Customs didn't even put out a press notice. The Home Office put out a press notice after we rang and said, 'What the hell is going on?' That day is burned in my brain, sitting in the office and realising that we had been completely screwed over by other departments. Our minister had written to their ministers and they had written back to say they would cooperate. But no stronger message could have been sent; 'you might be called the UKADCU, but we are in charge'. Ian McCartney [the junior Cabinet Office minister] went absolutely apeshit and it was the only time I have ever been shouted at by a minister in a meeting.

After that, I was speaking to a woman at the No. 10 Policy Unit and she said, 'Look, we want to do something on drugs to make it up to Keith.' I'd given her all the options about health and prevention programmes and what did she say? 'Couldn't we arrange for a police boat on the Thames or the police to kick somebody's door in?' I remember just sitting at my desk with my head in my hands.

Another indication of the status of UKADCU generally was the grades of the civil servants working in it – at best a grade five would be trying to do deals with a much higher-level grade two in other departments. A bit like a platoon lieutenant speaking to a general. If that unit was genuinely supposed to take over and run drug policy, it would have been headed up by at least a grade three with more staff and crucially it would have had the money.

By the end of 2000, it was clear that the czar experiment was dead in the water and Hellawell was already planning his exit. The public face of government disengagement was to announce that the czar would be the UK's roving ambassador, meeting enforcement colleagues around the world on a part-time basis – in effect, international gardening leave. Following the election in 2001, David Blunkett took over as Home Secretary and for the Home Office, normal service was resumed when the UKADCU was taken in-house and disbanded to be replaced by the newly created Drug Strategy Directorate. Once that happened, the drug strategy focused on developing ways to (in the buzz word of the day) 'grip' those using the most harmful drugs while (supposedly) committing most of the acquisitive crime. First though, an important prelude to the focus on drugs and crime.

Cannabis Huff and Puff

The dramatic increases in all kinds of drug use prompted a wave of commentary and analysis that the UK needed to do something different about the drug laws. The main focus since the 1960s had been cannabis. Various cannabis campaign groups came and went while Release always had drug law reform on its agenda. In 1979, ISDD published a book, *Cannabis: Options for Control,* predicated on the idea that it was time to investigate alternatives to blanket prohibition, while the ACMD had recommended the reclassification of cannabis from Class B to C. In 1991, the law reform and human rights organisation Justice published a report on drugs and the law, which made several recommendations including that a distinction should be made between commercial and social supply. None of this activity over many years had the least impact on successive governments.

Some retiring Chief Constables had suggested reform was needed but in 1999, the Cleveland force, now led by Barry Shaw, became the first to warn the government in a public report (endorsed by the county police authority) that the police were not winning the drugs war. It went beyond cannabis reform to recommend it was time to consider 'the legalisation and regulation of some or all drugs'.[13]

Back in 1997, Ruth Runciman, chair of the ACMD sub-committees that had published such seminal reports on drug policy, was frustrated in her attempt to persuade the ACMD to review the whole of the Misuse of Drugs Act. She approached social psychologist Dr Barrie Irving, founder of the Police Foundation, an independent research group set up in 1980 to make policing more effective. Irving gained the trust of senior police officers as somebody who could give constructive criticism concerning policing policy and practice. ACPO had produced a paper in 1996 recommending a thorough review of drug controls and this helped Irving persuade the other Foundation trustees to back Ruth Runciman's application so long as Irving could raise the necessary funds. Nine other trusts and foundations joined in and £500,000 was raised, which paid for extensive additional research covering young people's drug use, asset confiscation, comparisons with other EU countries, plus a public opinion poll, none of which the ACMD could have commissioned as it had no research budget. Thirteen highly experienced commissioners were appointed and over a 30-month period, they held 28 meetings, hearing evidence from 34 expert witnesses and receiving more than 100 written submissions.

Published on 21 March 2000, this first comprehensive review of the working of the Misuse of Drugs Act, which became known as the Runciman Report, made more than 80 recommendations covering many aspects of how the drug laws were enforced. It again included a recommendation that there should be a new penalty for not-for-profit social supply. However, the main recommendations were that MDMA and LSD should be moved from Class A to B and cannabis from B to C on the basis that the classification system should reflect the scientific evidence of comparative harms. Ruth Runciman went to the Home Office three days before publication to present it to Home Secretary Jack Straw. He dismissed it out of hand, prompting Mo Mowlam to suggest it might be an idea to read it first.

The government got in with early rebuttals over the weekend prior to Monday publication, with all the major Sunday newspapers carrying the government position that nothing was going to change. Jack Straw had calculated, not unreasonably, that the report would be slated by the press, with headlines like 'Dope Smokers' Charter'. In fact, he was caught on the back foot. Ruth Runciman had boxed clever; in advance she had briefed both *Daily Mail* editor Paul Dacre and *Daily Telegraph* editor Charles Moore, newspapers where she could expect the most hostility to the report– and it paid off. The *Mail on Sunday* declared 'We should all join in the drug debate' and on the evidence of the UK's premier league position in Europe as number one for young people trying drugs, reluctantly concluded that enforcement was failing (*Mail on Sunday*, 27 March). *The Daily Mail* (29 March) placed an extract of its editorial on the front page: 'Despite this paper's instinctive reservations over a more relaxed approach to drugs, we believe that the issue deserves a mature and rational debate.' There was more support from the *Mail*'s stable companion, the *London Evening Standard*, and calls for a proper debate on the drugs from the pages of *The Daily Telegraph*. It is possible that one reason for such an unexpected response from Conservative-supporting media outlets was simply a chance to embarrass the government for dismissing the report before publication, while knowing full well there would not be any law changes – especially with a general election only a year away. After all, calling for a 'mature debate' was hardly a big ask. It is also likely that middle-class university-educated editors might have more sympathy than their predecessors about youthful experimentation with drugs, especially if they were parents too.

There was a certain amount of government back-pedalling over the next few days but with an election looming, Tony Blair was determined there should be no ammunition for the Conservatives to lob a charge of being 'soft on drugs' at them, as beleaguered Tory leader William Hague had done in the weeks before the report was published. Attempting to win back traditional Tory support, Hague declared a Tory government would get tough on drugs and jail anybody caught in possession of any drugs (including cannabis) within 400 metres of a school. In the next move in the game of rapid-response politics, Blair invited the parents of Leah Betts to No. 10, insisting that Mo Mowlam and Keith Hellawell attend. The equally beleaguered drug czar was made to announce that he was 'misquoted' in the *Observer* suggesting that the effort against cannabis should be relaxed.[14]

Ironically, it was William Hague who was undone on cannabis. At the 2000 annual Conservative Party conference Ann Widdecombe, the shadow Home Secretary, announced her intention, should she become Home Secretary after the 2001 election, to introduce a £100 fixed-penalty fine for cannabis possession and prison for a second offence. Visions of smokers being frogmarched down to cash machines were invoked and mocked, but even more damaging to her doomed plan, eight of her (presumably enemy) shadow Cabinet colleagues admitted to smoking cannabis as students. She was slaughtered in the popular press while the police declared the scheme unworkable. These dismal examples of the political tit-for-tat war of words were to nobody's credit.

Doing the Lambeth Walk

The government was beginning to drill down to determine what had to be done to break the link between drugs and crime. It became clear that most of the increase in crime in the late-1990s/early-2000s was acquisitive and many of the perpetrators were people with heroin and crack problems. The figures were disputed though. Some police put the number at above 50 per cent, but most of the crimes committed by drug users were shoplifting and low-level dealing rather than burglary and street robbery. This led some researchers to conclude the national figure might not exceed 20 per cent, although it was probably much higher in hot-spot areas like Merseyside and parts of London.

From the government's point of view, this meant reallocating more resources to tackling the drugs causing the most problems and paying less attention to cannabis. While Jack Straw was Home Secretary (and indicative of the difference between public statements and private conversations), the ACPO lead on drugs, Chief Constable Peter Hampson of West Mercia, met with a senior Home Office official who asked him about regrading; the Home Office and the UKADCU were fed up with time spent on dealing with letters from the public about cannabis. A staff officer at the meeting told me, 'She said it doesn't matter what we do, it always comes back to cannabis.' The feeling was that a regrading would help shut down the argument. Peter Hampson did not object.

Cannabis came into focus for the Metropolitan Police (the Met) in late 1999 when its study sampled the amount of time taken to process cannabis arrests in three London divisions. In May 2000 it produced a report entitled 'Clearing the Decks' written by Deputy Assistant Commissioner Mike Fuller and Inspector Stuart Dark from the Met's Drugs Directorate. The report suggested ways in which police time could be saved in order to divert resources to areas of 'high priority'. It explored alternatives to arrest for some minor crimes, including possession of cannabis. But the Met's board rejected the idea.

Then in January 2001, Brian Paddick became Lambeth Borough Commander based at Brixton police station. According to the Inspectorate of Constabulary, Lambeth was one of the busiest commands in the country with high crime rates and emergency call-outs while it was short of 100 officers. Paddick determined that his officers were spending too much time processing cannabis arrests. He had another cannabis problem too.

Officers had been confiscating cannabis on the street and then disposing of it without any record of the encounter. One Brixton officer faced various charges in connection with cannabis, including one which related to unlawful disposal. He was eventually sacked; angry officers responded by threatening to arrest everybody for cannabis possession and swamp Brixton station.

Paddick began to investigate what the local response might be should his officers reduce or stop cannabis arrests to deal with higher-priority crimes. He shared his thoughts with *Evening Standard* crime reporter Ken Hyder who splashed the story over the front pages in March 2001. This did not go down well with the Met's top brass, but eventually a pilot scheme was sanctioned by Commissioner Sir John Stevens starting on 4 July 2001 and due to end in December. Anybody caught in possession of cannabis would be given a warning and not arrested. As the scheme progressed, the Police Foundation commissioned a poll of residents and found 83 per cent were in favour – either fully or on the condition more serious crimes were dealt with.

Off the back of this favourable poll, the Met decided to extend the pilot scheme, but the tide began to turn. The amount of cannabis warnings rose significantly, which underlined growing community concerns about drug tourism, provoking hostile responses from local press and politicians. However, in its review of the scheme, published in September 2002, the Metropolitan Police Authority could find no evidence that more young people were using cannabis or that there was a general perception cannabis was now legal. What might have created that impression was David Blunkett's announcement on 10 July 2002 of his intention to reclassify cannabis from Class B to Class C. The Lambeth scheme ended on 31 July: after that Lambeth police had the discretion to arrest for cannabis possession.

In 2014, a detailed analysis was published evaluating the scheme in terms of its success in focusing police resources elsewhere.[15] Previous research had concluded that thousands of police hours had been saved, but what was the impact of the time saved? The 2014 report concluded there was no significant increase in arrests for Class A drug offences, but the scheme did impact on arrests for non-drug crime.

When David Blunkett took over as Home Secretary in June 2001, he would have been briefed that the police had no objection in principle to the idea of some kind of law reform – this would give political cover to the police relaxing efforts on cannabis possession especially as the money released by the Treasury would allow for a more intense focus on delivering on the drugs–crime agenda. Blunkett also had in his back pocket the intellectual ballast of the Runciman Report (despite government rejection of all the main recommendations) but even more important politically, the sympathetic media responses. There was also a sense that David Blunkett was more independently minded than Jack Straw, that he wanted to make his mark by not necessarily toeing the Home Office line. A modest tweak to the drug laws – and the publicity it would receive – would help stake his claim.

Before the Lambeth scheme got under way, Blunkett received a visit from Chris Mullin MP, newly elected chair of the Home Affairs Select Committee (HASC) who expressed a wish that HASC's first inquiry would be to examine the workings of the government's drug strategy. Blunkett told Mullin that reclassification was being considered, a thought further cemented when he visited Brixton police and other stations. 'It was clear that police were already prioritising the pushers, so why not align policy with practice on the ground?'[16] He even told Mullin he was prepared 'to contemplate legalising and regulating the sale of heroin, 'although I don't accept it's benign'.[17] David Blunkett was no liberal, but he did take the view that 'being tough as the Home Secretary allows you to do things you wouldn't otherwise be able to do because you have provided yourself with some broad cover in terms of the fact that you haven't lost your marbles and gone soft. The classic example was Richard Nixon's visit to China which no Democrat could have pulled off.'[18]

The HASC started taking evidence on 30 October 2001 when David Blunkett publicly stated he favoured cannabis reclassification. His officials were less comfortable. Chris Mullin in his memoir recounted that,

> the witnesses were various officials from the government's anti-drugs apparatus, including the 'Tsar' Keith Hellawell, who seemed depressed. We ambled along predictably for the first 90 minutes or so. It was only when I inquired why their written evidence had not addressed decriminalisation – half our terms of reference – that things livened up. The officials seemed to be in a state of denial … [about the public debate post-Runciman]. Round and round we went, but they seemed reluctant even to address the issue…The poor woman from the Home Office was distraught. When I suggested she go away and provide us, by Thursday, with a paper rebutting the arguments for decriminalisation her forehead actually touched the table.[19]

The final HASC report published in May 2002 recommended ecstasy be reclassified to Class B and cannabis to C and, for the third time in a report, recommended a new not-for-profit social supply offence. It also favoured a heroin prescribing trial, the introduction of drug consumption rooms and urged the government to review the international drug control legislation with a view to investigating alternatives. Only one member of the committee refused to sign up to the recommendations, but the MP for Witney was on board – David Cameron.

Blunkett asked the ACMD to effectively endorse his view and he announced the decision to reclassify in July 2002 while simultaneously rejecting the proposals to reclassify MDMA and open safer injecting rooms. However, when interviewed for *Druglink* in 2003 he said he would countenance the ideas if they were linked to a supervised heroin prescribing regime rather than people bringing in drugs off the street into what the media called 'shooting galleries'. The decision to reclassify cannabis provoked a futile gesture from Keith Hellawell, who 'resigned' in protest.

Despite having announced the decision in July 2002, it took until January 2004 for the regrading to pass into law. There was the normal problem of finding parliamentary time within a packed legislative agenda, but Blunkett also ran into trouble with the Met and was visited by Mike Fuller in charge of drug policy and Deputy Commissioner Ian Blair. In very simple terms involving various sections of the Police and Criminal Evidence Act, they were concerned that as the law stood, if cannabis was reclassified to Class C, the police would lose the power of arrest. In that situation they would not, for example, be able to search the premises of somebody arrested for possession to see if other offences had been committed. The upshot was that the reclassification went through without the changes to policing procedure the police feared. However, the police also persuaded David Blunkett not to reduce the penalties for cannabis trafficking because, at least in London, they were seeing the very earliest examples of more commercial cannabis growing and Blunkett did not want any law change to make it easier for those supplying cannabis.

If anybody in the Home Office thought reclassification would derail the debate, they were sorely mistaken. A report published in 2003 by the Joseph Rowntree Foundation confirmed police intelligence and revealed the increase in a home-grown market for cannabis that was beginning to overtake imports of Moroccan hashish. The purpose of the report was to push for reform of the law to allow for cultivation for personal use to be treated no differently than possession. It also found that to escape detection, cannabis was being grown indoors, in water and under strong lights rather than soil. Using imported seeds from Holland, the plants produced a higher level of THC than normally found in hash and went under the name skunk.[20]

Once the existence of stronger cannabis became public knowledge, and without any forensic information to back it up, the media were full of wild stories about cannabis being anything up to 100 times stronger than it used to be and causing a significant surge in referrals to psychiatric units. Once the analysis was done and published it appeared that on average the strength of skunk was only about twice that of hash,[21] although there were stronger strains mainly used by cannabis cognoscenti – and there were always people who should never have smoked cannabis in the first place whatever the strength. Consultant psychiatrists, who only ever see the worst cases, backed by some mental health charities and anti-drug campaigners, were blaming the regrading for sparking increased use when all the official surveys of drug use, including cannabis, showed a downward trend from about 2000 onwards.

However, taking his revenge for past clashes with Tony Blair over drugs, Conservative Party leader Michael Howard attacked Labour in the run-up to the 2005 General Election for being soft on drugs and causing a wave of mental health problems. Tony Blair kicked the issue into the long grass by referring it back to the ACMD. The ACMD recommended to Home Secretary Charles Clarke that there was no evidence to support a change. When it looked as if Clarke would ignore this, the no-nonsense ACMD chair Sir Michael Rawlins threatened mass resignations and Clarke backed down. Then Clarke did a strange thing; early in 2006, he announced in the Commons that cannabis would remain a Class C drug, but that he had ordered a review of the Misuse of Drugs Act. It's not clear what was behind the announcement and the review never happened because Clarke was replaced in May 2006 by John Reid in the wake of the scandal about 85 serious foreign offenders released from prison without being considered for deportation, and now on the run. A 50-page draft consultation paper was drawn up prior to Clarke's departure, but never published, only coming to light in 2010 following a Freedom of Information (FOI) request. The paper did not allow for law reform as an option, but instead suggested different ways of configuring the Misuse of Drugs Act because as the Ministerial foreword stressed, 'having a clear and readily understood classification system on which to base messages which are realistic, relevant and credible is essential'.[22] On the basis that the review would now not happen under John Reid as he had other priorities to worry about, the Parliamentary Science and Technology Committee weighed in with its own analysis of the classification system. In its report, *Drug classification: making a hash of it?*, published in July 2006, the conclusion was, in the phrase *de jour*, that like the Immigration Department, it too 'was not fit for purpose' and the government was attacked for using the Act to send out messages rather than actually delineating drugs according to the scientific and clinical evidence of harm.

The issue came up again when Gordon Brown took over as Prime Minister in July 2007. One of his very early statements was his intention to return cannabis to its Class B status. He had to refer this to the ACMD, which stuck to its guns, but the PM was not to be denied and Home Secretary Jacqui Smith announced the re-regrading in 2009. Some observers put Brown's decision down to a very traditional and dour view on drugs (a view shared by his advisers), but others believed he did a deal with Paul Dacre (the *Daily Mail's* brief flirtation with a sensible drug debate being over) that in exchange for support, Brown would regrade cannabis and also tackle immigration and scrap proposals for super casinos.

***

Clearing the smoke back to 2000, the political drive towards encouraging less focus on cannabis was simply to signal a more concerted effort on the drugs and the users perceived to be causing the most community harm. At the start of the millennium, the political atmosphere around drugs seemed almost frantic. In 2000 Ann Widdecombe was banging the drum for an unworkable drug crackdown. At the Labour Party spring conference of 2001, Tony Blair announced a similarly unworkable plan, apparently cooked up with a Scottish MP over dinner, to start a register of drug dealers similar to the register of sex offenders. He told delegates that anyone freed from jail and liable to deal in drugs would go onto the register, so unusual bank transactions and changes of address would be monitored. Apart from the fact that police and customs already had detailed criminal records of those convicted of dealing, most drug dealing was carried out at street level involving small amounts of drugs sold by users to fund future purchases – people who rarely had bank accounts or permanent addresses. Politicians seemed to be thrashing around trying to 'out tough' each other.

In 2002, after five years in charge, the PM's drugs–crime agenda was in trouble. Several policy strands were happening at once to address the perceived delivery deficiencies either thought through – or thought up on the hoof – trying to stimulate action or at least to be seen by the outside world as 'doing something'.

There were three main strands of the policy in place or being piloted for reducing drug-related crime: Drug Testing and Treatment Orders (DTTOs), Arrest Referral, and the prison-based Counselling, Assessment, Referral, Advice and Throughcare (CARAT) programme. But in the early period of trying to build the treatment system, relatively few people were turning up at treatment services from the criminal justice system while there was no proper linking of care for drug-using offenders coming out of prison and wanting a community drug service. The first few days of release for those who had been using heroin before they went inside were the most dangerous. Many went back to using at their pre-jail dose straight away and died within the first week or so due to diminished tolerance levels. Even if somebody did arrive at the treatment gates from the criminal justice system, they were shown to the back of a very long queue. There was an overriding imperative to build capacity in the drug treatment service.

The atmosphere inside government at the time regarding drugs and crime is best summed up by this conversation. I asked a senior Home Office official if he had seen *The Thick of It,* which first aired in May 2005. Somewhat wearily he said, 'I watched the first episode, but it was too much like a day at the office.' Referring to David Blunkett, he commented: 'He was a five-initiatives a day sort of person. It was a bit nightmarish because you'd come in and find he'd slept on a few ideas and wanted to launch them that day.'

The PM and his advisors remained convinced that much street crime was caused by drug users looking to fund their habit – cue the launch of the Street Crime Initiative in 2002. This too failed to get users into treatment. The Criminal Justice Joint Inspection report on the initiative found that most perpetrators were not problematic drug users and nearly half of the recorded street robberies were caused by youth-driven mobile phone theft, not crime to pay for drugs.

The Performance and Innovation Unit mentioned above became the PM's Strategy Unit in 2002, headed by Geoff Mulgan, while the Delivery Unit was led by Sir Michael Barber. The Strategy Unit's role was to present strategy advice and policy analysis on key priorities and the first item on the agenda was drugs. Former BBC Director-General John Birt was brought in and tasked to do some radical 'blue-sky thinking' (brainstorming with no limits, trying out ideas which do not have to be practical as one idea begets others until an innovative solution is uncovered).

Birt and his team produced two reports in 2003. They confirmed what they termed 'High Harm Users' were using the most damaging drugs and committing most of the associated crime to fund drug purchases. However, the unit was there to come up with radical thoughts – not tell the PM what he already knew. They concluded trying to stop heroin coming into the country was a waste of time; whatever the enforcement agencies achieved in terms of seizures and arrests failed to dent the supply. The answer, they said, was to make heroin *use* illegal (not just possession and supply) and then make heroin widely available across the NHS. The thinking behind this was you need not bother with all the stuff about drugs and crime; it didn't matter whether you had committed an acquisitive crime or not – using heroin (and just having track marks would be deemed evidence enough) meant a referral into treatment. Time and money saved. The reports were never formally published and only appeared following a FOI request in 2005. The press had a field day, but rain poured down on the blue-sky thinking and that was that. How so?

There was a concern that not enough drug-using offenders were entering treatment. However, the doctors refused to sign up to heroin use as an offence on ethical and human rights grounds, while the police saw major problems trying to enforce the law on the streets. Logically crack use should have been banned as well, but there was no treatment for crack and supplying it on the NHS was, shall we say, unlikely. In general terms, it was all too radical for all the relevant ministers, their civil servants and most importantly Sir Michael Barber. Everyone had signed up to an incremental process for delivering this top political priority. Treatment was viewed as the key to success, so all eyes turned to the National Treatment Agency.

In the Thick of It

In 2001, Mike Trace was transferred over from the UKADCU to set up the NTA until Paul Hayes took over as CEO while Trace became Director of Performance. Hayes was in a unique position of being in the cabinet room with Tony Blair and Secretaries of State, a privilege denied even to most junior ministers, which gives an indication where drugs stood in the pecking order. Hayes' suggestion was to join up all the existing (and failing) interventions and then deliver the necessary crime reduction dividend through building the treatment system. From this emerged the Criminal Justice Interventions Programme running initially in 30 pilot areas. It was later renamed the Drug Interventions Programme (DIP) because Caroline Flint, who became the drugs minister in June 2003, thought the name should be more drug specific as everything the Home Office did was concerned with criminal justice. Paul Hayes got the nods of agreement around the table; offstage he was told to deliver or else. The first order of business was to shake up the treatment system.

On 19 October 1999, *The Guardian* published a damning article on the state of some drug treatment services. Like all health and social care workers, most staff working in drug treatment services wanted to do their best for those in their care. But as we know from past and present hospital and residential care scandals, there will always be exceptions. The drug treatment system was no different. In some ways, drug users were more vulnerable than most people. Many of the scandals in mainstream services only come to light because of a critical mass of complaints from family and friends or whistle-blowers. Drug users facing those staff who take judgemental and uncaring attitudes are usually isolated from these networks and fear being kicked off a programme if they are identified as troublemakers. Whistle-blowing drug workers fared no better.

The Guardian article exposed some horror stories. One user was admitted to the psychiatric ward of his local hospital for a detox from methadone and Valium. While there, he had to contend with harassment from a naked psychiatric patient and witnessed two attempted suicides. Another user wanted to change the date of his clinic appointment as it clashed with a dental appointment and was told to bring the extracted tooth as proof, while another arrived late to find the door locked and a worker on the other side dangling his prescription in front of him before tearing it up. The problems went far deeper than the individual actions of those who should never been allowed within a country mile of a vulnerable person – including those I heard at the first NTA national conference in 2002, such as the 'virtue' of long waiting times as they demonstrate 'commitment'.

The Audit Commission produced a report on the state of drug treatment. Published in March 2002, *Changing Habits* did not make comfortable reading for services. The commission cited poor service planning, professional differences over 'what works', difficulties for users accessing treatment, long waiting times, failure to address individual needs and lack of coordination between services. The Department of Health published *Models of Care* to address the issues emerging from the findings which the Audit Commission noted 'provides a significant challenge for the drug treatment sector'. The document basically set out the structures, policies and procedures that were expected to deliver a decent treatment system.

The Drug Strategy had been updated in 2002 to re-emphasise the importance of the drug–crime agenda and with it came a substantial amount of extra funding for treatment. The Drug Intervention Programme went national in 2004, which helped the NTA fend off an attempt by the Department of Health to mainstream drug treatment services into the NHS. At the same time, the 'gripping' of drug-using offenders in treatment intensified.

At the start of *Trainspotting*, Renton goes through all the choices that life offers. None of them appeal. Who needs to make choices when you've got heroin? The government had another view. Choose Treatment or Choose Prison. These were the key elements of the Tough Choices programme launched as part of The Drugs Act 2005. Whereas some aspects of the Drugs Intervention Programme were voluntary, others were not. The Drugs Act 2005 majored on the coercive elements. Anybody committing a so-called trigger offence had to supply a urine sample. Failure to do so was an offence. So too was failure to attend a two-part assessment procedure for drug treatment. Both carried the potential for prison and fines. There was also a reversal of the presumption of bail for drug-using offenders. In effect it was a new law to swerve around the existing Bail Act. And all of this was on top of the Prolific and Other Priority Offenders scheme propelling the hard core of offenders, many of whom were drug users, towards the treatment 'choice'.[23]

When the NTA was created, it was agreed that formally the money would come down through the Department of Health to the primary care trusts with the Drug Action Teams responsible for commissioning the services. Thus, the NTA was not technically responsible for allocating the pooled treatment budget, but it played a key role in decision making at the centre. Yet in trying to determine how and where to best to spend the money, the NTA initially faced a similar problem to the UKADCU; there was very little reliable data on treatment. The 'Addicts Index' had been discontinued in 1996 to be replaced by the National Drug Treatment Monitoring System, which nobody bothered to fill in. There was a target to double the people in treatment by 2008, but no reliable baseline: 'We had no definition of "in treatment",' said Paul

Hayes, 'or even a definition of "in".' Another problem was the workforce – there wasn't enough of it. The Treasury wanted the sector to grow quickly to accommodate all those it projected would be referred by the criminal justice system. Adverts appeared in the press offering good salaries without any experience required. There was little or no training capacity; in 1995 the ACMD had produced a report, which was ignored, detailing the importance of training at a regional and national level.

However, driven by the NTA and as a result of what seemed like a bottomless money pot, between 2002–2004 the field expanded very quickly: treatment numbers grew as more service capacity came onstream and waiting times fell dramatically. Opioid substitute therapy became the gold-standard treatment and increasing numbers of GPs were now involved in treating users, caring for their primary health needs and prescribing under the auspices of 'shared care' arrangements where they had the support of local drug services. The creation of the Substance Misuse Management in General Practice support organisation also helped encourage the involvement of GPs in user care.

Another Audit Commission Report, *Drug misuse 2004: reducing the impact,* concluded there had been 'impressive progress' in all areas of treatment service delivery. Things were clearly moving in the right direction. There was a sting in the tail, however: spending millions of pounds of public money to 'protect' the public from a very unpopular sector of society demanded some serious accountability. There was a tension in New Labour which favoured dispensing power and responsibility to local communities, while demanding upward flow of accountability to justify the expenditure. This could easily tip over into panicky command and control management. In 2007, DrugScope went around the country to engage with its membership. It asked what members they thought were the best and worst developments of the previous decade. The NTA came top of both polls.

Pressure to deliver on the crime reduction dividend through treatment flowed from the very top. A senior Drug Strategy Directorate official said, 'I was seeing the PM to report on progress on a weekly basis. I saw him more than some of my Home Office colleagues.' Tony Blair personally chaired quarterly 'stocktake' meetings of all the departments involved in the drug strategy where again all eyes were on treatment. Why?

Although education and prevention, and domestic and foreign drug enforcement were given equal billing in the drug strategy, solid evidence of effectiveness was in short supply. During the course of Tony Blair's premiership, the British Crime Survey showed a steady decline in the general population using drugs, but it was impossible to determine the factors behind falling figures. The Birt Review had already determined that enforcement wasn't making any sustainable impact. Education and prevention programmes fared no better. Despite Tony Blair's commitment after the fall of the Taliban in 2002 that the UK would lead on opium eradication, still the heroin flowed out of Afghanistan in ever-increasing quantities.[24]

Regarding treatment, at least you could show local needs assessment reports, rising numbers coming in, falls in waiting times, evidence from the Audit Commission report citing demonstrable progress and map that against the overall decreases in acquisitive crime (although that was somewhat dubious in relation to drug users because there didn't seem to be specific falls in drug arrests or incidents of shoplifting). Even so it was enough to convince those who needed convincing.

Since the demise of the UKADCU, DAT coordinators had felt increasingly isolated from the centre. Each government department had regional offices and initially it was regional government officials who interceded in DAT business until the NTA took over with its own regional managers. There was pressure from the NTA headquarters on their team of regional managers and down to the DAT coordinators for rafts of data to be crunched by an expanding army of NTA number-crunchers to enable Paul Hayes to deliver the good news about the treatment to the Home Office and No 10. In truth, the NTA didn't really trust the DATs to deliver without constant scrutiny any more than the NHS were trusted to spend the money on drug treatment. Paul Hayes conceptualises the relationship as 'we'll put an arm around your shoulder, but we'll feel for the windpipe in case we need to find it'. Mike Trace readily admits that the NTA didn't get the balance right between guidance and supervision and that the demands for torrents of paperwork did get 'out of control'.

As public servants, DAT coordinators tended to keep their heads below the parapet and how they reacted to the rising tide of bureaucracy very much depended on their background. Some had been dyed-in-the-wool administrators and just got on with it, especially if they came from the NHS or social services whose employees were no strangers to mountains of paperwork. Once out of the job, it was different. In May 2003, *The Guardian's* Nick Davies wrote up a view from the trenches from one beleaguered coordinator who'd had enough:

Richard Elliott couldn't stand it anymore. For nearly two years, he had been acting as the government's drugs envoy in Bristol, running the city's drugs action team, handling millions of pounds a year, linking together police, health and social workers and voluntary agencies into one big drive against drugs, but earlier this year he realised he couldn't stand it anymore, so he quit.

In fact, for most of that time he wasn't supposed to be running the drugs action team (DAT), but his coordinator had quit a year earlier because she couldn't stand it anymore either and so Elliott, who was supposed to be the commissioning manager, had taken on her job as well.

He didn't want to do that; he knew of at least four other DAT coordinators in the area who had gone off sick in the previous 12 months. He did at least have some help but his new colleague was soon working so hard that he started getting chest pains and, when he carried on regardless, his left arm started tingling and going purple until finally he couldn't stand it anymore and went off sick. Then he quit too.

Elliott could no longer bear the waste. He had six staff and a budget of £3.5m a year. He had a potential client group of 25,000 recreational users of cocaine and amphetamine, ecstasy and cannabis; plus a further 12,500 chaotic drug users who buy heroin and crack cocaine on the city's open drugs market, centred on St Paul's. He focused on the 4,500 chaotic users who live in Bristol but at the end of all his work and all that public money, the total number of NHS detox beds which he was able to provide to help any of those users was five, one of which was reserved for those with mental illness.

Even more than that, what Elliott really couldn't stand was the bureaucracy – the 44 different funding streams, each one with its own detailed guidance and micro targets from the centre, each one with its own demand for a detailed business plan and quarterly reports back to the centre; the endless service agreements he had to sign with every local provider with their own micro targets and a demand for quarterly reports back to him so that he could collate them and pass them back to the centre; the new annual drugs availability report to the centre; the annual treatment plan to the centre over 68 pages and nine planning grids with 82 objectives (that's what Elliott's colleague was working on when his arm went purple); the funding announced too late for planning and then handed over too late to be spent and finally spent for spending's sake to prevent it being reclaimed by the centre; the staff hired and trained and then suddenly sacked when funding or targets were switched by the centre (or just quitting because they couldn't stand it anymore). He reckoned he and his staff spent only 40% of their time organising services for drug users – the rest of their time was consumed by producing paper plans and paper reports for Whitehall.

Elliott wrote a resignation memo for a colleague with the heading 'Ravings of a burned-out mind'. He described the culture of control in Whitehall, their 'monitoring fetish' and their short-term thinking, and he wrote: 'Monitoring has become almost religious in its status, as has centralised control ... The demand for quick hits and early wins is driven by a central desire analogous to the instant gratification demands made by drug users themselves ... The criminal gangs that control the market are laughing all the way to the bank and beyond, as we tie ourselves in knots with good practice guidelines and monitoring. It's like trying to fight with one hand tied behind your back, a boxing glove on the other and strict instructions not to punch.'

Initially the DAT coordinators had been successful in getting senior figures from across the local public sector agencies to their meetings, often chaired by the local authority chief executive. As time went on, however, those attending from other sectors dropped in seniority both because the focus was increasingly on treatment and because senior managers were getting tired of being told by NTA regional managers they were doing a bad job. The line was toed mainly because this was a ministerial and even a prime ministerial priority and nobody wanted to be publicly embarrassed for what, in primary care trust terms, were relatively small amounts of money. Small it might have been, but as the money eventually dried up from about 2007, they stopped coming altogether as more and more DATs were merged into local Crime and Disorder Reduction Partnerships.

The disquiet among some DAT coordinators exploded at a DAT conference in Blackpool. The keynote speaker from the Home Office tried an approach last seen in the sitcom *Are You Being Served* when the elderly owner of the department store periodically rocked up to tell the staff, 'You're all doing very well'. There were boos and some of the audience just turned away from the stage. As if to underline the general atmosphere of nausea, the hotel was hit by an outbreak of food poisoning. I met two Home Office officials on the train home who had turned to the bottle to blot out the horror.

There was also disquiet among some workers that harm reduction had been side-lined in pursuit of the crime agenda. Yet none of the money coming into the system had special criminal justice conditions attached. The expansion of the system was obviously crime driven but treatment led, providing little evidence that harm reduction was being air-brushed out of history. Nor was there any documented evidence to back the claim that the best chance of getting into treatment was to commit a crime. That said, lack of evidence simply provides an opportunity for plausible deniability: there were parallel lines of entry from the criminal justice system and the community, but anecdotal stories persisted across the country of two-tier triage once inside the treatment gates.

While NTA micro-management certainly helped drive down waiting times, expand service provision, improve access and attempt to drive up quality, some aspects were sacrificed on the altar of crime reduction. The government view seemed to be that the only harm worth talking about was the harm to society caused by drug-related crime. Despite lots of fine words from government about the importance of families and carers, little central funding and support ever materialised or was sustained. Most support groups were run on a shoestring, started by a desperate parent answering the phone in the back bedroom and holding local support group meetings.

The Effectiveness Review had acknowledged service users as stakeholders who should be involved in the development of services, similar to developments taking place among many mental health and learning disability groups. Opinions are divided on the success of this ambition. The NTA was criticised by some for just trying to control the agenda and tick boxes; others welcomed the funding to attend conferences and to establish local groups. How these fared very much depended on the enthusiasm of local service managers and regional NTA managers for meaningful engagement. Again, experiences were mixed. Service-user involvement tended to work better at a local level where users were trying to influence how the care of users was delivered. It was more difficult at a national level where aims were more policy-driven and so more diffuse, although the Methadone Alliance achieved some success acting as advocates for individual users trying to resolve treatment issues.

There is no doubt, however, that as the treatment system built up, it came to be regarded with some envy around the world. Over the years,

I have spoken to many people who have accessed services in all its manifestations from community drug teams to residential rehab, from interventions as diverse as counselling to prescribed heroin – as well as those who simply joined a peer support group outside the system like NA. Not only was it clear that we needed and still need the maximum diversity of options, but the system as a whole did help thousands of people: 'if it wasn't for [insert service type here] I wouldn't be here' was a refrain I heard regularly.

Yet while able to cough up some plausible facts and figures for the PM, these very facts and figures presented the NTA with a major presentational headache. From around 2005, it was becoming increasingly obvious that while the strategy for hitting targets for those in treatment was working, the system itself was silting up. Plenty were coming in, few were leaving. The government was not asking questions about people leaving treatment. The prime directive was to get people into treatment and then if you can keep them from dropping out for three months, the evidence showed they had a better chance of staying in treatment. The emphasis had been on building the system from a very low base of effectiveness and engagement.

In 2006, the NTA updated its document 'Models of Care'. In it, was a reference to a previous document detailing the NTA business plan 2005–2008 entitled 'Treatment Effectiveness Strategy'. It stated, 'For clients who wish to be drug-free, treatment systems need to be better configured to create better-planned exits from treatment.' It is possible that if the NTA had seen their plan through to 2008, there would have been more progress in properly planned exits from treatment. As it turned out, the NTA was overtaken by events.

In 2004, the Centre for Social Justice (CSJ) was established as a right-wing think tank by the then leader of the Conservative Party Iain Duncan Smith whose key adviser was Phillipa Stroud, a deeply committed Christian whose husband was a minister in the evangelical New Frontier Church. In December 2006, the CJS published a series of reports under the banner of 'Breakdown Britain' including one entitled 'Addicted Britain'. The main thrust of the 150-page report was to accuse the government of being little more than licensed drug dealers, to call for the methadone tap to be turned off and for the focus instead to be on a more abstinence-based treatment system, making the unsubstantiated claim that abstinence was 'the most effective form of treatment' when the Effectiveness Review from a decade earlier could find no evidence to support any one-size-fits-all solution. However, the report did start a hum in the mood music that would challenge the prevailing treatment agenda.

With bonfire night approaching in 2007, the BBC lit a slow-burning fuse under the NTA. Back in April, the NTA had commissioned a report into the use of contingency management in the treatment system, a way of incentivising people to change their drug-using habits. There was some evidence from the USA that this worked by reducing crack use among the heroin users engaged in methadone treatment by handing out vouchers, which were redeemable for food and other essentials, or methadone take-home privileges in exchange for a 'clean' urine sample.

However, there were no established ethical protocols in place and the UK research revealed some UK services offering or considering offers of rewards such as extra methadone.

BBC Home Affairs editor Mark Easton interviewed Paul Hayes at the NTA offices. Believing he had a good story to tell about the progress of drug treatment, Hayes (or rather the communications person) allowed the interview to continue for 2 hours. Towards the end, perhaps realising he had yet to find the story, Easton raised the issue of services providing extra methadone as a reward. Hayes had to admit he hadn't read the report but commented that such practices were unacceptable. The 'extra methadone' story was reported by the BBC on 18 October. At the bottom of the online report, however, Easton stated that based on NTA treatment figures, only 6 per cent had left treatment 'drug-free' (including methadone) in the past year. By 30 October that figure had come down to 3 per cent. Health Minister Dawn Primarolo stumbled through an interview on Radio 4 and after the row back at NTA HQ, Jon Hibbs, a senior communications manager, was drafted in from the Department of Health to ensure the minister was never blindsided again.

The figures were disputed (it was more like 11 per cent) but whichever way you cut the cake, from a public point of view, the return on what was by now a £400 million investment did not appear impressive. There was a disconnect between the government, who essentially viewed 'treatment' as simply a way of reducing crime, and the media and general public who expected treatment to deliver a 'cure'. And it was residential rehabilitation that most people associated with treatment, fuelled by regular media stories of celebrities going to rehab for a few weeks to be 'cured'. There was little independent evidence that rehab was any more successful over the longer term than many other interventions and some rehab establishments were run on very dubious ethical lines. No doubt though that public sector funding for residential treatment was in short supply because providing 24/7 care is expensive.

Within the drug treatment sector, buoyed by the CSJ report and the BBC reporting, the fireworks exploded. Those who had never supported methadone maintenance took this very public opportunity to call into question the whole treatment strategy. A major fault line opened between supporters of harm reduction on the one hand and abstinence on the other, driven by a hearts and minds debate over the definition of recovery. The mantra on one side was 'you can't recover if you are dead' contrasted with criticisms that people were 'parked on methadone' and that the system was nowhere near ambitious enough for drug users. Both sides of the argument had serious points to make, yet they were not mutually exclusive positions. Harm reduction interventions helped keep people alive to pursue their treatment journey wherever that might lead, including to a drug-free life. The debate played out on the pages of *Druglink* with my former colleague Mike Ashton penning a 16-page forensic examination of the arguments,[25] followed by articles both for and against the strategy. Views on both sides were aired at special DrugScope conferences. Before the debate began, Ruth Runciman had been instrumental in establishing the UK Drug Policy Commission (UKDPC) to provide independent analysis of drug policy and practice. Then in July 2008, the UKDPC produced a consensus statement on a vision of recovery which majored on the rights of the individual to self-determine recovery but that hardly settled the matter.

Even before the row broke out, the writing was on the wall for spending on drug treatment. With another NHS funding crisis looming, the Department for Health was pushing for no increase in the pooled treatment budget, a move fiercely resisted by the Home Office. However, in an NTA newsletter, Paul Hayes warned the sector that funding for treatment was running out of steam; increases of the sort the field had enjoyed since 2002 could not be guaranteed beyond 2008. The prescience of that comment became apparent when on 15 September 2008, Lehman Brothers collapsed, which sparked the global financial crisis and brought the treatment gravy train to a shuddering halt.

13

States of the Nation

During the election campaign of 2005, Conservative party leader Michael Howard announced there would be money for 25,000 extra beds for abstinence-oriented residential rehabilitation. The Centre for Social Justice led by Iain Duncan Smith, a prospective Cabinet minister, was also pushing for an abstinence-based approach. So, in the run-up to the 2010 General Election, service providers had high hopes of changing fortunes from an incoming Conservative government and were stalking the corridors of Whitehall seeking assurances. However, promises made in the shadows did not stand up to the harsh daylight of financial reality.

Meetings of the All-Party Parliamentary Group on Drugs were usually only modestly attended; the post-election meetings of 2010 were packed to the rafters by campaigners in a failed attempt to persuade first Home Office Minister James Brokenshire and then Health Minister Anne Milton to 'top-slice' the pooled treatment budget to boost funding for residential rehabilitation.

Under David Cameron, the drugs–crime agenda was being replaced by the recovery agenda. Before Labour came into power in 1997 promising to break the drugs–crime link, the process had already begun under the Conservatives. Similarly, the Labour government was already in recovery mode before Cameron's coalition government took office. In the 2008 drug strategy, never implemented, there was a pledge to move people through the treatment system more quickly with the necessary post-treatment policies in place to effect 're-integration'.

From 2010, the watchword was 'recovery', or rather 'Recovery', and there was a difference. It would be hard for anybody to argue that people should not be given every opportunity to move on from a chaotic and dangerous life as a street heroin or crack user. That would be recovery with a lower-case 'r'. What emerged was Recovery – less a practical intervention, more an ideology, that total abstinence from all substances was the only way forward for people with drug problems.

There were flies in the ointment of this thinking. Many people with serious drug problems had never been 'integrated' in the first place. They come from dysfunctional backgrounds and suffer what amounts to post-traumatic stress disorder, self-medicated over many years with drugs and alcohol. People accessing treatment in receipt of methadone prescriptions may well have been 'living better' while not necessarily yet 'getting better'. Even those who were ready to move on – move on to what? People need a decent place to live, a job or training, access to other health and social care services. Who was going to prioritise drug users? Many did, and do, find great comfort in peer support groups and the lucky few found fulfilment in some of the excellent recovery social enterprise schemes dotted around the country or volunteering (or employed) in drug treatment services. But for some there was/is as much danger of being 'trapped' in a Recovery feedback loop as 'parked' on methadone.

As Norman Fowler said, it would have been very hard to help drug users at risk of HIV if only that group were deemed to be at risk. The second wave of funding came simply to deliver the drugs–crime agenda. Fear was driving investment. Now the existential threat appeared diminished; now it was all about Recovery, to make drug users 'better'. Who was going to pay for that at all, let alone during a time of 'austerity'? The new political imperative was to save money, while attempting to construct a more ideologically driven drug strategy.

With all this in mind Iain Duncan Smith, now Secretary of State for Work and Pensions, initially tried to take over the drug strategy from the Home Office so he could link welfare benefits to treatment engagement. By all accounts Home Secretary Theresa May suggested he go run in a wheat field.

Civil servants at DH had managed to deflect ministers away from an end to methadone prescribing, but in the new political climate, it was important to base this evidence in the context of recovery. In 2012 an expert group chaired by John Strang did just that with their report whose findings concluded that 'well-delivered' medically assisted therapy 'provides a platform of stability and safety to protect people and creates the time and space for them to move forward in their personal recovery journeys'.[1] The findings were supported by two very influential architects of the US recovery establishment: Professor Thomas McLellan and William White. Writing for *Druglink*, they said, 'Why would we deny any patient attempting to recover from any disease, the ability to access an effective medication to aid them in their recovery?'[2]

Not to be denied, the Inter-Ministerial Group on Drugs published an unofficial document majoring on 'full recovery' – covered in departmental logos but disowned by civil servants. The Group commissioned the ACMD, which had formed a recovery sub-committee, to investigate time-limited treatment. The committee emphatically concluded that limiting the time people could be enrolled in treatment would increase the possibility of relapse and could lead to other 'significant unintended consequences', such as increased rates of overdose, blood-borne viruses and drug-related crime. Despite the assertion that much of the treatment population were 'parked' on methadone, the report found only around 10–15 per cent of service users received opioid substitute therapy (OST) for five years or more, a larger minority 'may not be in OST long enough to derive long-term benefit'. OST use is 'episodic and relatively short' for the majority of people, with nearly 40 per cent stopping within six months.[3]

Knocked back yet again, Iain Duncan Smith railed against the ACMD and the 'methadone industry' through the pages of the *Sunday Telegraph* (16 November 2014), but the recovery agenda did underpin the new government's approach to drug treatment as enshrined in the last two drug strategies published in 2010 and 2017. There were attempts to link welfare benefits to treatment engagement and an incentive scheme for treatment agencies called payment by results, both of which were quietly shelved as it became clear they were entirely unworkable and in the case of the second, hugely expensive to administer.

In the last few years of operation, DrugScope organised meetings of senior treatment sector staff to discuss matters of common interest, with government officials invited along to be questioned about government policy. Obviously, concerns over funding were high on the agenda; officials would admonish the group for what they called 'shroud waving', but there was every good reason to fear the spectre of austerity.

Since 2010, drug treatment (and drug policy generally) has slipped right down the political agenda to the point at which any arguments over harm reduction, abstinence and recovery (capitalised or otherwise) are now academic in the face of swingeing cuts in treatment and rehabilitation budgets. In 2013, the NTA was merged into Public Health England, staffed primarily by those who had come from Health Protection England, which focused on disease control. Its staff had little knowledge of wider addiction issues. The centrally administered pooled treatment budget disappeared to be replaced by a local authority-controlled ring-fenced public health grant. Drug treatment initially accounted for about a third of the grant, then the ring fence came off, leaving drug treatment budgets at the mercy of cash-strapped local authorities that were more focused on everything else, from adult social care to potholes.

The attitude of many local councillors with few insights into drug dependency was summed up by one councillor approached by the operations manager of a major voluntary sector treatment agency. When asked about funding, the reply was, 'Why should we fund a lifestyle choice?' Many local drug agencies have closed or merged into the larger agencies. They in turn are locked into tit-for-tat contract battles with each other over who runs the services around the country and are also taking hefty budget cuts. There are instances of treatment agencies refusing to tender for services because the money on offer is simply not enough. Residential services have been particularly hard hit. While not the magic recovery bullet some claim, nevertheless, the best services offer a safe environment, daily structure, a range of psychosocial interventions and accessible peer support for those unable to live independently in the community. Past studies have shown that for those who respond to the environment, the longer they stayed the better chance of avoiding relapse. Back in the 1970s, stays of 18 months or more were not unusual. In recent times, local authority funding might only last 6 months.

Some of the poorest parts of the country have the highest levels of need, yet these are areas where business rate income is very low, putting even greater pressure on local authority funding. NHS staff have also been squeezed out of services because of consultant psychiatrist and nursing costs. There are still approximately 300,000 people with a heroin and/or crack problem while drug-related deaths have been going up after a period of relative decline. Statistically, those at most risk are users in the older age group where years of drug and alcohol use and smoking begin to take their toll on the ageing body. However, many users are not in treatment, including around half of those dying of an overdose and anecdotally there are concerns that the treatment policies of some agencies (such as under-dosing) are discouraging attendance or causing early drop-out. Moreover, deaths have been rising across all age ranges and drug-use. Those needing treatment for alcohol problems are even more poorly served with fewer than 20 per cent in treatment. The Centre for Social Justice published a new report in 2019, 'The Road to Recovery', in which ironically, it called for the creation of a new national agency which it hoped would be a new champion for treatment and rehabilitation at the centre.

Drug treatment is one of the three main pillars of any drug strategy; the other two are education/prevention and enforcement. So how have these been faring?

Education, Education, Education

Wherever one sits along the spectrum of the drug policy argument, there is a general agreement that drug education is 'a good thing'. Like enforcement, it remains one of those unassailable policy fortresses. Below that top line, however, opinions are polarised between Just Say No shock/horror tactics through to giving young people accurate and credible information and letting them make their own judgements. A number of good practice guidelines have been issued by drug charities on how to deliver drug education in schools, but drug education (along with everything else under the banner of personal, social and health education) has never been a compulsory part of the national curriculum, although this is set to change in September 2020.

The situation to date has resulted in a complete ragbag of interventions including a policeman armed with a bag of drugs, with or without the sniffer dog on a leash; ex-users going into schools; theatre projects; US-style drug and peer resistance programmes; and cults offering free drug education. Not free was the Labour government's Blueprint pilot project. Adapted from another US school programme, it was a £5 million flop leaving officials blaming the researchers for faulty methodology.

Many schools have often been wary of delivering drug education lessons at all for fear of gaining a reputation of a school with a drug problem. Parents might be worried about drugs, but few turn up to school-based parental drug awareness sessions for fear of the stigma that might attach itself to the family.

Little or no training was offered to teachers expected to deliver drug education. Teachers often felt they knew nothing about drugs compared to their students, while students thought they knew everything. In any class of 30 young people, you might have every extreme from the child who would never try drugs to the kid who has drug dealers coming to the house supplying mum and dad. It has never been a level playing field of experience.

Drug education and prevention is less a solid fortress, more a bouncy castle; nobody wants to stick a very public knife in it, but at the back the air of funding has been slowly released until it is entirely deflated. Despite the political rhetoric about the virtues of drug education, the Department for Education itself has never really been committed to the subject. It has twice pulled funding for local drug advice for schools, once in the 1990s with Drug Education Coordinators and then again with District Drug Advisors. In 1992, the UK hosted the first European Drug Prevention Week. At the launch event, the chair reserved for the education minister remained empty. Recently the department has funded a school support drug education information service run by the charity Mentor UK. Both the service and the organisation are no more.

The essential problem with drug education in schools is that the bar is set too high – preventing young people from experimenting with drugs and effecting behaviour change in those who have started. No doubt those young people taking part in the activities, such as theatrical role-playing, had a good time and may have got something out of the experience. At a population level, however, there is no evidence that any programme can achieve such ideals with any level of measurable sustainability and so there is no incentive for government to fund programmes. Furthermore, no school heads, governors or PTAs are going to stand for anything other than the bad news about drugs. If they did, the local media would be all over them like a rash and the school intake would likely fall with resulting loss of income.

Intuitively, a better approach is not to isolate drugs as something outside normal experience, but instead incorporate any discussions into other areas concerning alcohol, smoking, relationships and sex, diet and nutrition, body image and bullying. There is evidence that many young people are increasingly suffering from depression and anxiety. This might explain why there is a fashion for tranquilliser drugs such as Xanax, bought through social media, which in turn is causing some of the mental health problems young people are facing, problems which are compounded by the desperate state of child and adolescent mental health services. Whether schools have the time and resources for a more holistic approach to health and well-being remains to be seen.

The National Drugs Helpline set up in the late 1990s morphed into the FRANK campaign launched in 2003. I was contacted by a very young-sounding marketing guy who said they were working on a campaign for government with a view to creating a brand suggesting an older brother or uncle you could confide in. 'We're thinking of calling it Keith. What do you think?' 'Err... do you know who the drug czar is?' 'No'. I sat in rooms with Bright Young Things who truly believed nobody had ever thought of engaging footballers and pop stars in anti-drug campaigns until the words 'Hostage' and 'Fortune' were uttered.

The overall campaign comprised a multimedia approach with printed materials, merchandise, billboards, print and broadcast advertising. In terms of brand recognition, it was a great success. The early TV advertising was promising as it contained humorous elements. I once attended a drugs conference where the keynote speaker began with, 'I usually start a speech with a joke, but there is nothing funny about drugs', which left me thinking 'why not?' Anything which is humorous is automatically less threatening, which in turn can allow more sensible and credible public health messages to be conveyed.

Unfortunately, government TV ads soon became silly and patronising: the Brain Warehouse where you swapped your cannabis-damaged brain for another one; a David Attenborough spoof where young people were viewed through a window at a house party as if they were some sort of wildlife. Then there was Pablo the dead dog – a head-in-hands moment. Why was it all so daft? Because whatever was proposed had to be signed off by ministers and they needed political cover. The English anti-cocaine campaign starring the doomed canine was put on hold for a while because the evaluation of the Scottish equivalent revealed that 12 per cent of respondents said they were more likely to try cocaine as a result of the campaign. Over time, FRANK gained increasing popularity with parents in proportion to declining interest from young people, but still provides signposts for treatment.

In 2012, John Strang and colleagues published an article in *The Lancet* summarising the effectiveness of a range of drug policies. They analysed many of the education and prevention interventions at both the classroom and community level and for the majority there was no evidence of effectiveness in preventing or delaying initiation into drug use either in the short or medium term.[4] For a comment piece in the *British Medical Journal*, Keith Humphreys and Peter Piot outlined the reasons why scientific evidence is only one arbiter of drug policy. Even so, they stated that where evidence is lacking, the net result 'can also lead to a massive waste of public resources (such as the billions of pounds spent worldwide on ineffective youth-oriented programmes to prevent drug use)'.[5]

Between a Cop and a Hard Place

There is an expectation among the public, politicians and the media that the enforcement agencies will do their utmost to act against drug traffickers, although it is unlikely these days that this expectation (albeit untested) extends fully to people carrying small amounts of drugs for personal use. Taking into account action by police, customs, border force (covering all the expense of often lengthy investigations and all the work required following an arrest) plus probation, courts and the prison service, enforcing the drug laws sucks up the lion's share of the budget to deliver the drug strategy. Yet evidence of effectiveness remains elusive.

The Birt Report concluded enforcement had no impact on the flow of heroin into the UK, although of course, the same charge could be levelled at most enforcement action against illegal goods and activities targeting the UK such as human trafficking. The unpublished government 'Drugs value for money' review (2007) said there was no way of even calculating if enforcement activity was value for money. The authors of the 2008 UKDPC report on UK drug markets could not find 'any comprehensive published UK evidence of the relative effectiveness of different law enforcement approaches'.[6] Certainly throwing more money at the problem was no guarantee of results. For their Home Office report on the economic aspects of the illicit drugs market, Wagstaff and Maynard quoted US research which concluded that, 'even large increases in expenditure on law enforcement, at any level of the market, would leave US cocaine and marijuana consumption relatively unchanged'.[7]

Politicians have been equally disappointed; during the 2003 *Druglink* interview, David Blunkett said that for all the heroin seized there was no dent in supply, while in 2009, the Home Affairs Select Committee report on the Serious and Organised Crime Agency expressed concern that only £1 was seized for every £15 in its budget.[8]

Police interventions such as Operation Welwyn which ran in the Kings Cross area of London in the early 1990s can reduce the problems associated with drug markets in certain areas, although there is always the risk of a 'balloon' effect – squeeze the air out of one area and you shift the problem somewhere else. In 2003, Avon and Somerset police successfully ended the Bristol turf war between Jamaican dealers and the local 'Aggi' gang, but the drug market remained intact creating an atmosphere of fear and intimidation which hung around the St Paul's area centred on the Black and White Café. Police at the time admitted they saw little hope of improvement despite hundreds of arrests.[9]

The number of times drugs are seized is not the only barometer for success; in fact, it is a highly unreliable measure of criminal activity let alone general drug prevalence. If the figures go up, does this mean better intelligence or more drugs coming into the country? If they go down, does this mean less drug use, more devious smuggling, or more enforcement success stopping drugs reaching UK borders, or what?

Usually front-line activity is more a measure of enforcement priorities often driven by local or national political pressure such as dealing with drug dealing hotspots, closing down crack houses or targeting cannabis farms. Apart from the number of times drugs have been seized and the number of arrests, other indicators of success might be street drug prices, drug purity or availability on the streets. Here again though, there is no evidence that enforcement has any sustainable impact.[10] So why has the effort to stem the flow of drugs into the UK proved so difficult?

One problem has been the 'pushme-pullyou' of political intervention in enforcement activities. Each incoming Home Secretary, especially following a change of government, promises that there will be 'no hiding place for drug dealers' as crackdown efforts will be increased. Political expectations can be followed by a reorganisation of those agencies involved in drug law enforcement, a process which can also be the result of internal power struggles. Over time, one lead agency has followed another; the Central Drug Intelligence Unit, the National Drugs Intelligence Unit, the National Crime Squad, the National Drug Intelligence Service (NCIS), the Serious Organised Crime Agency (itself an amalgamation of NCIS and parts of Customs & Excise) and now the National Crime Agency. Certainly since 9/11, the emphasis on drugs work has diminished. Officers I spoke to thought this was a big mistake; crime gangs have diversified into many other activities apart from drugs, such as human trafficking and cybercrime. But as one officer told me, 'The money from drugs underwrites all the other stuff.' Officers also became frustrated that every time a new agency was established, they began with new administrative and IT systems, different working practices and the merging of cultures with different priorities or approaches demanded from senior management. When SOCA was established, there was disbelief among some customs officers that it was headed up by Sir Stephen Lander, former head of MI5 signalling the entrance of a new player on the drug enforcement pitch, looking for a new role following the end of both the Cold War and IRA hostilities. One former customs officer thought that branding SOCA an 'intelligence-led agency' was ridiculous: 'What else could it possibly be?' he asked.

The agencies are very hierarchical, following strict chains of command leading to top-heavy bureaucracy and rigidity when faced with new challenges. Moreover, to bring successful prosecutions, enforcement agencies must have all their ducks in row; a single investigation can take months and needs to follow all the legal processes and procedures of intelligence gathering, operational execution and follow-up. Even when the intelligence is sound, the sophistication of concealments can soak up substantial time and effort. Former Assistant Chief Investigations Customs Officer Jim Fitzpatrick told me this story:

The case in point occurred in 1991/2 when most of the bulk heroin imported into the UK was controlled by Turkish criminal groups. A large two-step trailer (that's two trailers, one being a swan-neck) was targeted and searched. Around 100 kilos of heroin were found after an in-depth search, [lasting several days] welded into the chassis of the trailer. Some four months later, the trailers were searched again as part of a training exercise and after some considerable time a further 50 plus kilos was discovered split between the two trailers.

At the time these lorries and trailers were favoured for smuggling large quantities of heroin. Most concealments were very sophisticated often with the trailers built around the concealment pockets. Some even used reverse screw bolts to make it difficult to access areas; they would shear off when trying to undo them. Access was only possible using welding torches.

When it came to container ships used especially by cocaine traffickers from South America, unless the intelligence was most precise, it was almost impossible to find concealments. You could have an army of rummagers on such a vessel for weeks and not find half of it. It's like searching the Empire State Building or for a needle in a haystack.

At an ACPO conference concerning cannabis farms, during the breaks I heard that by and large all the police could do was 'tip and skip'. In other words, they would bust a 'farm' and assuming there was nobody there, would tear the place apart and dump everything into a skip. They said they didn't have the resources to mount an intelligence operation to see if there was any link to a farm they'd found on the other side of town. There was a presentation, though, in which police in the West Midlands did the sort of mobile phone mast triangulation exercise seen in *The Wire* and linked several farms to one individual.

Translate serious resource limitations to day-to-day community policing and it is no wonder that serving Chief Constables and Police and Crime Commissioners are saying publicly they do not have the capacity to go chasing after people carrying small amounts of drugs or even very low level street dealers, many of whom, the police acknowledge, are users who the police are keen to steer into treatment.

Some go further. Richard Brunstrom, when he was Chief Constable of North Wales, and more recently Mike Barton, Chief Constable of Durham, made their views known about the need for law change. The former Chief Constable of Cambridgeshire Tom Lloyd is now an active reform campaigner.

But what do officers in the front line think about the value of the work they do when it comes to managing local drug markets? Little information finds its way into the public domain about the detail of drug enforcement beyond media reports of big hauls at ports of entry and the high-energy depictions in film and TV. The reality is far more mundane, certainly at street level. You can get a sense of what is going on here through the many 'police interceptor' reality TV shows, with the obvious health warning that 'reality' is always compromised by the presence of cameras.

In an idle moment, I tuned in to one such programme just as a patrol car was into hour five of sitting by the roadside unable to respond to any other calls based on intelligence that a local drug 'kingpin' would drive by. Eventually a scruffy VW is spotted and the chase is on. Well, not really a chase; as soon as the blues and twos light up, the guy pulls over. The car is searched but nothing found. The car is impounded and taken to bits until the team triumphantly unearth a couple of bags of cannabis and cocaine stuffed inside two Kinder eggs. Hardly Pablo Escobar but the apocalyptic voice-over trumpets another victory in the war against drugs. Except the local 'kingpin' is back on the streets in short order. At least for the benefit of the cameras, the police seemed to think it was another job well done although assessing the cost of that one incident could be revealing.

If the police are understandably reticent about discussing day-to-day operations, not much has emerged from the academic world either, probably because of access issues. The first study of British drug operations was *Police, Drugs and Community* by the late Mike Collison, a criminology lecturer at Keele University. In 1990, Collison embedded himself for a year with a drug squad in a northern non-metropolitan town.

In 2016, criminologist Matthew Bacon from Sheffield University published *Taking Care of Business: Police Detectives, Drug Law Enforcement and Proactive Investigation*. Between April 2008 and May 2010, Bacon spent a total of 96 days with two specialist teams of drug enforcement detectives in two Basic Command Units, one in the north of England and the other in the south. Bacon takes us on a trip through the world of the drug detectives, some of whom aspire to that 'outlaw' image of tackling the bad guys and how they can feel constrained (or not) by modern policing imperatives where drugs work is invariably intelligence-led, and dominated by the processes and procedures of managerialism and the restrictions imposed by organisational priorities. In his concluding remarks, Bacon states:

> While detectives rarely questioned the authority of the law, believing they were making a positive difference and remained motivated by operational successes on a case-by-case basis, their efforts were accompanied by a sense of futility and doubt. Many officers had a cynical outlook, they were defeatist, pessimistic about the future of policing drugs... [However] the majority of police officers remained faithful supporters of the status quo and resistant to change. Prohibition was viewed as the only morally legitimate and feasible policy option... Arguments for reform ... were generally viewed with scepticism or given zero weight ... the detectives were particularly dismissive of claims that enforcement was a waste of resources and exacerbated drug problems.[11]

However, he goes on to say that a 'significant minority' were very much of a different view and if Bacon had interviewed him, Neil Woods would have been right at the heart of that group.

In his study from the early 1990s, Mike Collison noted that drug enforcement undercover work was very restricted: it was viewed as almost impossible to manage and could lead officers into situations where they could be corrupted or even become users themselves to maintain cover. Former Detective Sergeant Neil Woods puts graphic flesh on Collison's observation in his autobiography *Good Cop, Bad War.*

When he joined the police in 1989, Woods found he had a knack for interviewing suspects and getting them to talk, a talent recognised by superiors who in 1993 asked him to go undercover posing as a street heroin user. So began a career lasting until 2007 developing his technique in various locations, primarily in some of the grimmer, poverty-stricken outposts of the north west, Black Country and the Midlands. Woods says he was proud of the murderous thugs he helped put away, but this was undermined by the disappointment, disillusionment and disgust that seemed to dog his tracks. While he has praise for some of his colleagues, he displays growing contempt for other individuals and the culture itself; inter-squad rivalries, short-sighted obsessions with buy/bust numbers; examples of blatant corruption and managerial failings which in some instances, he says, put his life at risk.

Woods increasingly saw the drugs war as an arms race; the more undercover operations took place, the more clued-up the gangs became and the people who suffered most were the very vulnerable street users (some of whom Woods befriended) who became human shields, commanded to do the street deals under threat of extreme violence. For Woods, this reached the nadir when he was posted to an operation in Brighton which had the dubious honour of being the heroin overdose capital of England. Although no cases were ever followed through, Woods was led to believe that rather than shoot a heroin user for messing up, they would be given a hot shot (an intentionally lethal dose of the drug). Heroin users lived in fear that their next hit would be their last. In the view of some of his colleagues it was a case of 'who cares about another dead junkie?' In the end, Woods resigned and now campaigns for drug law reform.

Looking at the issue from custom officers' perspective, they rarely see the fallout on the streets as they mainly deal with the higher end of the trade. Peter Walsh interviewed many former customs officers for his book *Drug War: The Secret History*. He was quite surprised to find the overwhelming majority still supported prohibition even though they knew it was a war they could never win. At least, they thought, they could do what they could to limit supplies. Just how difficult a job that is is shown by the nature of a drug market so very different from the structures within which the enforcement agencies operate.

There was an old model promoted by criminologists that viewed drug markets as a distinct pyramid structure – a group of Mr Big high-end importers with international connections at the top, under which operated a group of middle-markets dealers who in turn sold to dealers on the street. Enforcement press releases can give the impression of *Soprano*-style organised crime groups with a similar internal pyramid structure. Rank and file specialist officers are less convinced even though in the early stages of a negotiated drug deal there is usually one person or persons taking charge – planning, financing, capable and willing to exploit links to foreign counterparts.

Some crime 'families' with ethnic links outside the UK still exist, but even UK 'kingpins' such as Curtis Warren are rarely seen nowadays. The main reason is that the much larger group inhabiting the middle market, between importers and street dealers, are now making overseas links of their own. We are in a world of disorganised crime these days, but 'twas ever thus – in the late 1980s and early 1990s, when John Grieve was a Detective Superintendent in the Met drug squad, he was calling so-called organised crime 'a threadbare patchwork quilt of alliances and hatred'. He pointed out that the link between a Liverpool dealer and a Colombian cartel boss could be 'four handshakes'. The doyen of drug policy analysis, Peter Reuter, was writing about 'disorganised crime' back in the early 1980s.

For a long time, the police could not work out how cannabis under the control of Vietnamese gangs was finding its way to buyers as nobody was seen buying directly from growers. Before white British gangs became involved, the answer was (and still is to some extent) middlemen who could speak both Vietnamese and English bridging the gap between farm and street. At the 2009 annual meeting of ACPO, I asked a question at the end of a presentation about tackling dealing from the street level and up the chain. The presenter said there was much that was unknown about the drug market. 'What don't the police understand?' I asked. There was an embarrassed silence on the platform until one officer in the audience muttered, 'How long have you got?'

Any seemingly legitimate high street business could be a front to launder drug money; a takeaway, hair salon, nail bar or restaurant. The heroin and crack markets are in the hands of criminals, but when it comes to cannabis, the supply chain is more democratic. As we know from the tragic deaths of Vietnamese citizens in 2019 who died in the back of a lorry, commercial cannabis farms are often staffed by individuals trafficked from that country by gangsters. But anybody from a university student trying to earn living expenses to a tradesman making a bit on the side growing their own or renting an attic or basement to a grower can be involved in the trade. In their book about the UK drug trade, *Narcomania*, Max Daly and Steve Sampson mention a milkman who delivered cannabis with the gold top to his elderly customers to ease their aches and pains.

Variations on long-standing distribution networks have come into play. Looking to expand markets and move out of the big cities which were becoming increasingly violent, gangs were turning up in smaller cities and towns to sell to local dealers and then return home. They called it 'going country'. As business was brisk with less chance of turf wars, the gangs decided to stay and take over the local dealing network basing themselves in the flat of a user or other vulnerable person. This became known as 'county lines' with a new twist. By either bribing or threatening young people, the dealers could distance themselves from the product, sending teenagers far from home to conduct business. A teenager just riding around on their bike was less likely to get caught and if they did, so what?

Police and customs still make large hauls; many of the key players do get caught to serve long sentences or at least spend a lifetime looking over their shoulder expecting a rival (or even 'trusted' gang member) to turn up one day with a gun. Few get to live out their lives to enjoy the proceeds of crime.

Yet because the web of dealing is now so complex and impossible to unravel, the trade has woven itself into the warp and weft of everyday life in the UK even if largely hidden from public view. Globalisation, cheap air travel and our 24/7 leisure economy (the UK's fifth-biggest industry, accounting for at least 8 per cent of the UK's employment and annual revenues of £66bn)[12] have all played a significant role in expanding the opportunities at all levels of the trade from field to street. Arguably though, the real drug supply game changer of the past decade has been the internet – the war on drugs has moved into cyberspace.

The World Wired Web

Throughout our story, there have been moments or tipping points that propelled non-medical drug use into new and often more dangerous areas, sometimes as an unwitting consequence of medical progress: the isolation of morphine and cocaine from the plant base, the development of the hypodermic syringe, and the creation of synthetic mood-altering pharmaceutical drugs, but also the adaptations of existing drugs such as heroin and cocaine to smokable forms. Each has signalled a new era in the history of psychoactive drug use. The latest innovations fall into two categories. The first are what have become known as 'legal highs'. They were originally tagged as 'designer drugs' as they were and remain designed to mimic the effects of prohibited drugs, but through a tweak of molecules, they sit outside the law: to bring a prosecution, the charge has to be substance-specific. You cannot be charged with possession of a drug 'related to MDMA' for example. However, the rapid pace of product development, distribution and consumption of these new (and existing) drugs would have been severely hampered without the precursors to a truly global drug network – the internet and the world wide web.

The first legal highs were plant-based drugs such as salvia, yohimbe, kava kava, morning glory seeds and plants branded as 'herbal ecstasy' often of unknown derivation, but possibly ephedra, the plant root of the stimulant ephedrine. They were mainly advertised in drug subculture magazines, the very early online bulletin boards and chatrooms, and sold in head shops like Dr Herman's in Manchester under names such as Love Doves, Druid's Dream and Mind Bandits. And then…

There is an oft-quoted adage that if you arrest a murderer, that's one less murderer; if you arrest a drug dealer, you create a job opportunity. That may sound facetious but it carries with it the substance of truth. Taking out a drug dealer or gang (unlike a killer), still leaves the business you are trying to disrupt intact, allowing new players into the fray. Projected globally, the end of the French Connection presented new opportunities for heroin production in Colombia and Mexico with much-reduced costs of getting the drug into the USA. The break-up of the Medellin and Cali cartels saw a proliferation of smaller operators, soaring production rates and the movement of cocaine into new and expanding European markets.

In the late 1990s, there was a heroin drought in Australia and New Zealand caused in large part by a government drive to end opium production in northern Thailand. Unfortunately, drug traffickers abhor a vacuum every bit as much as nature, and into that drug vacuum came laboratories equipped to manufacture methamphetamine initially utilising the skills of chemists from eastern Europe and Taiwan. Methamphetamine, both in its smokable form, known as yabba, and injectable crystal meth, swept across the Pacific rim region and into Australia and New Zealand.

New Zealand musician and 'psychonaut' Matt Bowden, after the death of a cousin from an ecstasy overdose and because ecstasy was expensive for a drug-using community well away from the main global drug-trading routes, asked underground chemist associates to find a stimulant drug that could be promoted as safer and cheaper than either ecstasy or methamphetamine. They came up with benzylpiperazine or BZP, which had been developed but never marketed in the 1950s as an animal worming tablet. BZP re-emerged in clinical trials as a possible new antidepressant, but research stopped when amphetamine-like effects were noted. Bowden began selling BZP locally through the internet but was soon overwhelmed by orders from all over the world because the problem of making online micro-payments was solved by the launch of Paypal in 2001.

The spread of still-legal BZP started a gold rush of underground pharmaceutical activity to develop new generations of drugs – 'research chemicals' not controlled under national or international drug laws, creating a new version of 'whack-a-mole' – control one chemical and a near relative legal derivative appears almost immediately.

Writing about the future of designer drugs in the *Journal of Forensic Science* as long ago as March 1988, associate professor at the University of

California School of Medicine Gary Henderson predicted that, 'In the view of this author, it is likely that the future drugs of abuse will be synthetics rather than plant products. They will be synthesized from readily available chemicals, may be derivatives of pharmaceuticals, will be very potent, and often very selective in their action. In addition, they will be marketed very cleverly.'[13] How right he was.

Rapidly expanding global communications revolutionised the legal high drug scene. Chatrooms and bulletin boards allowed for information exchange about drug effects and sources of supply. Research chemicals aptly described the new chemical landscape; individuals willing to try out untested drugs and then report online what happened. Underground chemists scoured the web looking for drug patents lodged by companies but never brought to market.

Pharmacologist Professor David Nichols spent years working on psychoactive compounds and as long ago as 2001, he noticed that amateur chemists were watching his papers online. He synthesised a version of MDMA called MTA, which he thought might be helpful in the development of treatments for depression. It was clear to anybody who knew what they were doing that this drug had the potential to release dangerous levels of serotonin. Too much of the chemical causes symptoms that can range from mild, resulting in shivering and diarrhoea, to severe, as in muscle rigidity, fever and seizures. Severe serotonin syndrome can be fatal if not treated. MTA tablets, appropriately enough called 'flatliners', hit the streets with some UK deaths recorded in the early 2000s.[14]

Using encrypted e-mails, wholesalers bought finished products or the base chemicals from thousands of Chinese manufacturing outlets. Finally, consumers could simply go online and buy whatever they wanted using a credit card. The enforcement agencies got wise to this practice; in 2004, Operation Ismene (UK) and Operation Web Tryp (USA) ended with the credit card details and transactions being seized and the arrest of dozens of people who had bought already controlled drugs.[15] Yet a nascent Dark Web allowed the web-savvy drug customer to buy illegal drugs, a process made easier by the invention of Bitcoin in 2009. Police, customs and state security personnel around the world use sophisticated surveillance and tracking equipment to close both the drug sites and the Dark Web portals such as DeepDotWeb as they appear, but there are no signs yet of the authorities getting ahead of the game. Two drugs in particular impacted on the UK drug scene: mephedrone and the catchily titled synthetic cannabinoid receptor agonists, SCRAs but generally known simply as spice.

Feline Frenzy

The primary precursor chemical for manufacturing ecstasy is safrole made from sassafras, a plant found in East Asia. In June 2008, authorities in Cambodia seized 33 tons of safrole, enough to manufacture an estimated 245 million pills. The haul caused an ecstasy drought across Europe.

Lacking access to safrole, which was in any case a controlled precursor chemical, underground chemists turned to a legal variant, anethole. The result was PMA, another drug in the MDMA family but like MTA, more dangerous because while the drug was more toxic, the chemical was released more slowly in the body which led some users to increase the dose. Sold as ecstasy, the pills caused a cluster of UK deaths in 2013.

Following the safrole haul, ecstasy became much harder to obtain in the UK; the drugs still being produced not containing PMA were of very poor quality. Purity levels of cocaine too, hit an all-time low, down to 2 per cent in some places.[16] The government had also announced the planned banning of BZP, so stimulant users were looking for an alternative.

Cathinones are a group of synthetic stimulant drugs related to amphetamines whose plant root is khat, grown in parts of Africa and the Middle East. The primary drug in this group is mephedrone, which appeared in Israel in 2004 under the name 'hagigat' (party) and put several people in hospital; it was banned in 2008. Following deaths in Denmark and Sweden, the drug was banned there too. In the UK, the parent drug cathinone was a Class C drug under the Misuse of Drugs Act, but not derivatives such as mephedrone. Early adopters were buying the drug online from about 2007, but when the quality of stimulant drugs plummeted, interest in mephedrone soared, packing an amphetamine/MDMA punch yet entirely legal. Mephedrone, M-CAT or (through the alleged invention of a *Sun* reporter), 'meow, meow', attracted many of those who would never have dreamt of using let alone dealing illegal drugs.

Through 2009 and into 2010, M-CAT created a media firestorm but the lack of the predicted body-count left journalists clutching at straws. A ludicrous story alleged that a whole classroom of girls had been sent home, ill from the effects of mephedrone. The death of 14-year-old Gabriella Price turned out to be due to natural causes, while a bout of feline frenzy gripped the media involving the tragic deaths of two teenagers in Scunthorpe until the coroner revealed that the deaths had been caused by a combination of alcohol and methadone, information which did not make the front pages. Official statistics implicated only a handful of deaths, but they were all of people who had taken other drugs in combination, with the exception of one individual who died after repeated mephedrone injecting.[17]

The mephedrone story was a good example of 'damned if you do, damned if you don't'. The government was criticised for taking months to ban the drug and when it did, to get the ban through ahead of the 2010 General Election, criticised for a 'knee-jerk reaction'. The consequences of the ban reverberated over the next five years with the ACMD and Home Office legislators playing catch-up with the chemists, who kept pumping out new cathinones every time one was controlled.

MDMA was re-established, but now containing escalating doses with some pills containing upwards of 200mg, double or more of what would be regarded as a 'normal' dose. Without any supporting evidence, the best guess would be that the arrival of 'super strength' ecstasy was prompted by MDMA producers trying to wrest back the market from the new generation of stimulant drugs after the drought. This resulted in a potentially lethal game of who can produce the strongest drug, which has seen a rise in MDMA deaths from only 8 in 2010 to 92 in 2018 (including those related to PMA), the highest on record. The cathinone variants were mainly favoured by those on the festival and club scene; very different from those attracted to spice.

Not the Spice of Life

Beginning in 1984, John William Huffman, an American professor of organic chemistry, with his team synthesised the first of more than 400 synthetic cannabinoid receptor agonists (SCRAs) to examine the role of a new generation of drugs that might target the brain's natural cannabinoid receptors to aid medical research into HIV/AIDS, chemotherapy and multiple sclerosis. For a drug to work in the brain it must lock into brain receptors the way keys fit into locks. Natural cannabis fits like a loose key in the lock of the relevant cannabinoid CB1 and CB2 receptors giving a more mellow experience, at least at moderate levels of THC. The effect of these new substances was more like somebody kicking the door in. Huffman's research stalled because of the problem of separating out the desired medical effects such as pain relief from the unwanted psychoactive effects.

SCRAs first appeared in Germany in the late 2000s, marketed as K2 and Spice (also the name of a strong strain of cannabis). When asked about the fate of his invention, Huffman said, 'I figured once it got started in Germany it was going to spread. I'm concerned that it could hurt people. I think this was something that was more or less inevitable. It bothers me that people are so stupid as to use this stuff.'[18] The chemicals were usually sourced from China, sprayed onto plant material (usually herbs) and sold online and into UK head shops tagged with names clearly signalling what the user could expect: Annihilation, Psyclone, Kronic, Black Mamba and Exodus Damnation, to name just a few. The websites and shops displayed SCRAs in shiny, coloured packets, marketed to attract, just as Gary Henderson predicted.

SCRAs rapidly proliferated; the European Monitoring Centre for Drugs and Drugs Addiction identified seven main groups including one carrying Dr Huffman's initials, JWH, but with an endless array of variants under each group. Tests proved that substances in identical packets could contain different spice compounds. In truth, the precise nature of the compound hardly seemed to matter: they all produced dramatic physical symptoms including racing heart and difficulty breathing accompanied by mental conditions from catatonic states to violence and self-harming.

SCRAs were never party drugs; from the start the main customers were street heroin and crack users. Back in 2016, the BBC launched a series called *Drugs Map of Britain*. Episode one featured a street heroin user trying to come off spice, a drug which he said 'knocks the bollocks off heroin'. Spice caused (and continues to cause) serious problems for street drug users, prison inmates and therefore staff in prisons. From 2015 onwards, the prisons inspectorate expressed growing concerns over the use of spice in prisons and in 2017 devoted a whole report to the issue. Methods of getting spice into prisons range from drones to impregnated legal letters (often fake) to inmates, which staff are not allowed to inspect. Ambulance services from around the country reported a constant stream of calls to take homeless people and inmates to hospital. Some services reportedly had a 'mambulance', as dubbed by inmates at one prison, on standby.

Two generations of SCRAs were controlled under the Misuse of Drugs Act in 2009 and 2012, but like the cathinones, the legislation could not keep up with the proliferation of legal highs. Attempts were made to prosecute sellers under trading standards, consumer and anti-solvents legislation, leading to vendor claims that the pre-ban mephedrone they were selling was plant food. There were some instances of police simply pressuring sellers to clear their shelves. Legal highs could be bought in a range of retail outlets including garages, corner shops, pet shops, takeaways and mobile food vans.

Temporary Control Orders were introduced under the Misuse of Drugs Act enabling substances to be banned while the ACMD considered the evidence of harm. All this was however too slow a process for government; politically there was no way the government was going to continue allowing high street sales of drugs with effects like MDMA, amphetamine, ketamine and the nuclear end of cannabis. So in 2014, the Home Office established an expert group which while it contained ACMD members (and others like myself) primarily comprised criminal justice and forensic science personnel with the express brief to find the most effective way of legislating against the totality of what were officially known as novel psychoactive substances (NPS).

There were four legislative options on the table. The first was generic legislation in which a compound is banned with any chemically similar compound – essentially how the Misuse of Drugs Act operates. Secondly, American-style analogue legislation in which a compound is banned with any other compound that has similar effects, irrespective of its pharmacology. There was the option of a blanket ban as existed in Ireland and Poland whereby all products would be banned now and in the future. The most radical option was a proposal from New Zealand to have a regulated market whereby the onus would be on the manufacturer to demonstrate, following payment of an expensive licence, that a product posed minimal risk before it was allowed to be sold. In the end, there were no licence applications and the whole plan dropped because of protests from New Zealand animal rights groups opposed to product testing on animals. There was an amusing episode though when the UK drugs minister Liberal Democrat Norman Baker (always the more enthusiastic of the main parties for drug law reform) told the press he was not ruling out any course of action including introducing legislation to allow for a legal market. Cue hurried rebuttals from the Home Office.

In truth, government was opting for a blanket ban already in force in Ireland. The legal market was obviously a political non-starter; the generic approach was already failing in the UK to deal with NPS while it was felt the US-style analogue option would result in a field day for lawyers arguing over whether Drug A had the same effects as Drug B. The Psychoactive Substances Act (PSA) was introduced in 2016 covering any substance which delivered a psychoactive effect, excluding alcohol, tobacco, food and medicines.

There was no possession offence, unless on prison estate premises (covering inmates, staff and visitors), but a significant debate (both inside the panel meetings and subsequently) as to the definition of psychoactive. There can be no objective 'external' test based as it is on the subjective experience of the individual; however, the expected plethora of legal arguments did not materialise. As originally formulated, the PSA also covered amyl nitrate (poppers) and nitrous oxide. The first is primarily used as a muscle relaxant on the gay scene; the second is 'laughing gas' where the contents of small canisters are released into balloons and inhaled. Eventually, poppers were exempted as any psychoactive effect was secondary to why the drug was used recreationally. Nitrous oxide was not exempted. Despite being a commercial product – the gas used to propel cream from a pressurised can and a medical gas for anaesthesia – the small commercial gas whippets were being used for group hilarity, with some rare deaths, linked in one case to somebody inhaling directly from a large gas cylinder.

Once the Act was announced, many head shops had a sale to clear stocks. Some closed while others moved online. There is an escalating scale of warning sanctions under the PSA which culminates in a court appearance. The majority of prosecutions have been brought against nitrous oxide sellers.

Officials were warned that legislation would not of itself deal with currently available substances; spice is still causing significant problems for the most vulnerable, although use of most other drugs labelled as NPS are not significant. There were also warnings that once spice became a street drug, users would be more at risk in two respects; existing heroin and crack dealers would add spice to the menu and that the drugs themselves would be stronger.

The first concern played out and there were also examples of solo spice dealers offering the product to homeless people simply for whatever money they had in their pocket. The concerns about stronger spice was highlighted by widely distributed smartphone footage of users on the street in a catatonic state, helpfully tagged by the media as 'zombies', hearkening back to the earliest media drug fiend tropes. It is not clear if this state was the result of new strains or had simply gone unrecorded, but the question of SCRA toxicity is complex.

In 1986, Richard Cowan from the National Organisation for the Reform of the Marijuana Laws (NORML) coined the phrase, 'the iron law of prohibition', which states that the tougher the drug laws, the more potent street drugs become. This rule could be applied to cannabis; from outside growing plant, to indoor plant with higher THC content and to SCRAs – from weed to skunk to spice.

In respect of the chemicals themselves, there is a continuing, but now much slower, evolution of the more commonly encountered SCRAs. These are almost all now 'third generation' materials with high potency compared to the original 'first generation' SCRAs, although the process of developing more potent SCRAs was underway before the passing of the PSA. The cost of synthesising the more potent spice materials is similar to less potent variants, but a greater effect is produced from the same amount of product, so more bangs for bucks for both seller and user. Apart from the toxicity of the chemical themselves, there is a question mark over the amount of spice added to the smoking materials. In the pre-control days, when branded and pre-packaged materials were available in retail outlets, there was a small element of quality control in the large-scale commercial production process. Current materials tend to be distributed in small, unlabelled grip-sealed bags, probably put together in small production facilities, where powdered spice is dissolved in solvent and added to herbal material, using simple equipment (kitchen scales, buckets, cement mixers, etc.). In those circumstances, mixing errors and uneven distribution within batches can lead to problems. A spate of users in Greater Manchester suffering catatonic states was traced back to batches of smoking material which contained 10 times more spice than normally encountered.[19]

The PSA was criticised for the very broad definition of psychoactive and the blanket nature of the ban which fails to distinguish the relative harms of different substances.[20] But this was a move less concerned with science and more to do with politics. The boxes that needed to be ticked were duly ticked.

Pills and Ills

We have seen that pharmaceuticals – amphetamine, barbiturates, Diconal and to a lesser extent methaqualone – had a significant role in the diversification of the UK drug scene. During the 1970s, barbiturates were gradually phased out in general practice to be replaced by benzodiazepine tranquillisers, which provided a much higher threshold between therapeutic and lethal overdose. However, the new generation of drugs – most famously Valium – heavily marketed by pharmaceutical companies such as Hoffman La Roche, brought their own problems – dependence and withdrawal symptoms which were life-threatening if not medically managed.

As street drugs, benzodiazepine tranquillisers initially found favour with Scottish drug users because they are a cheap substitute for heroin, which in the early days of the heroin epidemic could be in short supply in some Scottish cities due to the distance from main ports of entry. Once the dealing networks across the UK became established, heroin supply was less of a problem, but tranquillisers remained readily available, both legitimately from doctors as well as from regular patients willing in hard times to sell on part of their prescription. That enabled tranquillisers to become embedded on the Scottish drug scene.

In the 1980s, one drug in the family, Temazepam, was available as a liquid in a green capsule; users in Scotland and elsewhere broke open the capsules and injected the liquid. The company responded by reformulating the liquid into a gel (known as 'jellies') only for users to then melt the gel for injecting. The gel solidified in veins causing gangrene and amputations.

The latter-day generic version of Valium, diazepam, continued to feature significantly on the drug scene. In 2010–2011, the UK experienced a heroin drought caused by poppy blight in Afghanistan, the opening up of a heroin market in Russia, and an enforcement crackdown in Turkey. Another theory suggested that as heroin prices had been falling in the UK, this was an attempt to cause a price hike by stockpiling. In any event, heroin was in short supply and in some places, purity levels dropped to an unprecedented UK low of 13 per cent.[21] The shortage created expanded markets for diazepam, fulfilled by significant importation of the drug from countries in Europe where pharmaceutical regulations were more lax than the UK.

There have been some new developments in benzodiazepine production; the discovery of illicit diazepam laboratories in the UK and the arrival of designer benzodiazepines, the main type being etizolam with currently about a dozen others. Notwithstanding the control of etizolam under the Misuse of Drugs Act in 2017, Wedinos, the Welsh drug testing agency (part of Public Health Wales), had this to say about benzodiazepines in its July–September 2019 newsletter:

> Since the launch of WEDINOS [in 2013] the programme has identified numerous benzodiazepine-type NPS and through previous reports evidenced their growing prevalence amongst samples analysed. Over the past twelve months benzodiazepines as a group have been the most commonly identified substances by WEDINOS, and this quarter continues that trend. Etizolam was not only the most commonly identified benzodiazepine, but also the most commonly identified substance, followed by diazepam. Alprazolam and Fualprazolam also featured amongst the top ten most commonly identified substances.

There have been several reports of young people using Alprazolam marketed as Xanax, purchasing the drug through social media and combining over-the-counter opiate-based cough medicines[22] with soft drinks or fruit to create a concoction known as purple drank or lean. Although there seems to be no direct link to the drug effects and the music scene (unlike MDMA and rave), these sedative-type drugs have been promoted by some American rap artists. Use of Xanax and similar drugs by young people which appear so readily available may be a transitory drug fashion. However, there is much concern these days about the levels of self-harm and suicide among young people. Lack of action here could see more young people self-medicating with these drugs. Mention of opioid-based medicines takes us to a brief consideration of the current trends in the use of opioid painkillers.

All Pain, No Gain

In recent years, the USA and Canada have been overwhelmed by an epidemic of opioid painkiller addiction and overdose deaths, driven primarily by overprescribing and underpinned by aggressive commercial marketing. In brief, there was a time when the fear of addiction among American doctors was so great that they could be called opiophobic, even when it came to relieving terminal cancer pain where the 'threat' of addiction was somewhat irrelevant. Then in January 1980, a letter was published in the influential *New England Journal of Medicine* suggesting that patients who were prescribed morphine in hospital would not become desperate heroin users when they returned home.[23] This encouraged more widespread prescribing for non-cancer pain, but there were two key developments which sparked the current problems. One was the marketing of Oxycontin. The claim was that because the drug was released 'continuously' (rather than a more immediate opiate 'hit') there was far less chance of addiction. The other factor was a re-run of the UK's heroin epidemic of the 1980s; painkiller use soared in white, working-class, mid-west towns that had suffered severe economic decline through industrial closures. Many people turned to painkillers to relieve stress rather than pain – and there were many doctors (often those who had been struck off the medical register) more than happy to swap prescriptions for cash, operating out of so-called 'pill mills'. When people could no longer afford to pay for prescriptions, they turned to much cheaper heroin coming in from Mexico.

In the UK, the highest levels of prescribing have also been in areas of highest social and economic deprivation such as the north-east of England and south Wales. Drug workers in these areas have reported that painkillers have become the new 'mother's little helpers'; 'codeine housewives' are using these drugs to take the edges off rough lives. Like the use of sedative drugs by young people, the lines between 'therapeutic' and 'recreational' drug use can become very blurred, making these distinctions distinctly meaningless. Northern Ireland has seen a problem with a different sort of painkillers – the gabapentins – which deal with nerve pain (and depression) rather than that associated with joint pain. The drugs gabapentin and pregabalin have become street drugs in Northern Ireland and are rife in prisons.

As the UK population ages and the pressures on GP services increase, prescriptions for painkillers (and antidepressants) have risen dramatically.[24] We have little idea about the numbers of people who might be dependent on opioid painkillers, but we do know there is no national network of services dedicated to helping those dependent on painkillers, antidepressants or tranquillisers.

The media likes nothing better than a new drug on the block; I have spent many years killing stories about the impending crystal meth 'epidemic' which thankfully has yet to materialise. Equally there is another drug we could do without which has the potential to be another different kind of global game changer – fentanyl.

Developed in the USA in 1960, fentanyl is a synthetic opioid widely used in anaesthesia and pain management. However, the drug is active in very small microgram doses; the main fentanyl molecule is 100 times stronger than morphine, with a whole range of even more potent analogues culminating in carfentanyl (used to sedate large mammals for surgery), calculated to be a 1,000 times more potent than morphine. Illicitly manufactured fentanyl has found its way into American street heroin with devastating effects. So far, only sporadic examples of the drug have shown up in the UK, but it has the potential to change the nature of the illicit heroin trade.[25] To bring heroin to the UK market requires a business enterprise stretching back 5,000 miles to the poppy fields of Afghanistan with all the costs and risks that entails. Contrast that with shipping in chemicals from overseas to an underground laboratory in the UK or elsewhere in Europe and producing a highly profitable opioid drug, active in minute doses and easy to smuggle. A kilo of fentanyl powder would be enough for 20 million doses. When a kilo of the even more potent carfentanyl was seized in Canada, it was calculated that it was sufficient to kill the entire population.[26]

* * *

When the first UK Dangerous Drugs Act was passed in 1920, the drug scene was limited to a handful of East London opium smokers and the morphine-injecting, cocaine-sniffing habitués of Soho's nightlife. By the end of the Second World War the scene had hardly changed, but from that point onwards the drug scene grew gradually, not as a smooth curve but categorised by step changes in youth culture, global trade, technology and the ability of criminal enterprises to cash in on these developments. Despite the hue and cry of the sixties, drugs only became an enduring political hot potato in the UK in the mid-1980s. As public, political and media interest and concern intensified, so the list of drugs grew into the pick 'n' mix drug culture of today. Of all the drugs to have graduated onto the drug scene since 1945, possibly only raw opium, barbiturates and methaqualone are now absent from the UK scene. LSD hauls actually increased in 2019 along with most other drugs controlled under the Misuse of Drugs Act.

In concert with the rest of the world, the UK drug 'problem' seems impervious to any kind of sustained government intervention. For many, the drug laws themselves are at the heart of our problems; reports from Parliamentary groups, think tanks, medical associations and campaigning groups each demanding a 'new approach' to drugs continue to pile up. To date, those in power are not listening. So, in the words of Vladimir Ilyich Ulyianov – better known as Lenin – what is to be done?

14

2020 Vision?

Apologies to anybody who has jumped to this last chapter hoping for the big reveal on how we tackle the drug problem in the future. At a most basic level, there is Gordian Knot of confusion over terminology and conflicting interpretations of international treaties, national laws and data sets. Even the concept of 'the drug problem' is a castle built on sand.

As Toby Seddon notes in his book *A History of Drugs: Drugs and Freedom in the Liberal Age*, the idea of these entities with a supposed life of their own called 'drugs' was only a product of the creation of the relatively recent regulatory system discussed in the Prologue. A subset of substances were designated as 'dangerous drugs', which in turn provoked a moral or political judgement on those people who used them. The substances themselves – whether cocaine, heroin or ecstasy – are drugs by any scientific or clinical definition and in that respect no different from alcohol, nicotine or caffeine. Other clearly problematic drugs such as opioid painkillers and tranquillisers are otherwise designated as medicines. Therefore, the idea of 'dangerous drugs' as we understand it is nothing more than a legalistic construct.

Popular perceptions of 'the drug problem' relate to the health problems caused by a proscribed set of substances and dealing with the problems caused by criminals trading in these substances. But what about the problems caused by the drug laws themselves? It seems that in many parts of the world there are as many 'intended' consequences as 'unintended' when it comes to State-sponsored violence and discrimination against certain sectors of society. What about the problem caused by global financial institutions turning a blind eye to the torrent of drug money flowing through the world banking systems? Or the problems caused to farmers with little opportunity to feed their families in war-ravaged countries other than by growing coca or poppies only to see their crops sprayed out of existence, or the problems for countries dragged to the brink of narco-statehood? How about the problems for street drug users unable to access primary health care, housing or mental health services? The drug problem is not one political, social or cultural issue. In which case, where do you start? Just a cursory dip into the subject does at least reveal one thing – that the complexities of drug policy go beyond simply (but by no means simple) questions of law reform, although globally the debate over reform increasingly takes centre stage.

Until the early 1990s, the international consensus among UN member states appeared to hold firm that the only way to deal with the non-medical use of drugs was to tackle drug supply through the strictest interpretation of the otherwise vaguely drawn enforcement provisions of the three UN treaties. Despite all the evidence that since the enactment of the Single Convention in 1961, increasing numbers of people had been using a growing array of more powerful drugs in more dangerous ways, the response of the main UN agencies with the drugs brief – the Commission on Narcotic Drugs (CND) and the International Narcotics Control Board (INCB) – has been to simply parrot, 'Come on chaps, we just have to try harder.'

The consensus fault lines appeared along two parallel tracks; there were increasing protests from producer countries like Mexico, Colombia and Bolivia who were getting fed-up with taking the blame for the drug situation, mainly from the USA, when the major western consumer countries were failing miserably to reduce demand. The mantra of the Latin American countries was – and continues to be – 'shared responsibility'. Then there were those countries beginning to push for a more pragmatic and balanced approach to use and possession of drugs, either within the latitude allowed for within the treaties or even outside it. Some members states were particularly unhappy that unlike the 1961 and 1971 Conventions, the 1988 Convention demanded of states that they criminalise possession. The history of the Conventions going back to those very early days before the First World War was all about controlling the international trade between countries. Drug control within countries was supposed to be a matter for domestic legislation.

The Dutch were the first to break ranks; cannabis possession and even low-level street selling had been unofficially tolerated since the passing of the 1976 Opium Act, but in the early 1990s, the government issued the first regulations governing the sale of cannabis in restricted quantities to adults in designated premises called coffeeshops. At a UN meeting in 1996, the Dutch, having concluded as long ago as 1969 that there was no evidence of a gateway effect, defended its approach by arguing that as current strategies were neither realistic nor effective, solutions to the drug problem could only be found through a process of trial and error. While they had disproved the gateway theory, even so they said it was worth trying to keep as much distance as possible between the trade in cannabis and more dangerous drugs by relaxing the laws on cannabis. Despite wild accusations by the Americans and various anti-drug campaigning groups that Dutch youth had gone to hell in a handcart, there was no evidence of a significant increase in cannabis use among young people, who were barred from coffeeshops anyway, let alone a lemming-like hurtle into heroin use. The Dutch said unequivocally they were no longer prosecuting people caught in possession of cannabis for personal use. It has been wrongly asserted that the Dutch formally legalised cannabis. They never did, it was more of an administrative fudge; moreover, the person selling the cannabis to the coffeeshop owner could still be prosecuted for supply, especially if they took one toke over the line by dealing in other drugs.

And café owners were not allowed to use the bank to deposit their profits or secure loans because this would be in breach the 1988 Convention.[1]

From then on. many European countries, supported by Australia and Canada, were challenging the US-dominated international prohibitionist hegemony. Nobody was calling for legalisation, but the cautious language of diplomacy made it clear that the fault lines would not be papered over by, for example, the political declaration of the UN Special Session on Drugs in 1998 which trumpeted, 'A Drug Free World, We Can Do It'. In the wake of the spread of drug-related HIV/AIDS, delegates at UN meetings also began raising the validity of harm-reduction measures such as opioid substitute therapies and needle exchange. This caused another rift with opponents attacking harm reduction both on grounds of condoning drug use and being a stalking horse for legalisation.[2]

Over time, the UN has had to concede ground, as countries around the world have embraced harm reduction with methadone and (in Switzerland) heroin prescribing, needle exchanges, and medically supervised facilities for drug injecting. Yet even today, whatever the views of individual officials, in general, UN agencies appear supportive of the principle and practice of harm reduction but still refuse to allow the phrase 'harm reduction' to appear in official documents as it remains in their view encumbered with unwelcome political baggage.

In 1995 the WHO sparked American outrage with the previously mentioned cocaine report, published in March, which stated there was no evidence that occasional cocaine use was that harmful, and a further draft report on cannabis later the same year, which concluded the drug was less harmful than tobacco or alcohol. That section of the report was deleted prior to publication in 1997, the two-year delay indicative of the struggle behind the scenes.[3]

More UN shenanigans took place in 2000, when the Director of the UN Drug Control Programme, Pino Arlacchi, heavily censored the UN's second *World Drug Report 2000*. The first report had a section on the growing debate over regulation. Not only was that section now removed, but the whole report was skewed towards a more favourable picture of the world drug scene, no doubt to keep the Americans, who provided most of the programme's funding, on side. The report coordinator Francisco Thoumi resigned in protest.

> Arlacchi was very concerned because the original draft did not reflect his vision of the world drug situation. In particular, he argued that it was too pessimistic and that it failed to show the great advances in the fight on drugs that had taken place recently. He frequently argued that the world drug problem was on the verge of being solved and that there were only three countries that were real problems: Colombia, Afghanistan and Myanmar.[4]

Quite a few other staff members were forced to leave or resigned over differences with Arlacchi. There was a purge – not to say a witch-hunt – to cleanse the UN drug control system of suspected 'defeatist' elements that might further disrupt the 'spirit of togetherness'.[5]

UN drug reports should be treated with some scepticism because they are primarily political documents aimed at the major donor countries. Depending on the funding imperatives at the time, the report might paint either a pessimistic or optimistic picture. For example, there have been long-standing discrepancies between UN figures for hectares of poppy and coca crops under cultivation compared to those of other agencies such as the DEA because of differences in the way yields are monitored and calculated.

While forced to acknowledge the health benefits of harm reduction, the UN agencies are also now forced to wake up to the fact that several member states are engaged in what drug policy analyst Professor David Bewley-Taylor calls 'soft defection' away from the provisions of the treaties as they apply to minor drug offences. In response UN officials are taking every opportunity to point out that there is nothing in the treaties demanding member states imprison people for minor drug offences.[6] However, one official from the United Nations Office On Drugs and Crime (UNODC) took a step too far for the bosses by using the D word – decriminalisation.

In October 2015, news outlets reported on a leaked briefing paper from the UNODC, which outlined how the decriminalisation of drug use for personal use was a key element of the HIV response. Written by Dr Monica Beg, chief of the HIV/AIDS section of the UNODC, she argued that 'arrest and incarceration are disproportionate measures'. The agency-headed notepaper document stated that it 'clarifies the position of UNODC to inform country responses to promote a health and human-rights approach to drug policy... Treating drug use for non-medical purposes and possession for personal consumption as criminal offences has contributed to public health problems and induced negative consequences for safety, security, and human rights'. It was prepared for an international harm reduction conference in Malaysia, but according to the UNODC was never sanctioned by the organisation as policy. One senior figure within the agency described Dr Beg as 'a middle-ranking official' who was offering a professional viewpoint.[7]

Lining up at an international level to further challenge the UN is the Global Commission on Drug Policy. Established in 2011, it boasts in its ranks 14 former heads of state and other prominent leaders from the political, economic and cultural arenas who advocate for drug policies based on scientific evidence, human rights, public health and safety. One of its leading lights was the late Kofi Annan, the former UN Secretary General. Back in 1998, he had a very different take on world drug issues. He gave this toast at the UN 20th General Assembly Special Session on drugs where 'A Drug Free World, We Can Do It' was declared: 'Allow me to raise my glass in the hope that when we look back upon this meeting, we will remember it as a time when the test of our will became the testimony of our commitment. The time when we pledged to work together towards a family of nations free of drugs in the twenty-first century.' And closing the summit he highlighted the sense of a 'growing convergence of views' and a 'spirit of togetherness', hoping that the session would 'go down in history as a truly watershed event'.[8] Annan's change of heart spoke to the not unknown phenomenon of political support for prohibition while in public office and a very different view when out of the media spotlight.

Nowadays, several countries from all parts of the world are trying to rebalance their internal drug policies away from criminal sanctions for personal use, possession and (in some cases) cultivation of cannabis, or personal use of all drugs in accordance with variances in permitted threshold amounts which differ from country to country. Either lesser criminal sanctions are imposed, or civil sanctions such as fines or referral to treatment, for those identified with drug problems. From the policies of around 30 countries listed in the Release 2016 report 'A Quiet Revolution: Drug Decriminalisation Across the Globe', there is no agreed definition of 'decriminalisation', and in some cases, countries (not included in this report) say they have decriminalised use, but instead imposed draconian regimes of forced treatment. In others (like Russia), the threshold amounts for personal possession are so low as to be meaningless. Moreover, Russian drug users regularly face extortion and violence at the hands of police.

At a UN drug meeting in 1995, the Uruguayan delegate warned about the dangers of allowing dissent to be expressed at all about drug reforms: 'We have deep concern at the voices raised for liberalising drug consumption... The UN from its high position must be clear. Any doubt, hesitation, or unjustified review of the validity of goals will only undermine our commitment... Our goals are noble and inflexible. We cannot be successful if there are discordant voices. We cannot retreat, we must be steadfast in our goals.'⁹ Fast forward to 2013 and Uruguay became the first country in the world to legalise cannabis.

Describing events in Uruguay as a policy case study for the journal *Addiction*, Rosario Queirolo and colleagues observed 'Uruguay had neither strong social movements pushing for marijuana legalisation nor a majority of the population supporting legalization ... was made possible by the concurrence of specific events and political characteristics that ultimately connected marijuana legalization to public safety.'¹⁰ In fact, a 2012 public poll showed 66 per cent of the country was against law change. What happened can be explained by Professor John Kingdon of the University of Michigan in his classic work on political science, *Agendas, Alternatives and Public Policies*. His book says that for an issue to get on the political agenda, three streams need to meet: the problem, the solution and the political will. Effectively, if there is no solution to a problem, it would be impossible to get any political attention. Even if there is political will to solve a problem, but no solution is available, nothing will happen. Political will itself comes from both predictable elements such as delivering on post-election commitments and unpredictable ones such as natural disasters. What he calls individual 'policy entrepreneurs' are needed to build acceptance for solutions and to create the links between problems, solutions, and political will.

In Uruguay, there were significant public concerns – manifested in protest marches – about violence and public safety often linked by the media to drugs. That was the essence of the problem. There was already a head of steam about cannabis legislation with various proposals brought to Parliament but knocked back. Some of the advocates for reform became 'policy entrepreneurs' now in positions of power and influence under a left-wing government presided over by a liberal leader, President Mujica. What the government came up with was a very quickly assembled package of measures to address public concerns about security combining the tough (such as increased penalties for crack offences) with the soft including cannabis legalisation as a way of taking some of the sting out of drug turf wars. The pace at which the proposals were pushed through is another aspect of Kingdon's theory.

In any discussions about drug law reform, the context for each country is different. During his election campaign, Canadian Prime Minister Justin Trudeau promised to legalise cannabis, which had been available medically since 2001. Trudeau was clearly after the youth vote, but as a Liberal took the view that legalising cannabis was a way to reduce the burden of cannabis laws on the justice system, undercut the illicit market for the drug and have a way of restricting young peoples' access to the drug. There was no problem driven by public concerns for Trudeau to solve but he positioned himself as a policy entrepreneur with the political will to deliver on an election promise.

Although drugs have not been legalised in Portugal it has become the flagship country for drug law reform, heralded by campaigners as the model to follow. Portuguese drug policy has been the subject of much misunderstanding – praised as a resounding success by some and a complete disaster by others, views invariably coloured by existing political and moral standpoints on drugs.[11] Portugal was an authoritarian military dictatorship until 1974; the country was very isolated internationally with very little freedom for citizens. Then a bloodless coup led the way to greater democracy and freedoms but with it came an increase in drug use, especially heroin in the 1980s and the rise of organised crime. Heroin injecting brought HIV in its wake, but the law still criminalised drug *use* and possession – both of which were punishable by imprisonment of up to 3 months or a fine. If the quantity of drugs amounted to more than 3 days' worth, then jail time went up to 1 year. Fearful of the authorities, few people came forward for what limited abstinence-based treatment was available. Rates of drug-related HIV and overdose rose; by 1989 about 100,000 people were dependent on heroin. Ten years later, Portugal had the highest rate of drug-related HIV cases in the European Union. Along with a growth in injecting heroin use, open-air drug markets and public drug use proliferated. One district of Lisbon, Casal Ventoso, was dubbed the biggest drug supermarket in Europe.

This is what the Portuguese government were trying to deal with – the same problem faced by the UK around the same time, but because of the law and minimal treatment options, Portuguese heroin users were in a far worse position than their UK counterparts. But with a new political ethos, even by the early 1990s the government was beginning a process of rolling back an over-criminalised drug policy. A law passed in 1993 contained language emphasising treatment rather than punishment for drug users. Regarding the occasional user, the law stated that 'they should, above all, not be labelled or marginalised'. The 1993 law also contained explicit provisions providing for the remittance of penalties for the occasional user and allowed for the suspension of prosecution or sentence if an individual considered an 'addict' agreed to participate in a treatment programme.

In 1998, a government-appointed commission developed a comprehensive intervention strategy, adopted almost in full to form the basis of Portugal's National Strategy for the Fight Against Drugs. The National Strategy set out a series of guiding principles, objectives, and corresponding policies, of which the decriminalisation of personal drug consumption was a centrepiece. The National Strategy formally recognised the dependent drug user as somebody in need of treatment rather than punishment. It also recognised the inefficacy of criminal sanctioning in reducing drug use. In addition to the removal of criminal penalties for drug consumption, the National Strategy and subsequent Action Plan called for additional resources devoted to prevention, treatment, harm reduction, and the social reintegration of drug users, as well as enhanced enforcement of laws prohibiting drug trafficking and distribution.

However, although fines were the major disposal option during the 1990s as opposed to prison for those caught using or in possession of small amounts of drugs, drug *use* was still technically a criminal offence until law 30/2000 passed in 2001. The law decriminalised possession of drugs up to 10 days' supply for personal use. The quantities delineated were 1 gram of heroin, ecstasy, or amphetamines, 2 grams of cocaine, or 25 grams of cannabis. Amounts above these thresholds would be treated as a supply offence. Under the new law, drugs would be seized and the person ordered to attend one of 18 Dissuasion Committees (DCs) which had a number of options at their disposal ranging from no action (suspension), fines or referral into treatment, although the majority of those facing a DC were and still are cannabis users so in no need of treatment. The law is silent on what happens to repeat offenders; for example, there appears to be no official 'three strikes and you're out' rule, so presumably repeat appearances before a DC earns you escalating or repeat sanctions.

In terms of dealing with the problems which prompted the creation of a new infrastructure of support outside the criminal justice system, the results have not been miraculous but are positive nonetheless: numbers in treatment up, rates of drug-related blood-borne infection and overdoses down – benefits already achieved by the UK in the 1980s and 1990s – but no significant increases either in drug use among the general population, including young people.

However, the attraction of the Portuguese model around the world, especially in the USA from where most lavish praise has come, is symbolic as much as legal. Unlike most countries, the Ministry of Health is the lead agency responsible for drug policy rather than the Ministry of Justice. The strategy document itself uniquely specified eight principles, a set of values which would guide drug-related interventions. These included 'Humanism, for example, a recognition of the inalienable human dignity of citizens, including drug users... Pragmatism calls for the adoption of solutions and interventions that are based on scientific knowledge while "Participation" calls for the involvement of the community in drug policy and implementation.' It would be hard if not impossible to identify this level of explicit political endorsement of drug user human rights and civil liberties in most other national drug strategy documents – leaving aside the extremes of those governments engaged in State-sponsored murder and death penalty sentences. This an example of drug policy reform ultimately driven by top-down political will.

The situation in the USA regarding cannabis is very different; neither medicinal nor recreational use of cannabis is supported by the federal government. However, because of the States Rights provisions of the US constitution, individual states have autonomy in many areas of public policy, including drugs. Voter power in more than half of American states has seen cannabis use and supply legalised mainly for medicinal use but also increasingly for recreational use. There probably isn't another country in the world where regional policy wins over that of the national government, with officials at the centre legally powerless to act. In the UK it would be the equivalent of Yorkshire having a county referendum about legalising cannabis. As these changes are not enshrined in the US federal law, cannabis reforms do not technically position the USA outside the UN treaties.

Overall, the UN appears quite toothless in the face of a gradual balkanisation of global drug policy despite the INCB taking on a self-appointed role to publicly condemn any member state it perceives as stepping out of line. This is classic mission creep; the INCB was created as a technocratic body to receive the numbers from states of the amounts of licit opiates they require. INCB looks at those numbers and then determines what the supply is on the international market and reports back to the CND. The idea that the INCB are 'guardians of the Convention' is a purely political creation and not mandated under any international agreement. It may be that some smaller countries would be sensitive to INCB criticism in case the USA reacted with any kind of sanctions. For the major countries though, criticism from the INCB counts for little.

There appears to be something of a power vacuum at the heart of UN drug policy. The political authority of the USA has diminished both because of its focus on terrorism post 9/11 and because of cannabis law reform across the country. For the last decade, a Russian has led the UNODC[12] and Russia itself is implacably opposed to harm reduction and law reform. However, the diplomatic freeze against Russia since the invasion of Ukraine has neutralised its influence while the other major world power, China, appears altogether absent from the debate. However, despite all the talk about cracks in the idea of monolithic drug prohibition, it needs to be remembered that large sections of the UN membership in Africa, the Middle East, Far East and Asia – including quietly but highly influential China – and elsewhere in the world would not countenance treaty reform and so it could be that in some respects the treaties could wither on the vine.

Where does the UK sit in all this? First let's deal with definitions. Legalisation, decriminalisation, depenalisation, medicalisation, regulation and reclassification are often used interchangeably and confusingly.

The UK drug law expert in these matters is Professor Rudi Fortson QC who defines the major terms as follows: Legalisation is conduct which does not constitute either a breach of criminal or civil law. Within the terms of the regulation and control of tobacco and alcohol as consumer products, somebody who produces, sells, possesses or consumes tobacco or alcohol is not breaking any law. Of course, there are laws consequential on actions which arise from the legal availability of alcohol: selling to minors, drunk driving, drinking in alcohol-free zones, and alcohol-related public order offences. Laws also prohibit illegal importation of both legal products to avoid duty payments. Decriminalisation is conduct which is not a breach of the criminal law (such as speeding unless the driver causes an accident) and depenalisation where conduct is technically criminal but does not attract punishment handed down by a court – such as a police caution.

Interviewed for *Druglink* in 2014, John Collins, an international drug policy analyst from the LSE, talked about moving global policy towards 'de-escalating the drug war towards reallocating resources towards making sure we don't get a new generation of politicians coming in at the international level saying, "Let's push harder."' Asked about the UK, he suggested that unlike many countries, there wasn't a huge amount of wriggle room, not a lot of low-hanging policy fruit to pick off so that 'the end of the drug war in UK policy terms is far more problematic as to what that actually means because policy isn't that extreme'.[13] This is a point made by Geoff Monaghan and John Corkery in their paper for 'Police Insight' – a detailed analysis of what they too call 'de-escalation'.[14] On paper, the UK has some of the toughest drug laws in Europe, so for example, the maximum penalty for a Crown Court conviction for cannabis possession is 5 years imprisonment and/or an unlimited fine. Since the early 1970s, however, the only people to find themselves imprisoned for drug possession would be either guilty of multiple previous offences or they had also concurrently been convicted of a more serious offence.[15] To demonstrate 'de-escalation' in the UK context, Monaghan and Corkery detail the plethora of what are called out-of-court disposals, e.g. simple cautions, cannabis/khat warnings and penalty notices for disorder (PNDs) which over the years have put increasing distance between somebody caught in possession of small amounts of drugs and the courts. Some penalties – such as cautions – will give the person a criminal record which may or may not need to be disclosed.

The authors go further by listing a range of current drug offences that could be treated as minor drug offences including production of small numbers of cannabis plants, conversion of a drug from one formulation to another such as cocaine to crack for personal use; social or not-for-profit supply of drugs (there is already discretion under Sentencing Council Guidelines for a reduced sentence in these circumstances).

Notwithstanding the tough political rhetoric, there has always been significant discretion in how minor possession offences have been dealt with by police on the streets, back at the police station and in the courts. In their report into the policing of cannabis in North Yorkshire, Charlie Lloyd and colleagues from York University found significant variations in how police dealt with cannabis possession on the streets, including some of those caught in possession of cannabis being given repeated cannabis warnings rather than having the offence escalated.[16] In other research, Andrew Fraser and Michael George investigated the policing of raves and discovered with the impossibility of arresting everybody with drugs at or going to a rave, officers in a Home Counties force were taking no action against those found in possession of a totally arbitrary figure, 3 tablets of ecstasy.[17] I understand too that police disposal of confiscated drugs without the attendant recording and paperwork still takes place. This level of discretion benefits many drug users, but the very nature of discretion means it can easily tip over into discrimination especially where minority groups subject to stop-and-search tactics are concerned. Moreover, for all the existing out-of-court disposals and however they may or may not be dispensed, those with a criminal record for simple drug possession offences with no aggravating circumstances still face potential obstacles to both foreign travel and career prospects rather than having their offence dealt with by civil processes.

As we saw in Uruguay and Portugal, for more liberal drug policies to be enacted, there needs to be policy convergence. There are similar examples elsewhere; in Denmark and Switzerland there were public concerns about open drug markets and drug litter on the streets. The responses were, respectively, supervised injecting facilities and a heroin prescribing programme. In fact, there are two examples of similar drug policy convergence in the UK.

Back in the 1980s, the problem was the risk of drug-related HIV spreading through the wider community: the solution was harm reduction and Norman Fowler acted as the primary policy entrepreneur to rapidly push the policy through.

In 2018, the serious health problems of two young people were publicised by their parents. Billy Caldwell and Alfie Dingley suffer from multiple daily epileptic fits for which their parents insisted that only cannabis-based medication helped control the symptoms. This being illegal in the UK, they had to go abroad. Then, coming back into the UK, Billy's mother had her supplies confiscated by the Border Force, igniting a furore of public and political condemnation. In June, the then new Home Secretary Sajid Javid announced a review of medicinal cannabis. While under investigation by ACMD, the Chief Medical Officer appeared to pull an evidence review out of a hat and by November – from a legislative point of view, in the blink of an eye – cannabis was regraded from a Schedule 1 to a Schedule 2 drug under the Misuse of Drugs Act. As well as the A-B-C classifications, drugs are also listed according to their medical value. Schedule 1 drugs are designated as having no medical value and include LSD, MDMA and until recently cannabis. Opioid drugs like morphine and diamorphine (heroin) are in Schedule 2 because despite being Class A drugs for the purpose of non-medical use, they are essential medicines for the treatment of chronic and terminal pain. I once asked a member of the Home Office legislative team by what process a drug could be moved from Schedule 1 to 2. The answer was that the Medicines and Health products Regulatory Agency (MHRA) would first have to have approved a pharmaceutical product coming to market. That certainly did not happen with cannabis oil; the government acted ahead of any approved products being available.

There are still severe restrictions on prescribing and the current law change goes nowhere near far enough towards a wider official acceptance of the drug for a range of medical conditions. Sufferers from degenerative diseases such as multiple sclerosis have long argued the benefits of the drug to relieve symptoms and some have literally been prosecuted for their pains.

Even so, the events surrounding the cases of Alfie Dingley and Billy Caldwell underlines Kingdon's central thesis, which I would slightly reconfigure into what I call a three-part stress test. Applying this just to drug policy, for change to happen in the UK it would have to pass not just the test of science and clinical evidence but also the test of public opinion often expressed through our particularly challenging national media and finally the political expediency test.

A decade ago, proposals for a legalised market in cannabis could be discounted by saying it would be a leap in the dark. Well, developments elsewhere have begun to shine a light – just because we don't know everything, doesn't mean we don't know anything. Picking through some early reports from the USA and Canada, cannabis use goes up when more widely available but not necessarily by a significant amount. In Western capitalist economies established industries like tobacco will stake a claim alongside new business while taxation might not be the predicted cash cow because a flood of cannabis onto the market depresses prices. A criminal market can still flourish because not all growers want to wade through official rules and regulations to be able to sell their product legally and because the illegal market may well sell a stronger product than that legally allowed. But the industries have yet to settle and due to differences in political, economic, social, legal and cultural traditions, what works in one country may not work in another or may work better.

Where does the British public currently stand just on cannabis reform? In 2018, an independent YouGov poll revealed 43 per cent were in favour of legalisation (mainly in the 18–24 age range), 41 per cent against (mainly in the 50–64 age range) while 15 per cent didn't know, although when you drill down into the detail it works out that if you include third-way options such as decriminalisation options, just over 50 per cent would back it. The public are probably more laid-back about cannabis these days than in the past, but after decades of information about cannabis being in the public domain still 15 per cent of those polled didn't know whether legalisation would be a good idea or not.

Recently a BBC radio producer contacted me and said, 'We're having a debate about drug legalisation and we wondered if you wanted to take part.' I replied, 'So you want me to say in thirty seconds whether we should or shouldn't.' 'I suppose so,' she laughed. I politely declined. This is typical of what passes for a 'debate about drugs'. My view is that there is no debate about drugs in the UK. My definition of a debate is an occasion when opposing sides of an issue have a serious discussion laying out their considered debating points in a coherent fashion. What happens in the UK is just one side of the argument utilising every possible communication platform – books, articles, op-eds, documentaries, conference speeches and getting out and about in the world of social networking – while from those against reform, apart from a couple of media commentators such as Peter Hitchens and Melanie Phillips, there is silence. Excepting a few Liberal Democrats and an outlier like the late Labour MP Paul Flynn, politicians too – especially those in government – stay quiet. And that silence reverberates through Whitehall. As one civil servant said to UKDPC researchers, there isn't much room for discussion about alternative approaches to tackling the problem. The solution was always to crack down. The headlines were we're going to toughen up the policy... it was the prevailing paradigm and the accepted view, and it was what prime ministers expected of home secretaries.[18]

Said one Home Secretary to the researchers about trying to take drugs out of politics,

getting political partisanship out of this is very difficult ... because politics is such a vicious activity that people really, really, really, do want to make whatever advantage they can out of areas of government. And getting to the state of affairs where you don't have that adversarial approach is very difficult.[19]

Perhaps it boils down to the question – what kind of drug policy do we want? It becomes an issue of societal values, morals and ethics rather than simply evidence. Incidentally, concepts such as morals and morality do carry with them the taint of narrow-minded faith-based puritanism. But I would contend that in relation to drug policy, the moral high ground, for example, is owned by those taking a humane and compassionate view of those with serious drug problems and who adopt policies and practices in that spirit.

It is said that you can judge a society by how it treats the most vulnerable. If we want a policy that helps the most vulnerable street drug users, then we would ensure we have a well-funded treatment and rehabilitation system allowing for the widest range of helping interventions; a well-funded mental and prison health service, decent housing and access to training and employment to give people something to strive for once they leave the treatment gates. All these improvements are possible without any drug law changes and most would clearly benefit a much wider cohort of those in need. If this is what society wants, then to help this process, part of the solution could be a rebalancing of the drug strategy budget. When the government reviewed the 2010 strategy in 2015, the only year they could quantify with any certainty was in 2014/15 when £1.6 billion was spent on all enforcement activities compared to £540 million on treatment.[20]

It was said in *The Wire* that if you follow the drugs, that's all you get; but if you follow the money, 'who knows where it may lead?'. Drugs is a cash business; stifle the money flow and traffickers would have a much harder life. But seizing actual cash yields only a fraction of what is out there because of the collusion of financial institutions with money laundering. All of Europe's top 10 banks, and 18 out of the 20 biggest, have been fined for money-laundering offences in the past decade.[21] So perhaps we want an all-out assault on global money laundering. In 2009 Antonio Maria Costa, then head of the UNODC, made an astonishing but nonetheless believable assertion that but for the drug money washing through the world's financial systems, keeping it all afloat, the financial crash of 2008 could have been a whole lot worse.[22] In those circumstances and given the strength of bank secrecy laws across the world, how likely is it that any serious inroads can be made to stem the tide of criminal cash? What are governments prepared to do to force the issue if the public clamour is loud enough? How many of those governments are already compromised by giving priority to developing financial services at the expense of due diligence?

Maybe we think a regulated and controlled market in all drugs is possible or even desirable. If so, then proponents of this solution have serious questions to answer including limiting access to young people, implementation of quality control, costs to health systems, issues around marketing and advertising, and denying organised crime access to legal markets. Those who support the criminalisation of drug users should answer the charge that natural justice is not being well served when tobacco and alcohol can be consumed with relative impunity, but not cannabis, especially as the conventions were forged internationally through a prism of class and racial discrimination and global diplomacy rather than public health. We live in an era of growing demands to recognise diversity across society, be it race, religion, gender and sexual identify. Maybe we should start acknowledging diversity of consciousness.

It could be instructive to have a proper nationwide debate on all these issues; Citizens' Assemblies could be an appropriate vehicle. Back in the 1990s, both Channel 4 and Lambeth Council independently ran Citizens Juries where a representative sample of the public was chosen to hear from experts and others about drug issues. Asked about drugs before the sessions and most had pretty hard and fast negative views that became far more nuanced once they heard a range of viewpoints. It would be interesting to give that idea a more comprehensive airing. What we don't need, by the way, is another 'My Big Fat Drug Report'.

In the meantime, while drug policy marks time, the drug scene itself will change; the search for altered states of consciousness will likely mutate as technology allows. Science fiction is reality ahead of schedule. In the 1960s, Arthur C. Clarke believed that we would live in a world in which we will be in instant contact with each other. He believed we would be able to contact our friends anywhere on earth, even if we didn't know their actual physical location. Now we have mobile phones, laptops, and the internet, all of which allow us to connect with people anywhere, and at any time. Clarke also predicted Artificial Intelligence (HAL in *2001*), 3D printing, remote surgery, communications satellites and tablet devices. We have them all.

A world of virtual drug experiences might become a reality; it was probably no coincidence that after his release from prison, Timothy Leary devoted his time to cyberspace developments. *The Matrix*, released in 1999, depicted an illegal online trade in pharmaceuticals and software predating the Dark Web, which was not made available to the world as open-sourced software by the US Government until 2004. There are current concerns about young people spending too much time engaged in online gaming. Again, back in 1999, the film *Existenz* posited the idea of being literally plugged into a game through a neural implant down which you could, in theory, stream any kind of drug experience. Central to Frank Herbert's SF series *Dune* was a fictitious drug called Melange or Spice, the most essential and valuable commodity in the universe. Spice prolonged life, increased vitality, heightened awareness and could also unlock prescience in some humans, depending upon the dosage and the consumer's physiology. Spice though, was highly addictive and withdrawal was fatal. Philip K. Dick (himself a prolific amphetamine user) invented Substance D in *A Scanner Darkly*. It produced an initial euphoria until the user finds out what D actually stands for – despair, desertion, dumbness, and in its final incarnation, death.

All stuff and nonsense? Maybe, although Gary Nicholson's 1988 prediction about the development and marketing of powerful synthetic drugs in shiny packets suggests otherwise. Perhaps Aldous Huxley's premonition was closer to a future reality with his 1932 dystopic novel *Brave New World* in which the population was drugged into blissful compliance with Soma. We already have unknown numbers of people levelling out the peaks and troughs of life on tranquillisers, antidepressants and painkillers. Who knows what might emerge once Big Pharma lock onto the current trials into the use of MDMA, LSD and ketamine to tackle depression, anxiety and post-traumatic stress disorder? Happiness pills for all?

In his book Toby Seddon quotes the Polish sociologist and philosopher Zymunt Bauman from his book *Freedom* about the possibilities of doing things differently in the future:

> The human condition is not pre-empted by its past. Human history is not pre-determined by its past stages. The fact that something has been the case for a very long time, is not proof that it will continue to be so. Each moment of history is a junction of tracks leading towards a number of futures. Being at the crossroads is the way human society exists. What appears in retrospect an 'inevitable' development began in its time stepping onto one road among many stretching ahead.[23]

At the moment, we don't seem to be learning much from the past history of drugs, but who knows what the future will bring except to say that if the Iron Law of Prohibition holds true, we might want to think hard in order to avoid some of the techno-drug scenarios of science fiction.

However, it does all come back to that crucial element of political will and there are no signs – unless some unforeseen policy confluence takes place – that the UK is going to divert from current policies and will instead continue down a road of damage limitation. Drug policy remains messy and controversial, 'often driven by a mix of reactivity, polarised position-driven analysis and campaigning interests, emotive media reporting, adversarial relationships between scientists, experts and policymakers along with a contested … evidence base'.[24]

And if all that gives you a headache, keep taking the tablets.

Notes

Prologue: Empires of the Senses

1. Thomas, *The Slave Trade*, p.150
2. Ibid, p.115
3. Moxham, *Tea*, p.155
4. Berridge, *Opium*, p.153
5. Stein, *International Diplomacy*, p.52

1 DORA, Billie and Freda

1. Kohn, *Dope Girls*, p.34
2. Berridge, *Opium*, p.249
3. Kamienski, *Shooting Up*, pp.97–98
4. Kohn, *Dope Girls*, p.41
5. The term 'narcotics' became the erroneous US and international shorthand for all illegal drugs including cocaine whereas it only applies to drugs which cause sleep (narcosis) such as opium, morphine and heroin.
6. Berridge, *Opium*, p.250
7. Renborg, Bertil, 'The Grand Old Men of the League of Nations', *Bulletin on Narcotics*, vol xvi, 4 (1964), p.9
8. Stein, *International Diplomacy*, p.65
9. Spear, *Heroin*, p.4
10. The supposed link between hashish and the cult of the Assassins is an early example of fake news. It was spread by opponents of Hasan ibn-Sabah, leader of a Shiite Muslim breakaway sect called the Nizari Ismaili. Hasan and his followers holed up in a remote castle in northern Iran, earning Hasan the nickname 'The Old Man of the Mountains'. From there he orchestrated a campaign of terror, ordering his followers to murder religious opponents. The derivation of the word 'assassin' remains obscure but there was no independent corroboration of the story that hashish ever played a part in providing 'Dutch courage' to psych up followers for the kill. The tale was picked up and spread first by the Crusaders and then Marco Polo. For an overview of the story see Booth, M., *Cannabis: A History*, pp.48–55.
11. Shapiro, *Shooting Stars*, pp.24–25

2 A Very British System

1. Spear, *Heroin*, p.21
2. Rolleston, p.18
3. Spear, *Heroin*, p.32
4. Parssinen, *Secret Passions*, p.197
5. Paul, *My First Life*, p.86
6. Spear, *Heroin*, p.52

3 The Light of the Charge Brigade

1. Mills, *Cannabis Britannica*, p.92
2. Indian Hemp Commission, Vol. 1 p.264
3. Thorp, *Viper*, p.25
4. Kohn, *Dope Girls*, p.26
5. McKay, *Circular Breathing*, p.107
6. Shapiro, *Waiting for the Man*, p.76
7. Thorp, *Viper*, p.30
8. Granger, *Up West*, p.297
9. Lyle, George. 'Dangerous Drugs Traffic in London', *British Journal of Addiction* 50, (1953), pp.47–58
10. Mills, *Cannabis Britannica*, p.74
11. Thorp, *Viper*, p.192
12. Harris, *Homegrown*, p.14
13. Spear, *Heroin*, p.114

4 Talkin' 'Bout My Generation

1. Kamienski, *Shooting Up*, p.121
2. Connell, *Amphetamine psychosis*, p.58
3. These undated news reports come from an unpublished manuscript called *Living for Kicks* by Lee Harris and his brother Mervyn who wrote about London's early sixties amphetamine subculture.
4. Shapiro, *Waiting for the Man*, p.123
5. Leech, *Keep the Faith*, p.11
6. Interview with Lee Harris
7. Shapiro, *Waiting for the Man*, p.123
8. Ibid, p.125

5 Long Strange Trips

1. Roberts, *Albion*, p.12
2. Ibid, p.22
3. Interview with Chris Green
4. On 2 September 1955, Labour MP Christopher Mayhew volunteered to be filmed by the BBC under the influence of mescaline. When questioned about his experience, he wasn't that coherent, leaving viewers somewhat bemused.
5. Melechi, *Psychedelia*, p.29
6. Miles, *London Calling*, p.175
7. Roberts, *Divine*, p.125
8. http://www.crimetime.co.uk/the-chelsea-girl-the-playboy-the-honest-cop-and-the-proven-lawyer/
9. Over the years, drug-related publications have run foul of the Obscene Publications Act. *Cain's Book* by Alex Trocchi was successfully prosecuted in 1965 on the basis that the pleasurable descriptions of drug use were likely to 'deprave and corrupt' in the words of the Act. The same principle was applied to drug books in the early 1980s, when police raided bookshops in seventeen locations around the country and cleared the shelves of books that described how to, for example, grow cannabis, or were seen to be promoting the enjoyment of drugs. Over 6,000 books were seized from one shop alone and 15 titles were presented in court on charges of inciting or conspiring to incite people to consume illegal drugs. The jury found the bookshop owner not guilty. A second trial involved a different shop and one title, *Attention Coke Lovers*, where the defendants were found guilty and fined. Police action led to concerns that harm reduction materials could be seized, although only one organisation was warned at the time – the Merseyside Drug Council withdrew a leaflet about

magic mushrooms. The issue was written up by ISDD's Nicholas Dorn in an unpublished report entitled *See You In Court* (1987).

In 1990, there was a later attempt under the Drug Trafficking Offences Act to prosecute Lee Harris, owner of the head shop *Alchemy* for selling items that could be used to consume drugs, such as bongs, scales and rolling papers. He was sentenced to 3 months in prison, released pending an appeal which he won.

10. This was a special issue edited by teenagers including rock journalist-to-be Charles Shaar Murray and prosecuted under the Obscene Publications Act with specific reference to a pornographic cartoon strip featuring Rupert the Bear. https://flashbak.com/schoolkids-oz-read-in-full-the-magazine-that-started-a-revolution-56985/#
11. Tendler, *Brotherhood*, p.121–122
12. https://datacide-magazine.com/dope-smuggling-lsd-manufacture-organised-crime-the-law-in-1960s-london/

6 Pot, Politics and Pilchards

1. Bruun, *Gentleman's Club*, p.196
2. Goode, *Marijuana*, p.x
3. Bruun, *Gentleman's Club*, p.202
4. Green, *Days in the Life*, p.132–133
5. Mills, *Cannabis Nation*, p.117–118
6. Wells, *Butterfly*, p.78
7. Green, *Days in the Life*, p.202
8. Wells, *Butterfly*, p.105
9. Mills, *Cannabis Nation*, p.119
10. Abrams, *Wootton*, p.2
11. Green, *Days in the Life*, p.192
12. Schofield, *Strange Case*, p.97
13. Young, J., 'Drugs and the Mass Media', *Drugs and Society*. 2, (1), (1971) pp.14–15.
14. Cohen, *Folk Devils*, p.9
15. Wootton, *Cannabis*, p.9
16. Moreland, *Art of Smuggling*, Kindle location 247
17. Ibid, 647
18. Enright *Dope*, p.174
19. Marks, *Mr Nice*, p.181–182

7 Too Much Monkey Business

1. Reed, *A Stranger*, p.97
2. Hallam, *Script Doctors*, p.136
3. Spear, *Heroin*, p.57
4. Ibid, p.56
5. Shapiro, *Waiting for the Man*, p.67
6. Judson, *Heroin Addiction*, p.36
7. Freemantle, *The Fix*, p.18
8. Judson, *Heroin Addiction*, p.50
9. Baker, *As Though*, p.97
10. Hewetson, J., *Anarchy*; 60 (1966), pp.33–39
11. Ollendorf, R., *Liverpool Journal of Psychiatry*, 4, (1966), pp.31–35
12. Spear, *Heroin*, p.141
13. Ibid, p.154
14. Ibid, p.154–155
15. Information about Dr Petro's interactions with the Home Office comes from Bing Spear's papers kindly supplied to me by his editor Joy Mott.

16. Leech, *Keep the Faith*, p.31–32
17. Tripp, M. 'Who speaks for Petro?', *Drugs and Society*: 3 (2) (1973), pp.12–17
18. Strang, *Heroin Addiction (2)*, p.36
19. Interview with Martin Mitcheson
20. Judson, *Heroin Addiction*, p.92
21. Freemantle, *The Fix*, p.31

8 Masterful Inactivity

1. Strang, *Heroin Addiction (2)*, p.28
2. Judson, *Heroin Addiction*, p.90
3. Ibid, p.41
4. Strang, *Heroin Addiction (2)*, p.31
5. Ibid, p.35
6. Stimson, *Heroin Addiction*, p.83
7. Ibid, p.205
8. Strang, *Heroin Addiction (2)*, p.39
9. Interview with Martin Mitcheson
10. Ibid
11. Stimson, *Heroin Addiction*, p.25
12. Walsh *Drug War*, p.91
13. Ibid, p.48
14. Interview with Martin Mitcheson
15. City Roads closed in 2019
16. Spear, *Heroin Addiction*, p.259
17. Personal communication, Geoff Monaghan
18. Wilson, *Northern Soul*, p.163
19. Burr, A. 'The Ideologies of Despair: a Symbolic Interpretation of Punks and Skinheads Usage of Barbiturates', *Soc.Sci.Med* 19, (9) (1984), pp.929–938
20. Walsh, *Drug War*, p.252
21. Stimson, *Heroin Addiction*, p.224

9 The Dark Side of the Spoon

1. *Druglink*: Spring (1984), p.18
2. Mars, *Politics*, p.189
3. Ibid, p.73
4. Salt, J., 'The Geography of Unemployment in the United Kingdom in the 1980s', *Espace Populations Sociétés Année* 2 (1985), pp.349–55
5. Walsh, *Drug War*, p.320. The best overview of the UK drug market of the early 1980s came from Wagstaff and Maynard's work for the Home Office published in 1988, *Economic Aspects of the Illicit Drug Market and Drug Enforcement Policies in the United Kingdom.*
6. Strang, *Heroin Addiction (1)*, p.82
7. Parker, *Living*, p.49
8. Walsh, *Drug War*, p.203
9. Interview with John Marks
10. Crick, *Militant*, Kindle location 1277
11. Walsh, *Drug War*, 279
12. Interview with John Marks
13. Mold, *Voluntary Action*, p.95
14. Personal communication, Geoff Monaghan
15. Walsh, *Drug War*, p.308
16. Andrew Irving Associates, *Anti-Heroin Misuse Campaign: Qualitative Evaluation Research Report*, 1986
17. Dorn, N., 'Media Campaigns', *Druglink*, 1 (2) (1986), pp.8–9

10 Smoke and Mirrors

1. Chronicled in forensic detail by Alfred McCoy in *The Politics of Heroin: CIA Complicity in the Global Drug Trade, Afghanistan, South-East Asia, Central America, Colombia.* Second revised edition Capella Books 2003
2. Streatfeild, *Cocaine,* p.216
3. Kamienski, *Shooting Up,* p.239
4. Walsh, *Drug War,* p.102
5. http://transform-drugs.blogspot.com/2009/06/report-they-didnt-want-you-to-see.html
6. Streatfeild, *Cocaine,* p.513
7. Williams, *Cocaine,* p.8
8. For another investigation into the CIA and cocaine, see Gary Webb's highly controversial book, *Dark Alliance: the CIA, the Contras and the Crack Cocaine Explosion* (Seven Stories, 1998)
9. Streatfeild, *Cocaine,* p.312–313
10. Koren, G et al. 'Bias Against the Null Hypothesis: the Reproductive Hazards of Cocaine', *Lancet,* December 16, (1989), pp.1440–1442
11. Streatfeild, *Cocaine,* p.315
12. House of Lords, Hansard, 15 June 1989

11 When Britain Ruled the Raves

1. Bussmann, *Once in a Lifetime,* p.43
2. Collin, *Altered States,* p.125
3. Silcott, *Book of E,* p.62–63
4. Ibid, p.56
5. Ibid, p.58
6. Ibid, p.59
7. Zobel, G., 'Chemical Reaction', *Druglink:* 24 (4) (2009), p.7
8. Silcott, *Book of E,* p.52
9. Couch, L., *et al.,* 'Variability in Content and Dissolution Profiles of MDMA Tablets Collected in the UK between 2001 and 2018 – A Potential Risk to Users?', *Drug Test Anal.* (2019), pp.1–11

12 Things Can Only Get Better

1. Silverman, *Crime,* p.2
2. Arnull, *Development and Implementation,* p.43
3. Ibid, p.191
4. Ashton, M., The Manners Matter Review', *Drug and Alcohol Findings,* Series of articles from 2004–2006
5. Strang, *Heroin Addiction,* p.191
6. Seddon, *Tough Choices,* p.58
7. Boulton, *Tony's Ten Years,* p.147
8. Silverman, *Crime,* p.4
9. Hellawell, *The Outsider,* p.298
10. Interview with Mike Trace
11. Hellawell, *The Outsider,* p.293
12. Dean, *Democracy,* p.195
13. Ibid, p.180
14. Ibid, p.196
15. Adda, J., *et al.* 'Crime and the Depenalization of Cannabis Possession: Evidence from a Policing Experiment', *Journal of Political Economy,* 122 (5) (2014), pp.1130–1202
16. Interview with David Blunkett

17. Mullin, *A View,* Kindle location 3417
18. Interview with David Blunkett
19. Mullin, *A View,* Kindle location 3825
20. Hough, M. et al. *The Domestic Cultivation of Cannabis* (York: Joseph Rowntree Foundation, 2003
21. Daly, M., 'Skunk: Potency Doubles', *Druglink,* 22 (5) (2007), p.3
22. *Review of the UK's Drugs Classification System – a Public Consultation.* Home Office, Crime and Drugs Directorate, May 2006.
23. In the autumn of 2004 and in classic Malcolm Tucker mode, as yet another General Election loomed, a Spad contacted the Home Office Drug Strategy Unit. 'Tony wants a drugs bill.' 'OK what does he want in it.' 'That's up to you.' In a bid to cobble together some legislation (and without proper consultation with the ACMD) the Drugs Act 2005 made the psilocybin 'magic' mushroom, that desperate driver of drug-related crime, a Class A drug. It was already an offence to try and extract the hallucinogenic chemical from the mushrooms by drying them out or brewing in tea, and now the mushroom itself was a controlled drug. London traders had started bagging up mushrooms and legally selling them exactly like the supermarkets sell mushrooms. Customs and Excise then determined that because the mushrooms were being sold for purposes other than a tasty addition to an omelette, they were liable to VAT. This whole nonsense reached its conclusion with the mushroom being banned despite growing wild in many parts of the country, including on the vast estates of our landed gentry.
24. In 2002, Tony Blair had committed the UK to try and stem the flow of heroin coming out of Afghanistan following the defeat of the Taliban in 2001. But the British and US diplomats were at odds over poppy eradication. The US Ambassador was William 'Chemical Bill' Wood who, as US Ambassador to Colombia, had favoured coca spraying. Initially, the British had been buying up the opium crop and destroying it. This was proving very expensive because the farmers quickly realised the more they grew, the more they got paid. The British officials on the ground wanted nothing to do with crop spraying as they wanted to adopt a 'hearts and minds' strategy to win over the poppy farmers against a resurgent Taliban. The Americans went in at ground level to destroy the crops while the British dropped leaflets saying, 'It's not us doing this' and went so far as to hand opium back to the farmers. The Americans were not best pleased. [Shapiro, H. 'The Politics of the Poppy', *Druglink,* 26 (6) (2011), pp.14–17).] The lack of enthusiasm for the 'war against heroin' went right to the heart of Whitehall. A senior customs official was in a meeting where Geoff Hoon, the Secretary of State for Defence, specifically ruled out British troops being involved in poppy eradication.
25. Ashton, Mike, 'The New Abstentionists', *Druglink,* special insert (23), 1 (2008)

13 States of the Nation

1. *Druglink*; 27, (5) (2012), p.2
2. Ibid, p.13
3. ACMD, *Time-limited opioid substitution therapy,* 2014
4. Strang, John, *et al.,* 'Drug Policy and the Public Good: Evidence for Effective Interventions', *Lancet,* 370 (2012), pp.71–83
5. Humphreys, K. and Piot, P. 'Scientific Evidence Alone Is Not Sufficient Basis for Health Policy', *British Medical Journal,* 344 (2012), p.24–25
6. McSweeney, *Tackling Drug Markets and Distribution Networks in the UK,* p.13
7 Maynard, *Economic Aspects,* p.56
8. https://www.express.co.uk/news/uk/109485/Soca-seized-163-1-for-every-163-15-spent
9. https://www.theguardian.com/uk/2003/feb/09/drugsandalcohol.tonythompson
10. King, *Test-purchase Database,* p.14
11. Bacon, p.245

12. https://www.bbc.co.uk/news/business-49348792
13. Henderson, G., 'Designer Drugs: Past History and Future Prospects,' *Journal* of *Forensic Sciences*, 33 (2) (1988), pp.569–575
14. Shapiro, H., 'Alphabet Soup', *Druglink*, 26 (3) (2011), p. 17
15. Power, M., 'World Wired Web', *Druglink*, 25 (1) (2010), p.11
16. Daly, M., 'Commercial Breakdown: Druglink Street Drug Survey 2009', *Druglink*, 24 (5) (2009), p.4
17. https://www.bbc.co.uk/news/10184803
18. Tatusov, M., *et al.*, '6 Things Every EP Needs to Know About K2/Spice & the Synthetic Cannabinoid Epidemic', *Emergency Physicians Monthly*, 23 October (2015)
19. Ric Treble, personal communication
20. Reuter, P. and Pardo, B., 'Can new psychoactive substances be regulated effectively? An assessment of the British Psychoactive Substances Bill', *Addiction*, 112 (2016), pp.25–31
21. Daly, M and Simonson, P., 'The Great Heroin Drought', *Druglink* (2011), p.17
22. The medicines used also contain promethazine and dextromethorphan, which have various psychoactive properties.
23. Quinones, *Dreamland*, p.16
24. For example, from 2006 to 2016, UK prescriptions for opioid painkillers rose 400 per cent according to Dr Jane Quinlan speaking at a meeting of the All Party Parliamentary Group on Prescribed Drug Dependence, 19 October 2016.
25. The number of recorded fentanyl and fentanyl analogue deaths in the UK rose from 7 in 2008 to 105 in 2018.
26. Ric Treble, personal communication

14 2020 Vision?

1. In selected Dutch coffeeshops, there is now a four-year trial underway looking at the feasibility of legal production and supply.
2. Bridge, J., *et al.*, 'Edging Forward: How the UN's language on drugs has advanced since 1990', IDPC Briefing Paper, 2017
3. Jelsma, M., 'The Unwritten History of the 1998 United Nations Assembly on Drugs', *International Journal of Drug Policy*, 14 (2003), p.190
4. Ibid. p.192
5. Ibid, p.193
6. For example, UNODC officials Chloe Carpenter and colleagues re-iterated this point in a reply to Wayne Hall's article in *Addiction*, 'The Future of the International Drug Control System and National Drug Prohibitions', 113 (2017), p. 1229.
7. https://www.bbc.co.uk/news/uk-34571609
8. Jelsma, p.181
9. Jelsma, ibid, p.186
10. Queirolo, R., *et al.*, 'Why Uruguay Legalized Marijuana? The Open Window of Public Insecurity', *Addiction*, 114 (2018), p.1313
11. For the most balanced assessments *see*: Hughes, C. and Stevens A., 'A Resounding Success or a Disastrous Failure: Re-examining the Interpretation of Evidence on the Portuguese Decriminalisation of Illicit Drugs', *Drugs and Alcohol Review*, 31 (2012), p.101–113; Laqueur, H., 'Uses and Abuses of Drug Decriminalization in Portugal', *Law and Social Inquiry*, 40 (3) (2015), pp.746–781; EMCDDA, *Portugal: Drug Policy Profiles*, EMCDDA 2011
12. At the time of writing, Ms Ghada Fathi Waly from Egypt, has been appointed as the new Director of UNODC.
13. Shapiro, H., Interview with John Collins, *Druglink*, 29 (3) (2014), p.18
14. Monaghan, G. and Corkery, J., 'The *Other* Quiet Revolution: Minor Drug Offences and De-escalation Law, Policies and Practices in the United Kingdom', *Policing Insight 2020*

15. Personal communication with Geoff Monaghan, who provided a table of those in prison 1990–2000 (source: Home Office) for a drug possession offence running concurrently with a more serious offence or because they had committed multiple previous possession offences. For cannabis the number averaged out at 150 people a year for that decade.

16. N8 Policing Research Partnership, *Policing Cannabis in North Yorkshire* (2018)

17. Fraser, A. and George, M., 'Southern England, Drugs and Music: Policing the Impossible' in Dorn, N., *et al.* (eds), *European Drug Policies and Enforcement* (MacMillan, 1996), pp.74–94

18. UKDPC, *How To Make Drug Policy Better*, p.13

19. Ibid, p.13

20. UK Government, *An Evaluation of the Government's Drug Strategy 2010* (2017)

21. https://glintpay.com/money-en_us/every-top-10-bank-fined-150-billion-laundered-annually/

22. https://www.theguardian.com/global/2009/dec/13/drug-money-banks-saved-un-cfief-claims

23. Seddon, *A History of Drugs*, p.135

24. UKDPC, *How To Make Drug Policy Better*, p.7

Bibliography

(Place of publication London unless otherwise stated)

Abrams, Steve. *The Wootton Report: the Decriminalisation of Cannabis in Britain.* (Unpublished, 1997)

Andrew Irving Associates. *Anti-Heroin Misuse Campaign: Qualitative Evaluation Research Report.* (AIA, 1986)

Arnull, Elaine. *The Development and Implementation of Drug Policy in England 1994–2004.* PhD Dissertation. (Middlesex University 2007)

Bacon, Matthew. *Taking Care of Business: Police Detectives, Drug Law Enforcement and Proactive Investigation.* (Oxford, Oxford University Press, 2016)

Baker, Bob. *The Druglink Guide to UK Drug Policy.* (DrugScope, 2004)

Baker, Chet. *As Though I Had Wings: the Lost Memoir.* (New York: St Martin's Press, 1997)

Bean, Philip. Ed. *Cocaine and Crack: Supply and Use.* (MacMillan, 1993)

Bean, Philip. *Legalising Drugs: Debates and Dilemmas.* (Policy Press, 2010)

Berridge, Virginia. *Opium and the People: Opiate Use and Drug Control Policy in Nineteenth and Early Twentieth Century England.* (Free Association Books, 1999)

Bingham, Adrian, and Conboy, Martin. *Tabloid Century: the Popular Press in Britain 1896 to the Present.* (Oxford, Peter Lang, 2015)

Boulton, Adam. *Tony's Ten Years: Memories of the Blair Administration.* (Simon & Schuster, 2009)

Bramley-Harker, Edward. *Sizing the UK Market for Illicit Drugs.* (Home Office, 2001)

Bruun, Kettil et al. *The Gentleman's Club: International Control of Drugs and Alcohol.* (Chicago: University of Chicago Press, 1975)

Burton, Kristen. *Intoxication and Empire: Distilled Spirits and the Creation of Addiction in the Early Modern British Atlantic.* PhD Dissertation. (University of Texas, 2015)

Bussmann, Jane. *Once in a Lifetime: the Crazy Days of Acid House and Afterwards.* (Paradise, 1998)

Campbell, Alastair. *Diaries Volume Three: Power and Responsibility* (Arrow, 2012)

Centre for Social Justice. *Breakthrough Britain: Addictions.* (CSJ, 2007)

Centre for Social Justice. *The Road to Recovery: Addiction in Our Society – the Case for Reform.* (CSJ, 2019)

Cohen, Stanley. *Folk Devils and Moral Panics: the Creation of the Mods and Rockers.* (MacGibbon & Kee, 1972)

Collin, Matthew. *Altered State: the Story of Ecstasy Culture and Acid House.* (Serpent's Tail, 1998)

Collins, John. *Regulations and Prohibitions: Anglo-American Relations and International Drug Control, 1939–1964.* PhD Dissertation. (London School of Economics, 2015)

Collison, Mike. *Police, Drugs and Community.* (Free Association Books, 1995)

Connell, Philip. *Amphetamine Psychosis.* (Chapman & Hall, 1958)

Cox, Barry, et al. *The Fall of Scotland Yard.* (Penguin, 1977)

Crick, Michael. *Militant.* (Faber, 1984)

Dally, Ann. *A Doctor's Story.* (MacMillan, 1990)

Daly, Max and Sampson, Steve. *Narcomania: a Journey Through Britain's Drug World.* (William Heinemann, 2012)

Dean, Malcolm. *Democracy Under Attack: How the Media Distort Policy and Politics.* (Policy Press, 2013)

Dorn, Nicholas et al. *Traffickers: Drug Markets and Law Enforcement.* (Routledge, 1992)

Dorn, Nicholas and Nigel South. *A Land Fit for Heroin? Drug Policies, Prevention and Practice.* (Macmillan, 1987).

Eastwood, Niamh. et al *A Quiet Revolution: Drug Decriminalisation Across the Globe.* (Release, 2016)

Ebenezer, Lyn. *Operation Julie: the World's Greatest LSD Bust.* (Talybont, yLolfa, 2010)

Edwards, Griffith. *Matters of Substance.* (Allen Lane, 2004)

Enright, Damien. *Dope in the Age of Innocence.* (Liberties Press, 2010)

Fielding, Leaf. *To Live Outside the Law.* (Serpents Tail, 2011)

Freemantle, Brian. *The Fix.* (Corgi, 1986)

Goode, Eric. *The Marijuana Smokers.* (New York: Basic Books, 1970)

Goodman, Jordan, et al. (eds). *Consuming Habits: Drugs in History and Anthropology.* (Routledge, 1995).

Granger, Pip. *Up West: Voices from the Streets of Post-War London.* (Corgi Books, 2009).

Green, Jonathan. *Days in the Life: Voices from the English Underground 1961–1971.* (Heinemann, 1998)

Hallam, Christopher. *Script Doctors and Vicious Addicts: Subcultures, Drugs and Regulations under the 'British System' c1917–c.1960.* PhD Dissertation. London School of Hygiene and Tropical Medicine, 2016. Published as *White Drug Cultures and Regulation in London 1916–1960.* (Palgrave MacMillan, 2018)

Harris, Lee. *Echoes of the Underground: a Foot Soldier's Tales.* (Barncott Press, 2014)

Harris, Lee and Render, Chris (eds). *The Best of Home Grown 1977–1981.* (Red Shift Books, 1994)

Hellawell, Keith. *The Outsider: the Autobiography of One of Britain's Most Controversial Policemen.* (HarperCollins, 2003)

Henman, Anthony et al. *Big Deal: the Politics of the Illicit Drugs Business.* (Pluto Press, 1985)

Herring, Jonathan, et al. (eds). *Intoxication and Society: Problematic Pleasures of Drugs and Alcohol.* (Palgrave MacMillan, 2013)

Hollingshead, Michael. *The Man Who Turned On the World.* (Blond & Briggs, 1973)

Honeycombe, Gordon. *Adam's Tale.* (Arrow, 1975)

Indian Hemp Commission Report 1893–94. (Simla; Central Government Printing Office, 1894–95)

Inglis, Brian. *The Forbidden Game: a Social History of Drugs.* (Coronet, 1975)

Judson, Horace. *Heroin Addiction in Britain.* (New York: Harcourt Brace Jovanovich, 1974)

Kamienski, Lukasz. *Shooting Up: a Short History of Drugs and War.* (Oxford: Oxford University Press, 2016)

Keay, John. *The Honourable Company: a History of the English East India Company.* (HarperCollins, 1993)

King, Les. *Forensic Chemistry of Substance Misuse: a Guide to Drug Control.* (Royal Society of Chemistry, 2009)

King, Les. *Test-purchase Database: Drug Type, Unit Prices and Purities in the Period 1992 to 2003.* (Metropolitan Police Specialist Crime Department, 2004)

Kleiman, Mark. *Against Excess: Drug Policy for Results.* (New York, Basic Books, 1993)

Klein, Axel. *Drugs and the World.* (Reaktion, 2008)

Kohn, Marek. *Dope Girls: the Birth of the British Drug Underworld.* (Lawrence & Wishart, 1992)

Kohn, Marek. *Narcomania: On Heroin.* (Faber, 1987)

Lee, Dick and Pratt, Colin. *Operation Julie: How the Undercover Police Team Smashed The World's Greatest Drug Ring.* (W. H. Allen, 1978)

Leech, Ken. *Keep the Faith Baby.* (SPCK, 1973)

Lenson, David. *On Drugs.* (Minneapolis, University of Minnesota Press, 1995)

Logan, Frank. ed. *Cannabis: Options for Control* (Quartermaine, 1979)

McAllister, William. *Drug Diplomacy in the Twentieth Century: an International History.* (Routledge, 2000)

MacCoun, Robert and Reuter, Peter. *Drug War Heresies: Learning from Other Vices, Times & Places.* (Cambridge; Cambridge University Press, 2001)

MacGregor, Susanne et al. *Drug Services in England and the Impact of the Central Funding Initiative.* (ISDD, 1991)

MacGregor, Susanne. *The Politics of Drugs: Perceptions, Power and Policies.* (Palgrave MacMillan, 2017)

McKay, George. *Circular Breathing: the Cultural Politics of Jazz in Britain.* (Durham: Duke University Press, 2005)

McKenna, Terence. *Food of the Gods: The Search for the Original Tree of Knowledge: A Radical History of Plants, Drugs and Human Evolution.* (Rider, 1999)

McSweeney, Tim et al. *Tackling Drug Markets and Distribution Networks in the UK.* (UKDPC, 2008)

Marks, Howard. *Mr Nice.* (Minerva, 1997)

Mars, Sarah. *The Politics of Addiction.* (Palgrave MacMillan, 2012)

Mills, James. *Cannabis Britannica: Empire, Trade and Prohibition 1800–1928.* (Oxford: Oxford University Press, 2003)

Mills, James. *Cannabis Nation: Control and Consumption in Britain 1928–2008.* (Oxford: Oxford University Press, 2013)

Matrix Knowledge Group. *The Illicit Drug Trade in the UK.* (Home Office, 2007)

Melechi, Antonio (ed). *Psychedelia Britannica: Hallucinogenic Drugs in Britain.* (Turnaround, 1997)

Miles, Barry. *London Calling: a Countercultural History of London Since 1945.* (Atlantic Books, 2010)

Mintz, Sidney. *Sweetness and Power: the Place of Sugar in Modern History.* (Penguin, 1986)

Mold, Alex and Berridge, Virginia. *Voluntary Action and Illegal Drugs: Health and Society in Britain Since the 1960s.* (Palgrave MacMillan, 2010)

Morgan, Nick. *The Heroin Epidemic of the 1980s and 1990s and Its Effect on Crime Trends – Then and Now.* (Home Office, 2014)

Morland, Francis. *The Art of Smuggling: the Gentlemen Drug Traffickers Who Turned Britain On.* (Milo Books, 2015)

Mowlam, Mo. *Momentum: the Struggle for Peace, Politics and the People.* (Hodder & Stoughton, 2003)

Moxham, Roy. *Tea: Addiction, Exploitation and Empire.* (Constable, 2003)

Mullin, Chris. *A View from the Foothills.* (Profile Books, 2010)

Musto, David. *The American Disease: Origins of Narcotic Control.* (Oxford, Oxford University Press, 1973)

Neville, Richard. *Playpower.* (Paladin, 1971)

Neville, Richard. *Hippie, Hippie, Shake.* (Bloomsbury, 1995)

Paddick, Brian. *Line of Fire.* (Pocket Books, 2008)

Parker, Edward and Yuan Wei. *Chinese Account of the Opium War.* [Reprint of original book from 1888 (Norderstedt, Hansebooks, 2019)

Parker, Howard et al. *Living with Heroin.* (Milton Keynes: Open University, 1988)

Parker, Matthew. *The Sugar Barons: Family, Corruption, Empire and War.* (Windmill, 2012)

Parssinen, Terry. *Secret Passions, Secret Remedies: Narcotic Drugs in British Society 1820–1930.* (Manchester: Manchester University Press, 1983)

Paul, Brenda, *My First Life: an Autobiography* (John Long,1935)

Pearson, Geoffrey. *The New Heroin Users.* (Oxford; Basil Blackwell, 1987)

Pearson, John. *The Cult of Violence: the Untold Story of the Krays.* (Orion, 2002)

The Police Foundation. *Drugs and the Law: Report of the Independent Inquiry into the Misuse of Drugs Act 1971.* (Runciman Report). (The Police Foundation, 2000)

Pryor, William. *Survival of the Coolest.* (Clear Press, 2003)

Quinones, Sam. *Dreamland: the True Tale of America's Opiate Epidemic.* (Bloomsbury, 2015)

Reed, Jeremy. *A Stranger On Earth; the Life and Work of Anna Kavan.* (Peter Owen, 2006)

Revie, Alastair. *I Came Back From Hell (The Story of Barrie Ellis) As Told To Alastair Revie.* (Brown, Watson, 1964)

Roberts, Andy. *Albion Dreaming: a Popular History of LSD in Britain.* (Marshall Cavendish, 2008)

Roberts, Andy. *Divine Rascal: On the Trail of LSD's Cosmic Courier Michael Hollingshead.* (Strange Attraction Press, 2019)

Saunders, Nicholas. *Ecstasy and the Dance Culture.* (Saunders, 1995)

Schivelbusch, Wolfgang. *Tastes of Paradise: a Social History of Spices, Stimulants and Intoxicants.* (New York: Vintage, 1993)

Schofield, Michael. *The Strange Case of Pot.* (Penguin, 1971)

Seddon, Toby. *A History of Drugs: Drugs and Freedom in the Liberal Age.* (Routledge, 2010)

Seddon, Toby. *Tough Choices: Risk, Security and the Criminalisation of Drug Policy.* (Oxford: Oxford University Press, 2012)

Shapiro, Harry. *Shooting Stars: Drugs, Hollywood and the Movies.* (Serpent's Tail, 2003)

Shapiro, Harry. *Waiting for the Man: the Story of Drugs and Popular Music.* Rev ed. (Helter Skelter, 2003)

Silcott, Push and Silcott, Mireille. *The Book of E: All About Ecstasy.* (Omnibus, 2000)

Silver, Gary. *The Dope Chronicles 1850–1950.* (New York: Harper & Row, 1979).

Silverman, Jon. *Crime, Policy and the Media.* (Routledge, 2011)

Spear, Henry. *Heroin Addiction Care and Control: the British System 1916–1984.* (DrugScope, 2002)

Stein, Stuart. *International Diplomacy, State Administration and Narcotics Control: the Origins of a Social Problem.* (Aldershot: Gower, 1985)

Stimson, Gerry and Oppenheimer, Edna. *Heroin Addiction: Treatment and Control in Britain.* (Tavistock, 1982)

Strang, John and Gossop, Michael (eds). *Heroin Addiction and the British System. Volume 2.* (Routledge, 2005.)

Streatfeild, Dominic. *Cocaine: a Definitive History.* (Virgin, 2002.)

Taylor, David. *Bright Young People: the Rise and Fall of a Generation 1918–1940.* (Vintage, 2008)

Taylor, Terry. *Baron's Court, All Change.* (Nottingham; New London Editions, 2011)

Tendler, Stewart and May, David. *The Brotherhood of Eternal Love: From Flower Power to Hippie Mafia: the Story of the LSD Counterculture.* (Panther 1984)

Thomas, Hugh. *The Slave Trade: the History of the Atlantic Slave Trade 1440–1870.* (Phoenix, 2006)

Thorp, Raymond. *Viper: The Confessions of a Drug Addict.* (Robert Hale, 1956)

Trocki, Carl. *Opium, Empire and the Global Political Economy.* (Routledge, 1999)

UK. Advisory Committee on Drug Dependence. *Cannabis: Report Prepared by the Sub-Committee on Hallucinogens.* (The Wootton Report). (HMSO, 1968)

UK Advisory Council on the Misuse of Drugs. *Treatment and Rehabilitation.* (HMSO, 1982)

UK Advisory Council on the Misuse of Drugs. *Prevention* (HMSO, 1984)

UK Advisory Council on the Misuse of Drugs. *Aids and Drug Misuse, Part One.* (HMSO, 1988)

UK Advisory Council on the Misuse of Drugs. *Aids and Drug Misuse, Part Two.* (HMSO,1989)

UK Advisory Council on the Misuse of Drugs. *Problem Drug Use: A Review of Training.* (HMSO, 1990).

UK Advisory Council on the Misuse of Drugs. *Aids and Drug Misuse Update.* (HMSO, 1993)

UK Advisory Council on the Misuse of Drugs. *Drug Misuser and the Criminal Justice System: Part II – Police, Drug Misusers and the Community.* (HMSO, 1994)

UK Advisory Council on the Misuse of Drugs. *Drug Misuse and the Environment.* (HMSO, 1998)

UK Advisory Council on the Misuse of Drugs. *Misuse of Fentanyl and Fentanyl Analogues* (Home Office, 2019)

UK Advisory Council on the Misuse of Drugs. UK. Anti-Drugs Coordinating Unit.

UK Advisory Council on the Misuse of Drugs. *Annual Report 1998/1999* (Central Office of Information, 1999)

UK Advisory Council on the Misuse of Drugs. *Annual Report 1999/2000* (Central Office of Information, 2000)

UK Advisory Council on the Misuse of Drugs. *Annual Report 2000/2001* (Central Office of Information 2001)

UK Advisory Council on the Misuse of Drugs. *Tackling Drugs To Build A Better Britain: The Government's Ten Year Strategy for Tacking Drugs Misuse.* (HMSO, 1998)

UK Audit Commission. *Changing Habits: The Commissioning and Management of Community Drug Treatment Services for Adults.* (Audit Commission, 2002)

UK Audit Commission. *Drug Misuse 2004: Reducing the Impact.* (Audit Commission 2004)

UK Drug Policy Commission. *How to Make Drug Policy Better: Key findings from UKDPC Research into Drug Policy Governance* (UKDPC 2012)

UK Home Office. *Tackling Drug Misuse: a Summary of Government's Strategy* (1985)

UK Home Office. Crime and Strategy Directorate. *Review of the UK's Classification System – a Public Consultation.* (Unpublished 2006)

UK Home Office. Drug Strategy Unit. *Drugs value for money review.* (Unpublished 2007)

UK House of Commons. Home Affairs Committee. *Crack: the Threat of Hard Drugs in the Next Decade.* (1989)

UK House of Commons. Home Affairs Committee. *The Government's Drug Policy: Is It Working?* (2002)

UK Ministry of Health. *Drug Addiction: Report of the Interdepartmental Committee.* (First Brain Report). (HMSO, 1961)

UK Ministry of Health. Departmental Committee on Morphine and Heroin Addiction. (Rolleston Report) 1926.

UK Ministry of Health. *Drug Addiction: the Second Report of the Interdepartmental Committee. (Second Brain Report.)* (HMSO, 1965)

UK Strategy Unit. *SU Drugs Project. Phase 1 Report: Understanding the Issues* (Unpublished 2002)

UK Strategy Unit. *SU Drugs Project. Phase 2 Report: Diagnosis and Recommendations.* (Unpublished 2002)

Wagstaff, Adam and Maynard, Alan. *Economic Aspects of the Illicit Drug Market and Drug Enforcement Policies in the United Kingdom.* (HMSO, 1988)

Walsh, Peter. *Drug War: The Secret History.* (Milo Books, 2018)

Williams, Terry. *The Cocaine Kids: the Inside Story of a Teenage Drug Ring.* (Bloomsbury, 1990)

Wilson, Andrew. *Northern Soul: Drugs, Music and Subcultural Identity.* (Routledge, 2007)

Wells, Simon. *Butterfly on a Wheel: The Great Rolling Stones Bust.* (Omnibus, 2011)

Woods, Neil. *Good Cop, Bad War: My Undercover Life Inside Britain's Drug Gangs.* (Ebury Press, 2016)

Young, Jock. *The Drugtakers: The Social Meaning of Drug Use.* (Paladin, 1971)

Index

Index